The Renaissance of Healing Art

Doctor Oljaca

ISBN-978-86-82984-00-9

Publisher: Published by Dragan Oljaca under the public name Doctor Oljaca

First edition, 2025.

www.doctoroljaca.com

Dedication

This book is dedicated to all my past and future patients, whose courage and trust inspire me to continually refine the art of healing.

I extend special gratitude to my fellow doctors, whose dedication to medicine and unending curiosity drive the continuous pursuit of knowledge and the sharing of insights.

This book is also dedicated to medical students, as well as my future students and participants of the Doctor Oljaca Academy, with the hope that they will find inspiration and guidance on their journey to serving the health and well-being of all.

I will praise thee; for I am fearfully and wonderfully made: marvellous are thy works; and that my soul knoweth right well.

Psalm 139:14 (KJV)

Preface

This book is not merely an informational document, but rather the culmination of my ten years of experience in the field of atlas vertebra realignment, shaped by the success stories of thousands of satisfied patients. Over the years, I have refined my methods and gathered invaluable insights that have transformed the lives of many.

However, this book serves an even deeper purpose. It has been crafted as a textbook for all my students at the Doctor Oljaca Academy. Every line, every illustration, and every case study is designed to guide future generations of doctors and therapists in continuing and advancing this important practice.

The purpose of writing this book is to share my knowledge and findings with fellow professionals, as well as with future medical students. Additionally, this book serves as an excellent resource for individuals who are keen on improving their personal health, offering them insights into techniques and principles that have proven essential for achieving optimal well-being.

I believe this book will become an indispensable resource for those dedicated to healing, whether through professional practice or through personal growth and health care.

Acknowledgments

I give all thanks and glory to the **Lord Jesus Christ** for guiding me in the writing of this book and for blessing my work.

Table of Contents

Introduction

Dear readers,

Welcome to the world of "The Renaissance of Healing Art"! This book is an invitation to a journey that will take you far beyond the usual boundaries of medicine and healthcare. At the heart of this approach is not only the treatment of symptoms but also the understanding of the deeper causes of our health challenges.

Through the lens of "The Renaissance of Healing Art," we will discover how correcting imbalances in the body, starting with the atlas vertebra, is crucial to achieving universal balance and healing. In this book, we will explore the power each of us holds within to transform our health and well-being.

This is an invitation to a journey towards inner harmony, vitality, and the universal beauty that surrounds us. I encourage you to embark on this journey with an open mind and heart, and to embrace the challenge of venturing into a new dimension of health and healing.

May this book be your guide and inspiration on the path to better health and a more fulfilling life.

With warm regards,

Doctor Oljaca

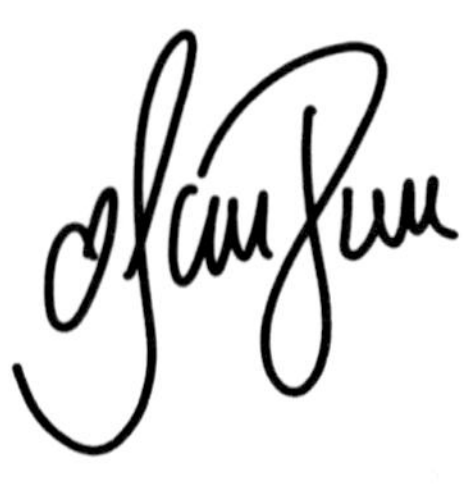

The Renaissance of Healing Art

True healing begins by addressing the root causes, not just the symptoms. The "Renaissance of Healing Art" guides you toward a holistic approach that nurtures both body and soul, leading to lasting well-being.

We often face challenges related to our health and well-being, experiencing symptoms such as back pain, headaches, dizziness, or general fatigue. However, we rarely devote enough attention to the root causes of these problems, often opting for superficial symptom relief rather than addressing the root cause. In today's world of fast-paced medicine, where the emphasis is often on instant symptom relief, the question arises - is there a deeper and more effective approach to healing that can take us beyond symptomatic treatment?

This book introduces us to the world of the "Renaissance of Healing Art", a revolutionary approach to health and well-being that shifts paradigms. At the heart of this approach lies the method of adjusting the atlas vertebra, a crucial part of the spine that plays a vital role in overall body health. Understanding the anatomy of the atlas vertebra and its role in the nervous system, circulatory system, lymphatic system, as well as its impact on the functioning of glands that influence fertility and the physical beauty of the skin, forms the foundation of this book.

Through the following chapters, readers will have the opportunity to delve deeper into the world of atlas adjustment methods. In addition to a detailed description of the anatomy of the atlas vertebra, we will explore the causes of problems related to this part of the spine. We will uncover the different types of atlas subluxations and their impact on an individual's health and well-being.

The central theme of the book will be the "Harmonic Balance" atlas adjustment method, which represents the integration of massage and therapy aimed at correcting imbalances in the atlas vertebra. Through detailed descriptions of the process of diagnosing a patient's condition, examining the patient, and preparing for treatment, readers will become familiar with the steps leading to the achievement of inner balance and healing.

Furthermore, the book will explore how atlas adjustment can improve not only physical health but also aesthetics and individual confidence. Through the lens of the "Renaissance of Healing Art", we will consider how this approach to healing contributes to overall well-being and universal beauty.

Through this exploration, we invite you to delve into deeper levels of health and beauty and discover the power each of us holds within to transform our health and well-being. "Renaissance of Healing Art" is not just a book but an invitation to a journey towards inner harmony, vitality, and the universal beauty that surrounds us.

"Wisdom is the principal thing; therefore get wisdom:
and with all thy getting get understanding."

(Proverbs 4:7)

Harmony of Body, Mind, and Spirit

In the midst of life's demands, restoring harmony between body, mind, and spirit is vital. This book guides you in reconnecting with your true self, offering tools for healing and balance.

In today's fast-paced world, where we're often juggling various commitments and challenges, we frequently forget to prioritize the harmony between body, mind, and spirit. This harmony isn't just an aesthetic ideal; it's a crucial component for our overall well-being and healing process.

This book, "The Renaissance of Healing Art," explores the deep connections among these three elements and how their harmony can be a catalyst for transformation and healing. Through the chapters of this book, we delve into various aspects of this theme, offering deeper insights and practical advice for achieving this harmony in everyday life.

The body, as our physical expression, is often the first point where imbalances in our inner being manifest. Physical symptoms may result not only from physical factors but also from emotional and mental states. Thus, it's important to treat the body as a whole, considering all aspects of our being.

Our mind, with its thoughts and emotions, plays a crucial role in our health. Stress, anxiety, and negative thoughts can have a profound impact on our physical state.

The spirit, as our essence and deeper being, is also an important factor in the healing process. Through the practice of spirituality, connecting with nature, and our unsurpassed Creator, Lord Jesus Christ, we can strengthen our inner strength and resilience. This can lift us above the challenges we face and help us find deeper meaning and purpose in life.

"The Renaissance of Healing Art" is a call to return to the roots of our being, to revitalize the connections among body, mind, and spirit. Through this book, we invite you to explore and practice various techniques and approaches that will help you achieve that harmony in everyday life.

This book is not just an informative guide but also an inspiration for personal development and growth. Through it, we hope you'll find inspiration and support for your journey toward health, happiness, and fulfillment.

"Bless the Lord, O my soul, and forget not all his benefits: Who forgives all your iniquities; who heals all your diseases."

(Psalm 103:2-3:)

Historical Context

The evolution of healing practices reflects humanity's enduring quest to understand health and alleviate suffering. This brief historical journey highlights the foundations of modern medicine and the integration of ancient wisdom.

Understanding the historical development of healing approaches throughout the ages provides valuable insights into the evolution of medical practices. From ancient civilizations to modern times, humanity has constantly sought methods to alleviate suffering and promote well-being. Traditional healing methods, rooted in ancient wisdom and cultural practices, have laid the foundation for contemporary medical innovations.

Ancient civilizations such as those in Egypt, Greece, and China developed sophisticated medical systems based on holistic principles. Herbal remedies, acupuncture, and spiritual rituals were integral components of their healing practices. These ancient traditions emphasized the interconnectedness of body, mind, and spirit, recognizing the importance of addressing the root causes of illness rather than merely treating symptoms.

The Middle Ages witnessed the rise of various medical traditions, including contributions from Jewish and Christian scholars in the fields of medicine and surgery. The establishment of medical schools and the translation of ancient texts paved the way for advancements in medical knowledge. However, this period was also marked by superstition and the limited understanding of disease, leading to the prevalence of ineffective treatments and practices.

The Renaissance period brought about a revival of interest in classical medical texts and a renewed focus on human anatomy and physiology. Pioneering figures such as Leonardo da Vinci made significant contributions to the understanding of the human body through meticulous anatomical studies. This era laid the groundwork for the scientific revolution and the emergence of modern medicine.

The 19th and 20th centuries witnessed unprecedented advancements in medical science, including the discovery of antibiotics and surgical techniques. These innovations revolutionized the treatment of diseases and significantly improved public health outcomes. However, alongside scientific progress, there has been a growing recognition of the limitations of conventional medicine and a renewed interest in holistic healing modalities.

Today, the field of medicine is characterized by a diverse array of approaches, ranging from conventional pharmaceutical interventions to alternative therapies such as acupuncture, chiropractic care, and mindfulness practices. Integrative medicine, which combines the best of both conventional and complementary approaches, has gained popularity as a comprehensive approach to health and wellness.

In exploring the historical context of healing practices, we gain a deeper appreciation for the rich tapestry of medical traditions that have shaped our understanding of health and healing. By recognizing the strengths and limitations of various approaches, we can embrace a more inclusive and holistic approach to healthcare that honors both tradition and innovation.

Personal Motivation

Driven by a deep belief in the body's self-healing power, I have explored atlas alignment as a key to achieving true health and harmony.

My personal motivation for researching and writing on this topic stems from a deep belief in the power of natural and holistic approaches to healing. I've always been fascinated by the complexity of the human body and its ability for self-healing when provided with appropriate support and care. I am convinced that harmony between the body, mind, and spirit plays a crucial role in maintaining health and well-being.

Throughout years of studying various medical approaches and traditions, I've discovered that the most effective treatments often consider the holistic picture of an individual's health, rather than solely focusing on disease symptoms. This realization has inspired me to explore revolutionary healing methods based on holistic principles, with a particular deep interest in the method of atlas alignment.

I believe that this topic is of paramount importance for the modern world, which is increasingly facing challenges related to stress, mental health, and prevalent health issues. In today's society, where quick-fix medicine has become the norm, deeper causes of illness and imbalances in the body are often overlooked. My goal is to highlight the significance of a holistic approach to healing and to demonstrate how the method of atlas alignment can provide effective and lasting solutions for numerous health problems.

By sharing my passion and motivation for this topic, I hope to inspire readers to consider new approaches to health and to open their minds to the potential benefits of holistic healing. I am confident that this topic is relevant to anyone who seeks better health, happiness, and harmony in their lives.

In my many years of practice as a medical professional, I have witnessed numerous cases where conventional approaches to treatment have not provided complete or lasting relief from issues. This motivated me to explore alternative methods that can complement or even surpass conventional therapies. In this process, I discovered atlas alignment as an extremely effective technique that not only addresses symptoms but also treats the root causes of problems.

My personal fascination with this topic stems from a deep understanding of the connection between the body's structure and its functional state. Through careful study of anatomy and biomechanics, I realized that even the slightest misalignment of the atlas can have a significant impact on overall health and well-being. This realization prompted me to delve deeper and discover how proper atlas alignment can contribute to improving overall health.

Additionally, I have personally witnessed the transformation of many patients who have undergone atlas alignment treatments. Their experiences testify to the incredible results that can be achieved when harmony is established between the spinal column and the nervous system. These testimonials not only confirm the effectiveness of the method but also serve as inspiration for further research and promotion of this holistic approach to healing.

By sharing my personal experiences and knowledge, I hope to encourage others to explore this topic and to embrace new approaches to health openly. I believe that this subject matter is relevant to all those who aspire to optimal health and wish to harness the full potential of their body and mind.

I hope, or I am almost certain, that the insights from this book, as the result of my ten years of experience in the field of practical application of atlas adjustment on over 3000+ patients and adjusted atlas vertebrae, will inspire colleagues worldwide to dedicate themselves to the method of atlas adjustment as a Renaissance in the art of healing.

"Wherever the art of medicine is loved, there is also a love of humanity."

(Hippocrates)

Chapter 1

Anatomy of the Atlas

Unique Shape and Function of the Atlas

The unique shape of the atlas vertebra plays a crucial role in supporting the head and enabling a wide range of motion in the neck. This specialized structure exemplifies the intricate design that enables both stability and flexibility in the upper spine.

The shape of the atlas vertebra represents a key characteristic that distinguishes it from other vertebrae in the spine. Its structure, which resembles a ring or loop, functions as a perfect mechanism that allows free movement while efficiently supporting the head [Image 1].

When discussing the atlas vertebra's shape, its exceptional structure, distinct from other vertebrae in the spine, cannot be overlooked. Instead of the typical body that characterizes most vertebrae, the atlas has a ring-shaped form adapted to its specific needs and functions. This unique form allows the atlas to move freely and support the head in various positions [Image 2].

It is important to emphasize that the shape of the atlas vertebra is perfectly adapted to its function within the spine. Thanks to the ring that constitutes its structure, the atlas allows the head to tilt forward-backward and left-right, which is essential for the mobility of the neck and head. This freedom of movement allows us to perform various activities and head movements without experiencing discomfort or restriction.

Additionally, the shape of the atlas vertebra gives it a unique ability to efficiently support the head's weight. A ring-like structure enables even distribution of the load, reducing pressure on the spine and facilitating the maintenance of neck stability.

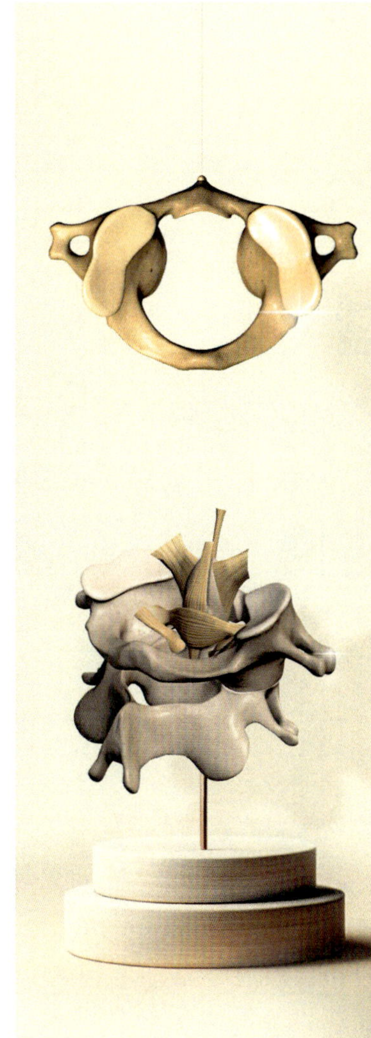

[Image 1] Structure

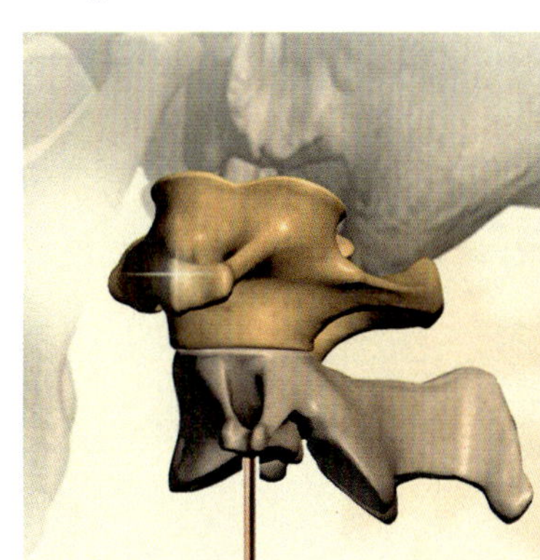

[Image 2] Position

Overall, the shape of the atlas vertebra represents a perfect example of anatomical adaptation that enables functionality and support of vital body parts. Understanding this characteristic helps us better comprehend the importance of the atlas in the spine and its role in supporting the head and neck [Image 1].

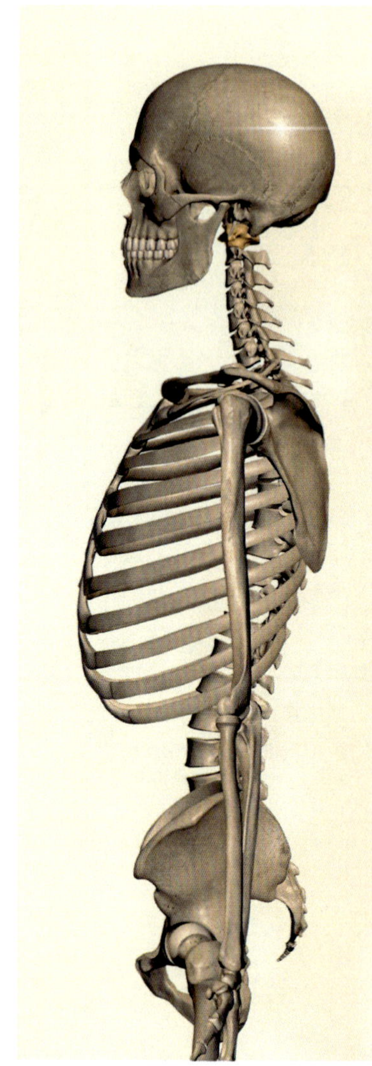

[Image 1] Atlas lateral view

"Simplicity is the ultimate sophistication."

(Leonardo da Vinci)

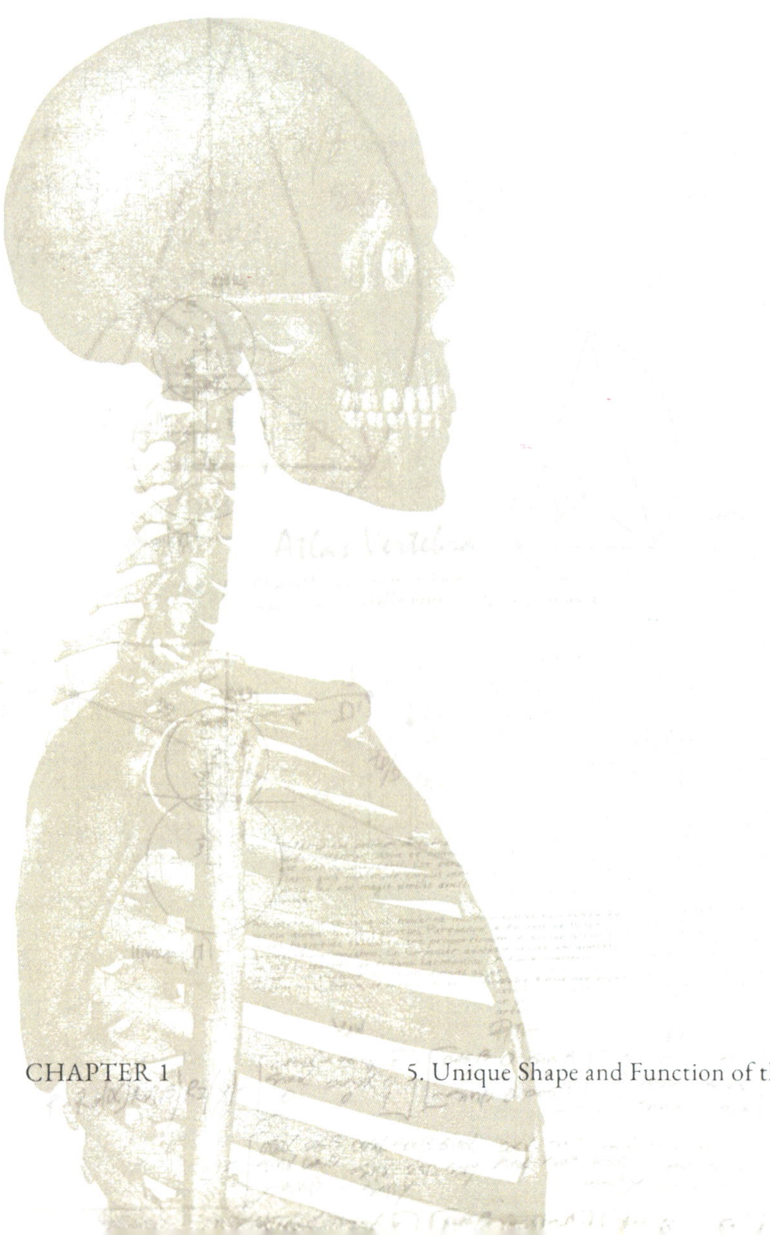

The Small but Mighty Atlas

Though small in size, the atlas vertebra plays a critical role in supporting the head and maintaining neck stability.

The size of the atlas vertebra, while relatively small compared to other vertebrae in the spine, is of essential significance for supporting the head and maintaining neck stability.

Despite its diminutive stature within the spinal column, the atlas vertebra plays a pivotal role in the structural integrity and functionality of the upper spine. As the first cervical vertebra, its compact dimensions are purposefully designed to fulfill its critical functions, particularly in supporting the weight of the head and facilitating its movement [Image 1].

While larger vertebrae provide substantial support for the torso and bear significant loads, the smaller size of the atlas allows for intricate movements and flexibility crucial for the mobility of the neck. This balance between size and functionality ensures that the atlas can perform its role effectively without impeding the range of motion required for various head movements and postures [Image 2].

Moreover, the relatively small size of the atlas vertebra contributes to the overall stability of the neck by minimizing bulkiness and reducing interference with adjacent structures. This streamlined design enables smooth articulation with the skull and neighboring vertebrae while optimizing biomechanical efficiency.

In summary, while the atlas vertebra may be diminutive in size, its importance cannot be overstated. Its compact dimensions are precisely tailored to support the head and maintain neck stability, showcasing the remarkable efficiency of anatomical adaptation in fulfilling vital physiological functions.

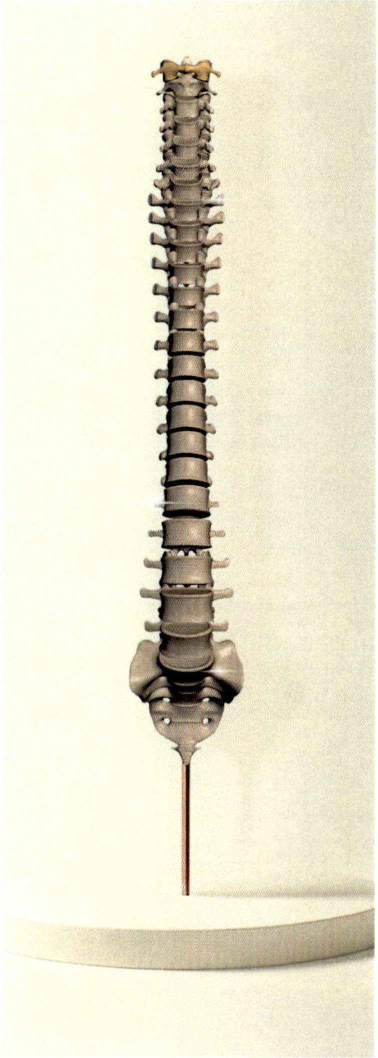

[Image 1] Atlas vs. larger vertebrae

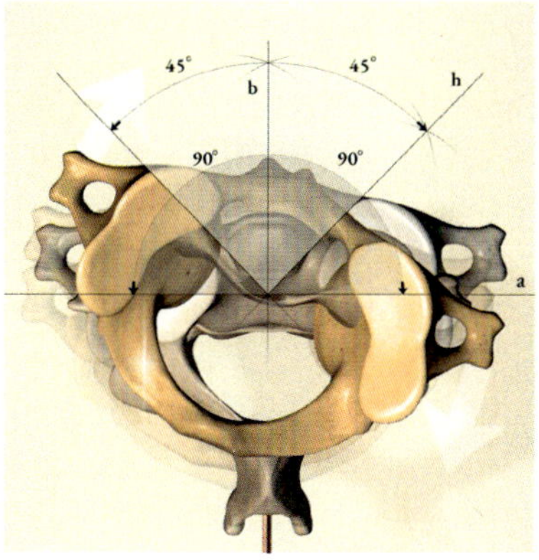

[Image 2] Atlas biomechanics

Key Structural Features of the Atlas

The atlas vertebra's structural components are intricately designed to ensure its functionality and connectivity within the spine.

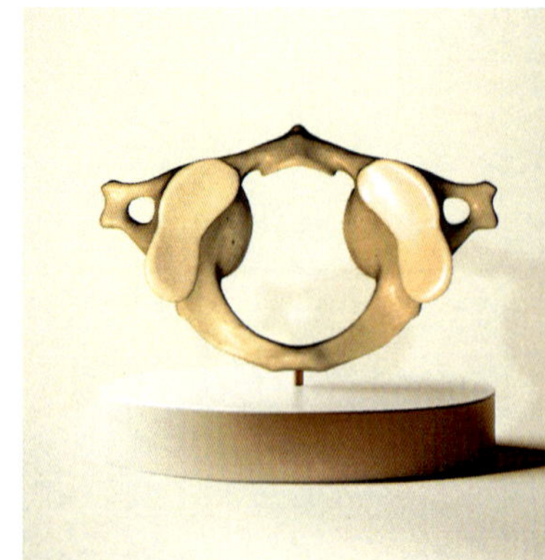

[Image 1] Atlas anatomy

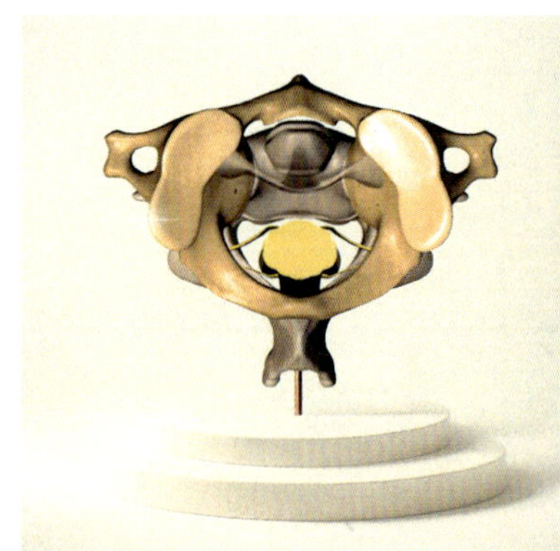

[Image 2] Atlas and spinal cord

General structural features of the atlas vertebra play a crucial role in its functionality and connectivity with surrounding structures.

The atlas vertebra consists of several key components that are essential for its function. Lateral mass processes, located on the sides of the atlas, provide stability and enable the atlas to connect with adjacent vertebrae and the skull [Image 1]. These processes are crucial for supporting the head and maintaining neck stability, as they allow the atlas to firmly attach to surrounding structures.

Additionally, the atlas vertebra possesses articular surfaces that allow it to move in conjunction with the skull and other vertebrae. These surfaces are smooth and articulating, facilitating smooth movements and head support during various neck movements.

One of the key structural features of the atlas vertebra is the vertebral foramen, located at the center of the vertebral structure. This opening is crucial for the passage of the spinal cord and provides a safe and protected passage for nervous tissue [Image 2]. Through this foramen, the spinal cord extends from the brain to the rest of the body, transmitting vital signals and information.

The structural features of the atlas vertebra are essential for its function, supporting the head, maintaining neck stability, and protecting the spinal cord, making it a vital component of the spinal and nervous systems.

Atlas in Head and Neck Support

The atlas vertebra plays a critical role in supporting the head and neck, ensuring their mobility and stability. Its unique structure allows for the even distribution of the head's weight, maintaining the functionality of these essential body parts.

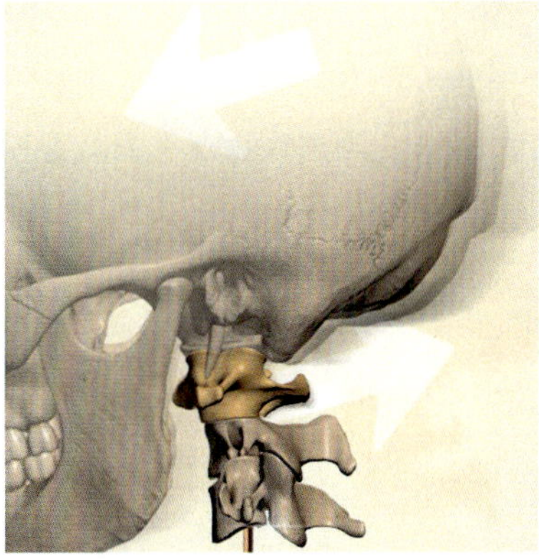

[Image 1] Atlas movement

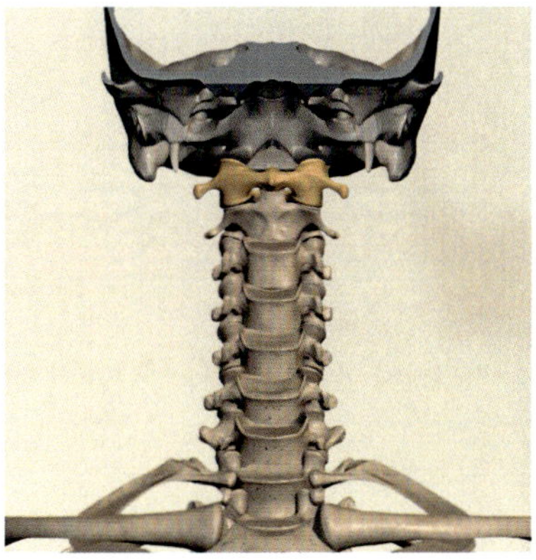

[Image 2] Atlas weight distribution

The role of the atlas vertebra in supporting the head and neck is crucial for maintaining mobility and functionality of these vital parts of the body.

The atlas vertebra plays a pivotal role in supporting the head and neck, enabling them to move and turn safely and without restrictions. Without the integrity of the atlas, the head would be unimaginably immobile, leading to serious issues with neck mobility and function. Due to its unique shape and structure, the atlas provides a stable foundation for the head, allowing it to tilt forward and backward and from side to side with ease [Image 1].

This support is essential for everyday activities such as turning the head, leaning forward or backward, or making lateral movements of the neck. Without proper atlas function, these activities would be limited or even impossible, seriously impairing normal body functions.

Additionally, the atlas vertebra plays a crucial role in maintaining the stability of the neck and head during movement and activities. Because of its ring-like structure, the atlas evenly distributes the weight of the head along the spine, reducing pressure on the cervical vertebrae and ligaments [Image 2]. This enables efficient support of the head even during dynamic activities.

In summary, the role of the atlas vertebra in supporting the head and neck is vital for maintaining normal mobility and functionality of these body parts. Understanding this role allows us to better comprehend the significance of the atlas in the complex spinal system and its contribution to overall health and well-being [Image 1].

"He who knows health, knows everything."

(Socrates)

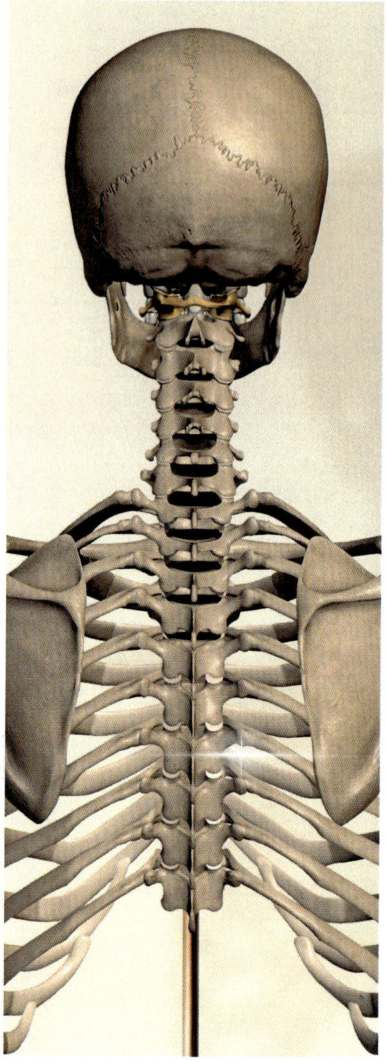

[Image 1] Atlas in spinal context

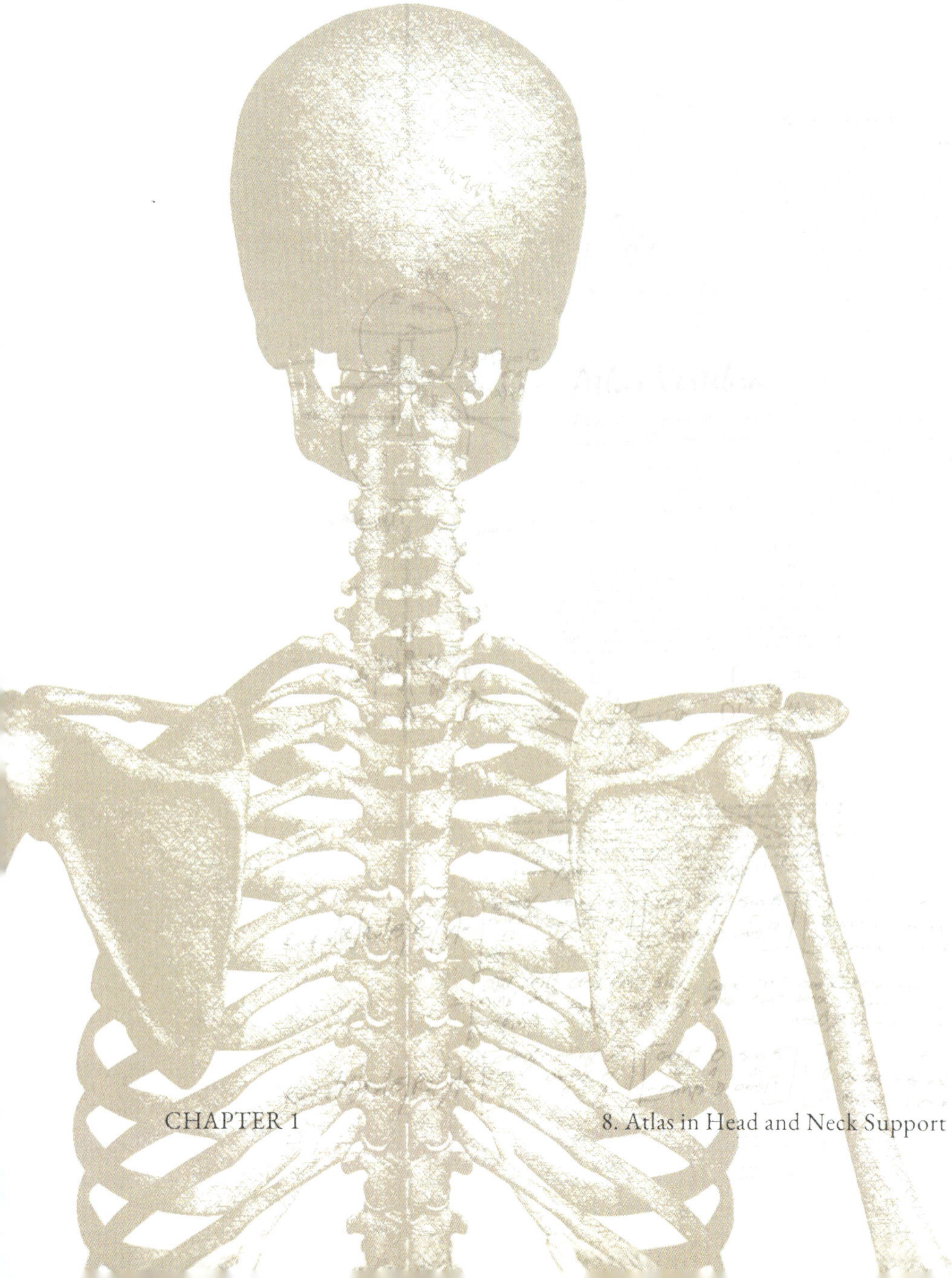

Distinct Structure and Role of the Atlas

The atlas vertebra's distinctive structure is essential for its unique role in supporting and mobilizing the head. Unlike other vertebrae, its ring-like shape allows for flexibility and rotation, making it a crucial component of the spine.

The atlas vertebra stands out with its unique structure, which is significantly different from other vertebrae in the spine. Instead of the typical vertebral body that characterizes most vertebrae, the atlas has a ring-like shape consisting of lateral masses and articular surfaces. This structure allows the atlas to move freely and rotate, providing flexibility and support to the head in various positions [Image 1].

In addition to its structural differences, the atlas vertebra also has a specific function that sets it apart from other vertebrae. Unlike other vertebrae that primarily provide support and protection to the spinal cord, the atlas is primarily responsible for supporting the head and enabling its various movements. This function makes the atlas a vital part of the spine, whose stability is crucial for normal body functioning.

Furthermore, the atlas differs from other vertebrae in its anatomy and position in the spine. It is located at the top of the spinal column, just below the skull, allowing it to directly support and connect the head to the rest of the body. This unique position makes the atlas a key part of the spine that influences the mobility and function of the head and neck [Image 2].

"The Lord by wisdom founded the earth; by understanding He established the heavens."

(Solomon, Proverbs 3:19)

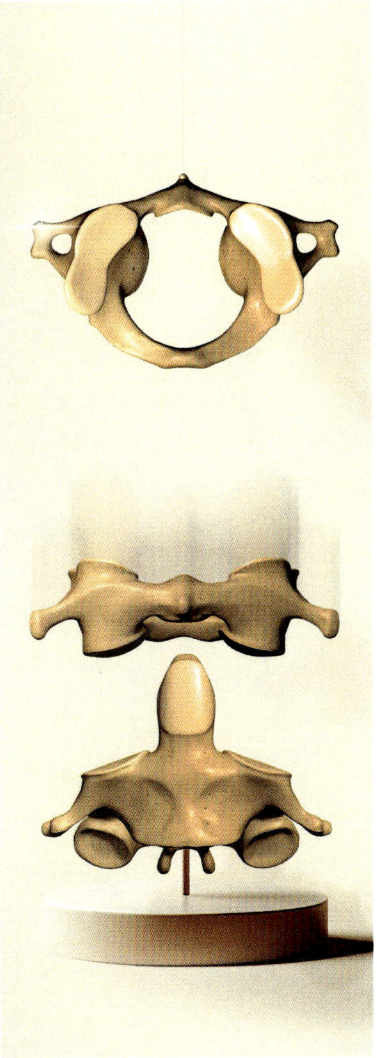

[Image 1] Atlas anatomy detail

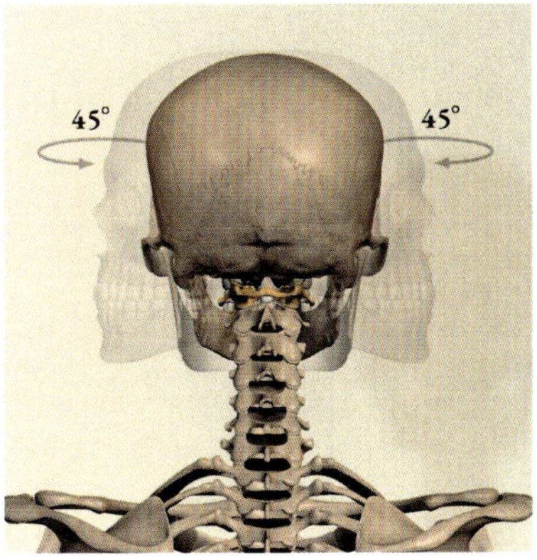

[Image 2] Atlas function with skull

Anatomy and Function of the Atlas

The atlas vertebra's unique bone structures are meticulously designed to support the head and facilitate smooth movement. Its articular surfaces and lateral masses play a critical role in ensuring the stability and functionality of the cervical spine.

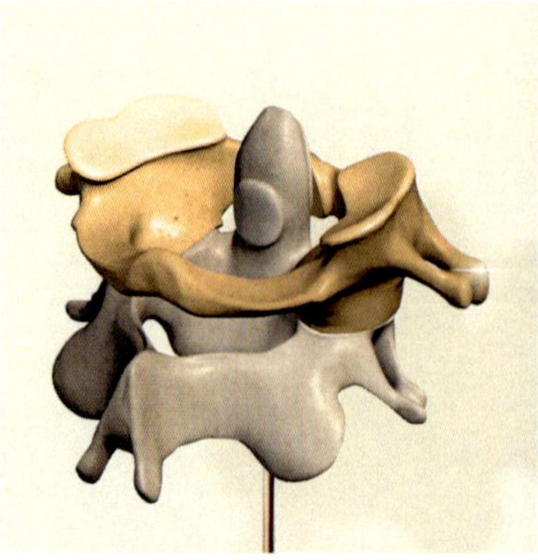

[Image 1] Atlas articular surfaces

The atlas vertebra is characterized by its unique bone structures, particularly its articular surfaces, which facilitate its articulation with adjacent vertebrae and the skull. These articular surfaces are finely crafted and precisely positioned to ensure smooth movement and stability of the cervical spine.

One of the key features of the atlas vertebra is its lateral masses, which serve as attachment points for ligaments and muscles that support the head and neck. These lateral masses provide strength and stability to the atlas, allowing it to withstand the weight of the skull and the forces exerted during movement [Image 1].

Additionally, the atlas vertebra features prominent processes and grooves that contribute to its overall structure and function. These processes include the transverse processes, which project laterally from the vertebra and serve as attachment sites for muscles and ligaments involved in head and neck movement. The grooves on the surface of the atlas accommodate nerves and blood vessels, ensuring their protection and unimpeded passage [Image 2].

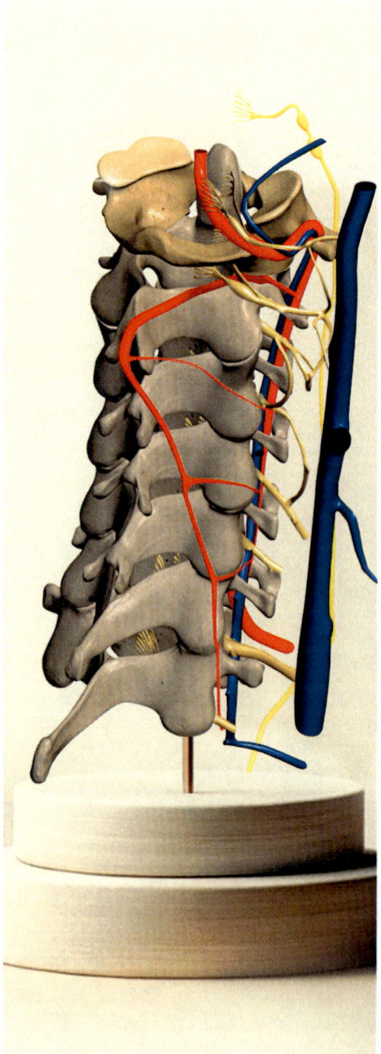

[Image 2] Atlas transverse processes

Furthermore, the bone characteristics of the atlas vertebra are essential for its role in supporting the head and facilitating movement. The bone density and composition of the atlas contribute to its strength and durability, allowing it to withstand the demands of daily activities and movements of the head and neck.

Key Components of the Atlas

The atlas vertebra consists of several characteristic parts, each of which plays a role in supporting the head and facilitating neck mobility. Here are some key parts of the atlas vertebra:

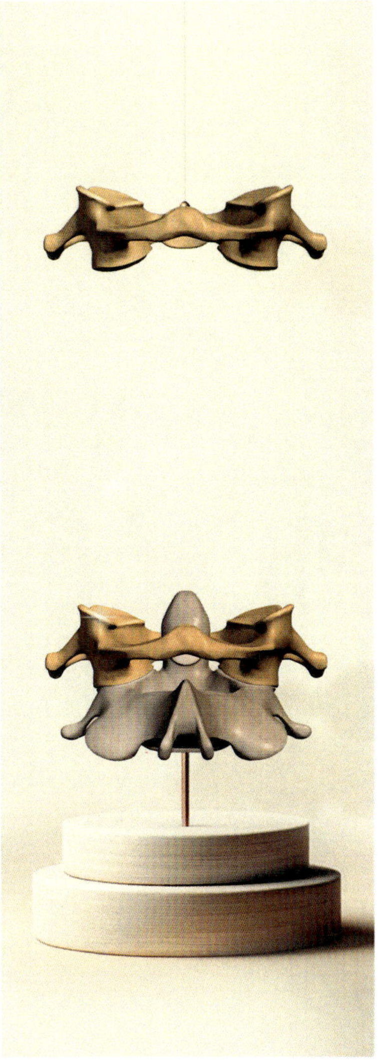

[Image 1] Atlas anatomy overview

1. Lateral Masses - (Lat. Processus lateralis) These are the lateral bulging parts of the atlas that provide support for the skull and allow for the attachment of muscles and ligaments that support the head.

2. Articular Surfaces - (Lat. Facies articularis) The articular surfaces of the atlas vertebra connect it to the skull and other vertebrae in the spine, facilitating movements of the neck and head.

3. Vertebral Foramen - (Lat. Foramen vertebrale) This is the central opening in the atlas vertebra through which the spinal cord passes.

4. Transverse Processes - (Lat. Processus transversus) These are the protruding parts that extend laterally from the atlas, providing points of attachment for muscles and ligaments of the neck.

5. Anterior Arch - (Lat. Arcus anterior) The anterior arch of the atlas is the curved part that extends forward, providing protection for the spinal cord.

6. Posterior Arch - (Lat. Arcus posterior) The posterior arch of the atlas is the curved part that extends backward, offering additional protection for the spinal cord.

All these parts work together to enable smooth movement and stability of the cervical spine, making the atlas a vital part of the human anatomy [Image 1].

Atlas - *Anterior Aspect*

1. **Anterior Arch** - Front arch of the atlas.

2. **Anterior Tubercle** - Small bump for ligament and muscle attachment.

3. **Transverse Processes** - Projections for muscle attachment.

4. **Transverse Foramina** - Holes for vertebral arteries, veins, and nerves.

5. **Facet for the Dens** - Surface for articulation with the dens of the axis.

6. **Lateral Masses** - Bulky portions supporting the skull

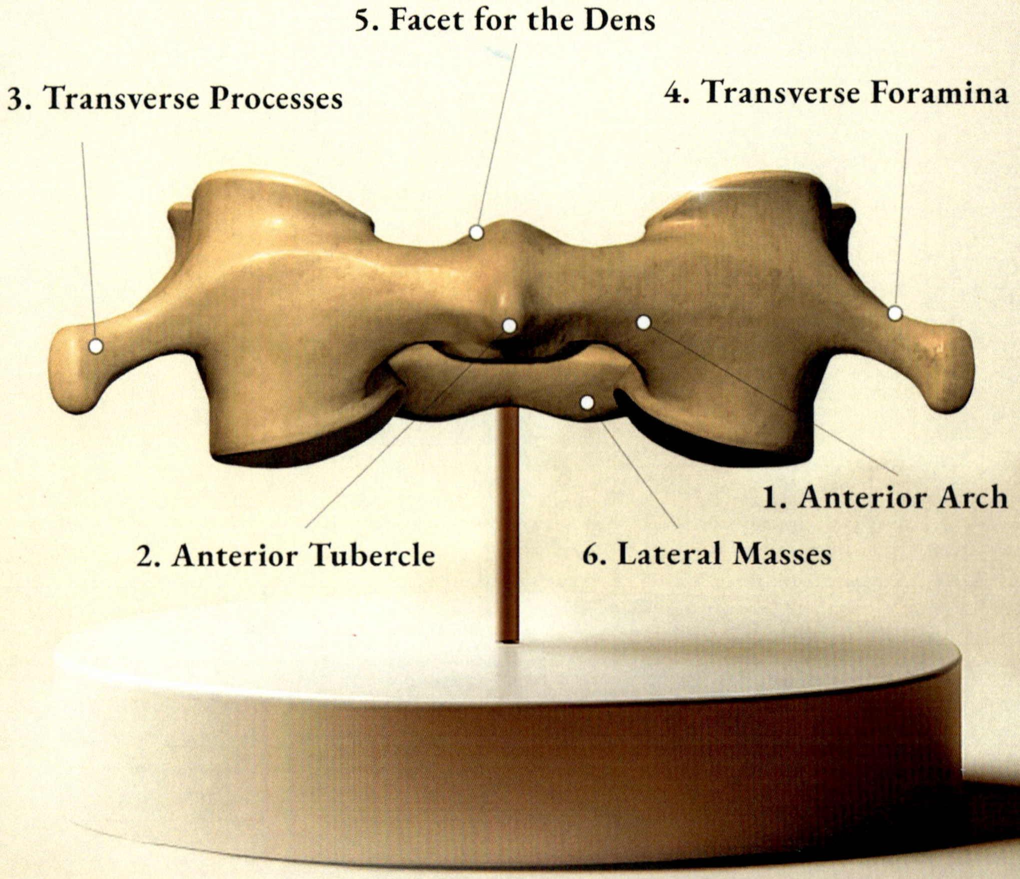

Atlas - *Posterior Aspect*

1. **Posterior Arch** - The rear arch of the atlas.

2. **Posterior Tubercle** - Small bump for ligament and muscle attachment.

3. **Transverse Processes** - Projections for muscle attachment.

4. **Transverse Foramina** - Openings for arteries, veins, and nerves.

5. **Superior Articular Facets** - Articulate with the occipital bone.

6. **Inferior Articular Facet** - Articulate with Axis C2.

7. **Vertebral Foramen** - Passageway for the spinal cord.

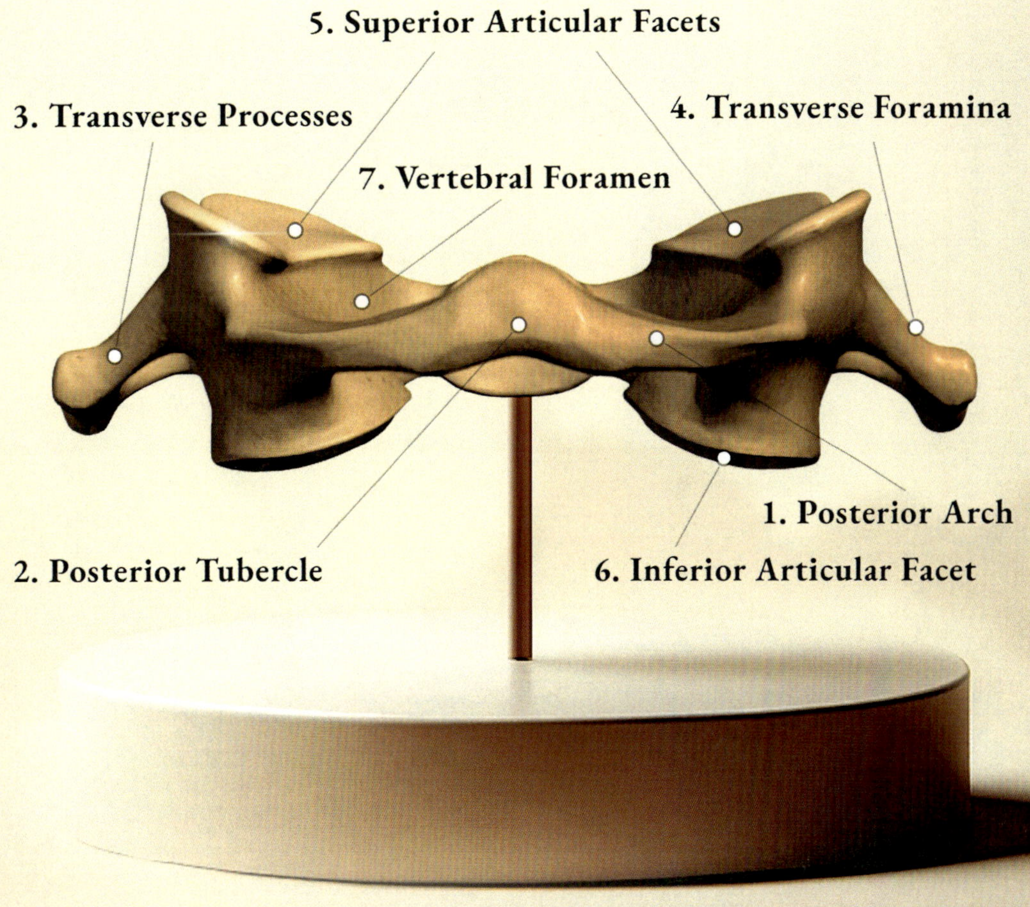

Atlas - *Superior Aspect*

1. **Anterior Arch** - Front arch of the atlas.
2. **Anterior Tubercle** - Small bump for ligament and muscle attachment.
3. **Transverse Processes** - Projections for muscle attachment.
4. **Transverse Foramina** - Openings for arteries, veins, and nerves.
5. **Superior Articular Facets** - Articulate with the occipital condyles.
6. **Lateral Masses** - Bulky portions supporting the skull.
7. **Posterior Arch** - Rear arch of the atlas.
8. **Posterior Tubercle** - Small bump for ligament and muscle attachment.
9. **Vertebral Foramen** - Passageway for the spinal cord.

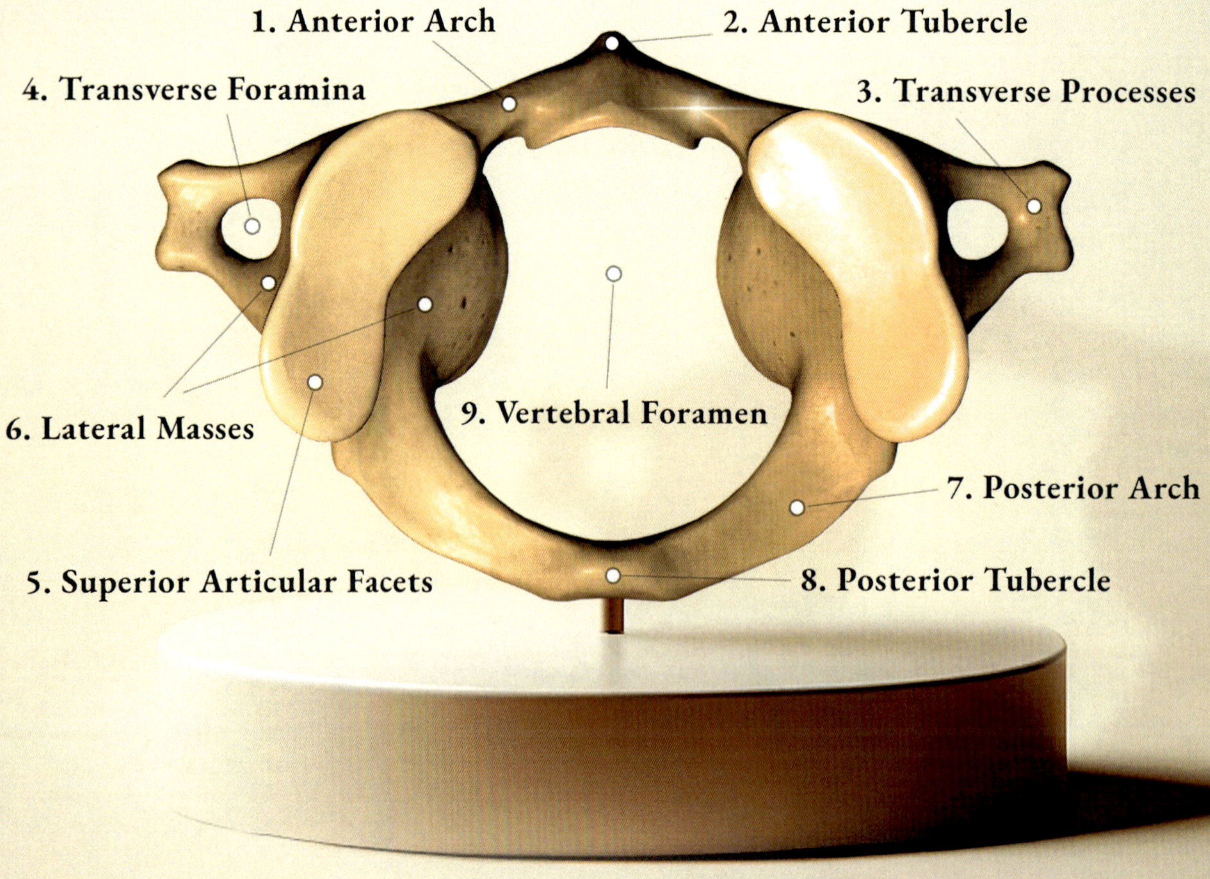

Axis - *Anterior Aspect*

1. **Dens (Odontoid Process)** - Bony projection that fits into the atlas.

2. **Body of Axis** - Central part of the axis.

3. **Transverse Processes** - Projections for muscle attachment.

4. **Transverse Foramina** - Openings for vertebral arteries and nerves.

5. **Superior Articular Facets** - Articulate with the atlas.

6. **Inferior Articular Facets** - Articulate with C3.

7. **Spinous Process** - Projection for muscle and ligament attachment.

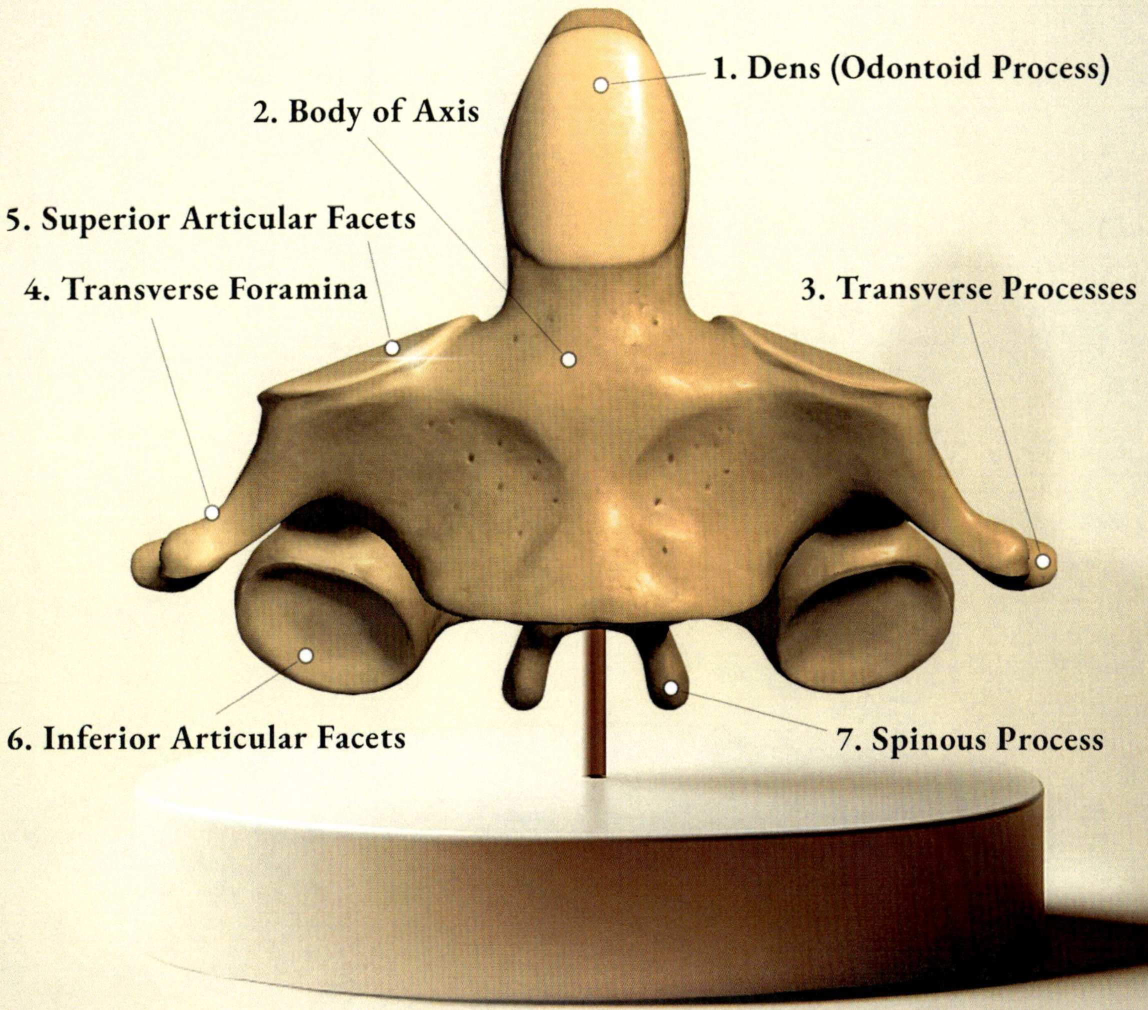

Axis - *Posterior Aspect*

1. **Dens (Odontoid Process)** - Bony projection that fits into the atlas.

2. **Transverse Processes** - Projections for muscle attachment.

3. **Transverse Foramina** - Openings for vertebral arteries and nerves.

4. **Superior Articular Facets** - Articulate with the atlas.

5. **Inferior Articular Facets** - Articulate with C3.

6. **Spinous Process** - Projection for muscle and ligament attachment.

7. **Lamina** - Between the spinous process and transverse process.

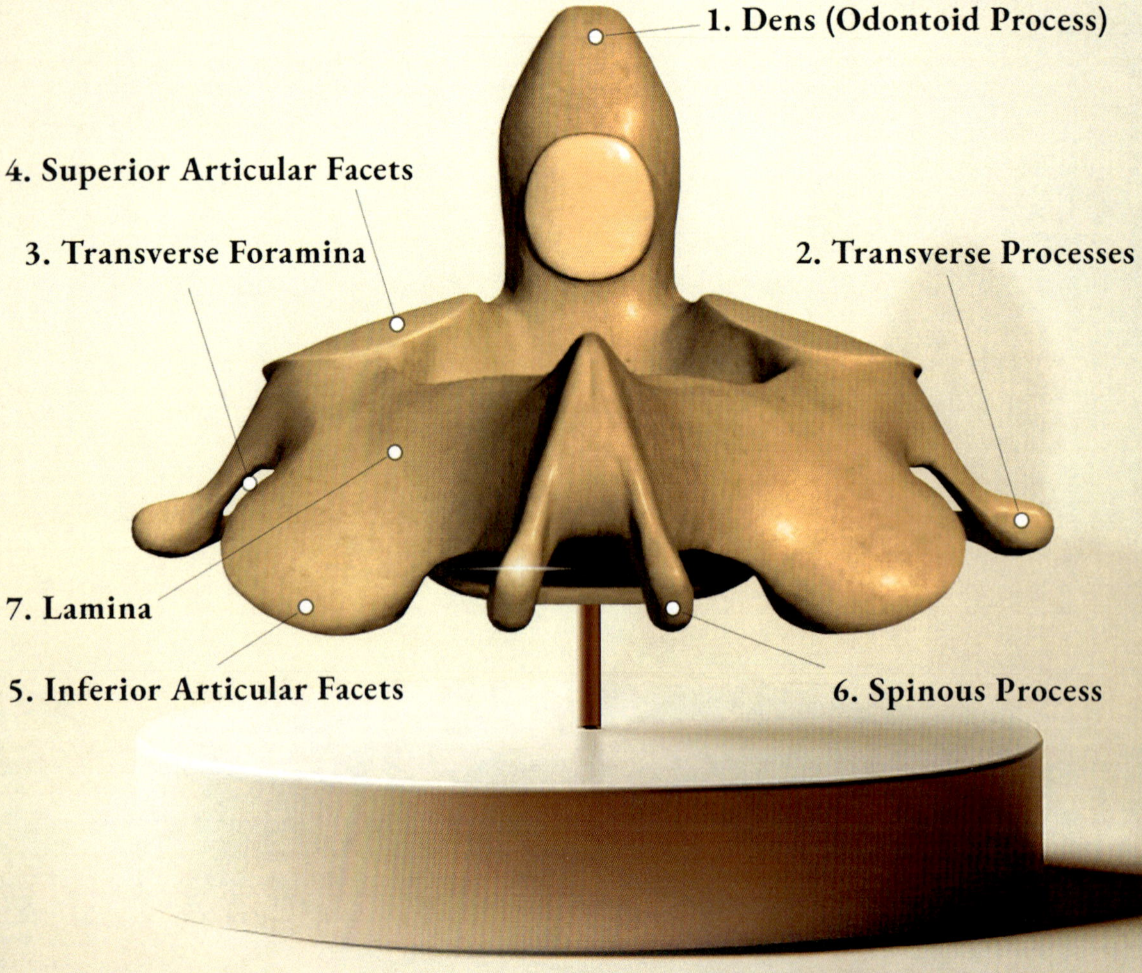

Axis - *Superior Aspect*

1. **Dens (Odontoid Process)** - Bony projection that fits into the atlas.
2. **Transverse Processes** - Projections for muscle attachment.
3. **Transverse Foramina** - Openings for vertebral arteries and nerves.
4. **Superior Articular Facets** - Articulate with the atlas.
5. **Lamina** - Between the spinous process and transverse process.
6. **Spinous Process** - Projection for muscle and ligament attachment.
7. **Pedicles** - Short bony projections that connect the body to the lamina.

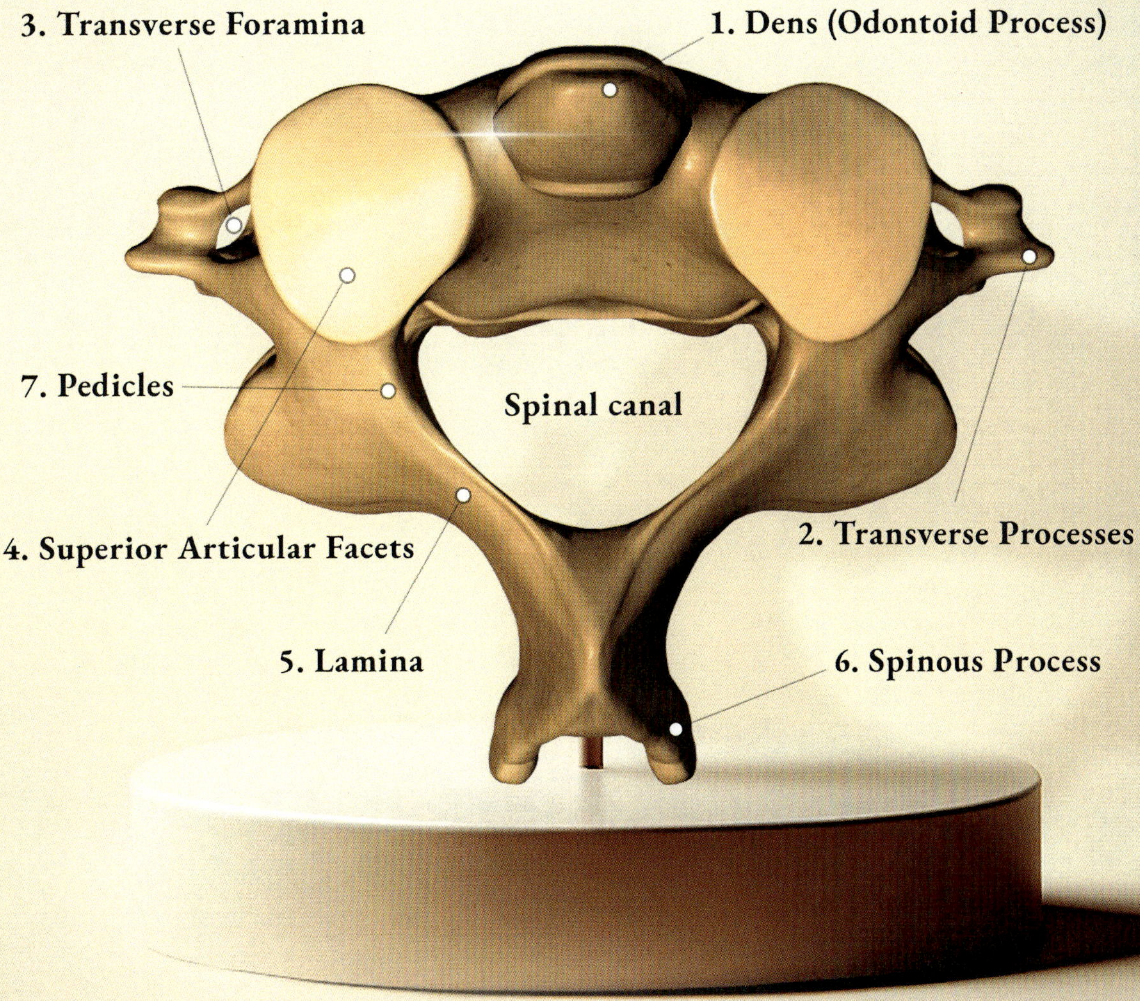

Atlas and Axis - *Atlanto-axial joint*

The joint between the atlas (C1) and axis (C2) vertebrae forms the atlanto-axial joint. This joint enables a significant range of motion for the head and neck. Here are the key functions of this joint:

1. Head Rotation: The atlanto-axial joint allows for the rotation of the head from side to side. About 50% of the total rotation of the head occurs at this joint.

2. Neck Stability: While it provides mobility, this joint also ensures the stability of the upper cervical spine.

3. Support for the Head: The atlas and axis together support the weight of the head and facilitate its proper positioning.

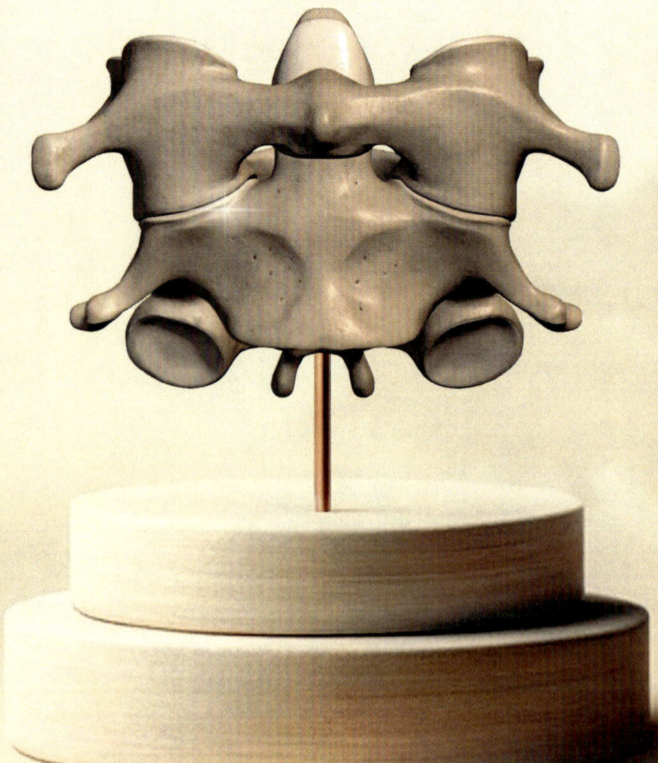

Atlas and Axis - *Three smaller joints*

This joint is crucial for the functionality and mobility of the neck, allowing for various head movements, including rotation, tilting, and flexion.

The atlanto-axial joint consists of three smaller joints:

The median atlanto-axial joint between the dens (odontoid process) of the axis and the anterior arch of the atlas.

Two lateral atlanto-axial joints between the inferior articular facets of the atlas and the superior articular facets of the axis.

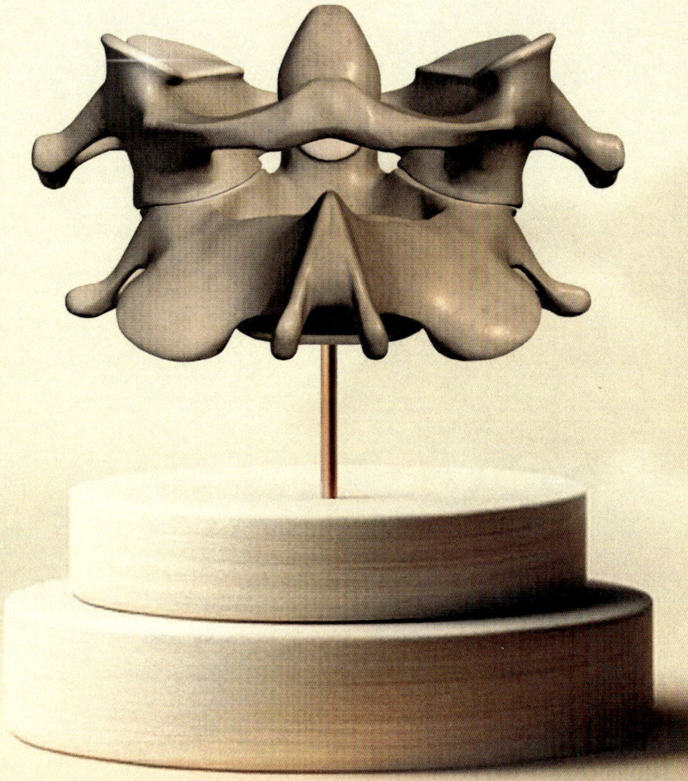

Atlas and Axis - ***Lateral View***

The lateral view of the Atlas (C1) and Axis (C2), particularly from the left side, plays a crucial role in diagnosing and analyzing these vertebrae. By utilizing advanced technologies, such as 3D scanners, it is possible to precisely assess anatomical relationships and detect atlantoaxial subluxation. This view provides detailed insight into the positioning and relationship between the Atlas and Axis, which is essential for accurate diagnosis and treatment planning.In clinical practice, the lateral view of the Atlas and Axis becomes an indispensable tool. It allows physicians to quickly and accurately identify structural abnormalities responsible for patient symptoms such as headaches, dizziness, neck pain, and neurological deficits.

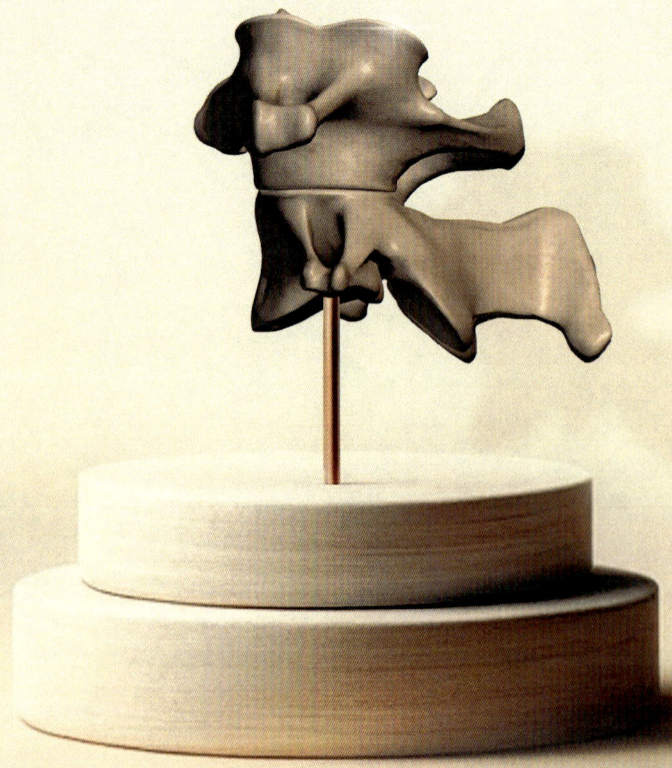

Impact of Atlas Changes

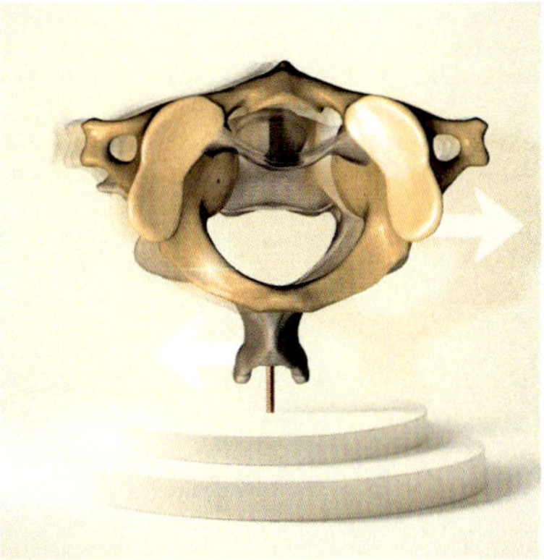

[Image 1] Atlas subluxation

Changes in the structure of the atlas can have a significant impact on the function of the spine and cervical region. These changes can be caused by various factors, including injuries, degenerative diseases, or congenital anomalies. When changes occur in the structure of the atlas, they can result in various health problems and limitations in mobility [Image 1].

Injuries to the atlas, such as fractures or dislocations, can lead to serious problems in the cervical spine. These traumas can disrupt the normal shape and integrity of the atlas, resulting in pain, limited movement, and neurological symptoms. In such cases, rehabilitation and treatments aimed at restoring the structure of the atlas and supporting the cervical spine can be essential for recovery and prevention of further complications.

Additionally, degenerative diseases such as osteoarthritis or disc degeneration can affect the structure of the atlas over time. Loss of cartilage tissue or increased bone mass can alter the shape and size of the atlas, leading to pain and reduced neck mobility. In such cases, therapies aimed at reducing inflammation, strengthening neck muscles, and preserving mobility can be crucial for managing symptoms and preserving function.

Congenital anomalies of the atlas, such as different shapes or sizes, can also lead to changes in structure and function. These anomalies may be present from birth and can cause problems in the development of the spine and cervical region. In some cases, surgical interventions may be necessary to correct these anomalies and prevent complications in the future.

Some of the most well-known medical research on changes in the structure of the atlas relate to the causes and consequences of degenerative changes in the atlas, the long-term effects and therapeutic approaches of traumatic injuries to the atlas, the clinical manifestations and therapeutic challenges of congenital anomalies of the atlas, perspectives on preventing degenerative changes due to the effects of aging on the structure of the atlas, and the results and complications of surgical approaches to correcting anomalies of the atlas [Image 1].

"Above all else, guard your heart, for everything you do flows from it."

(Solomon, Proverbs 4:23)

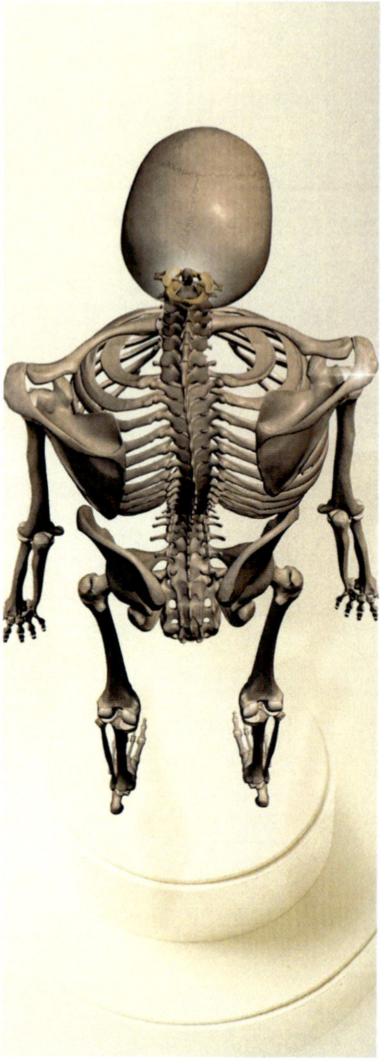

[Image 1] Consequence - scoliosis

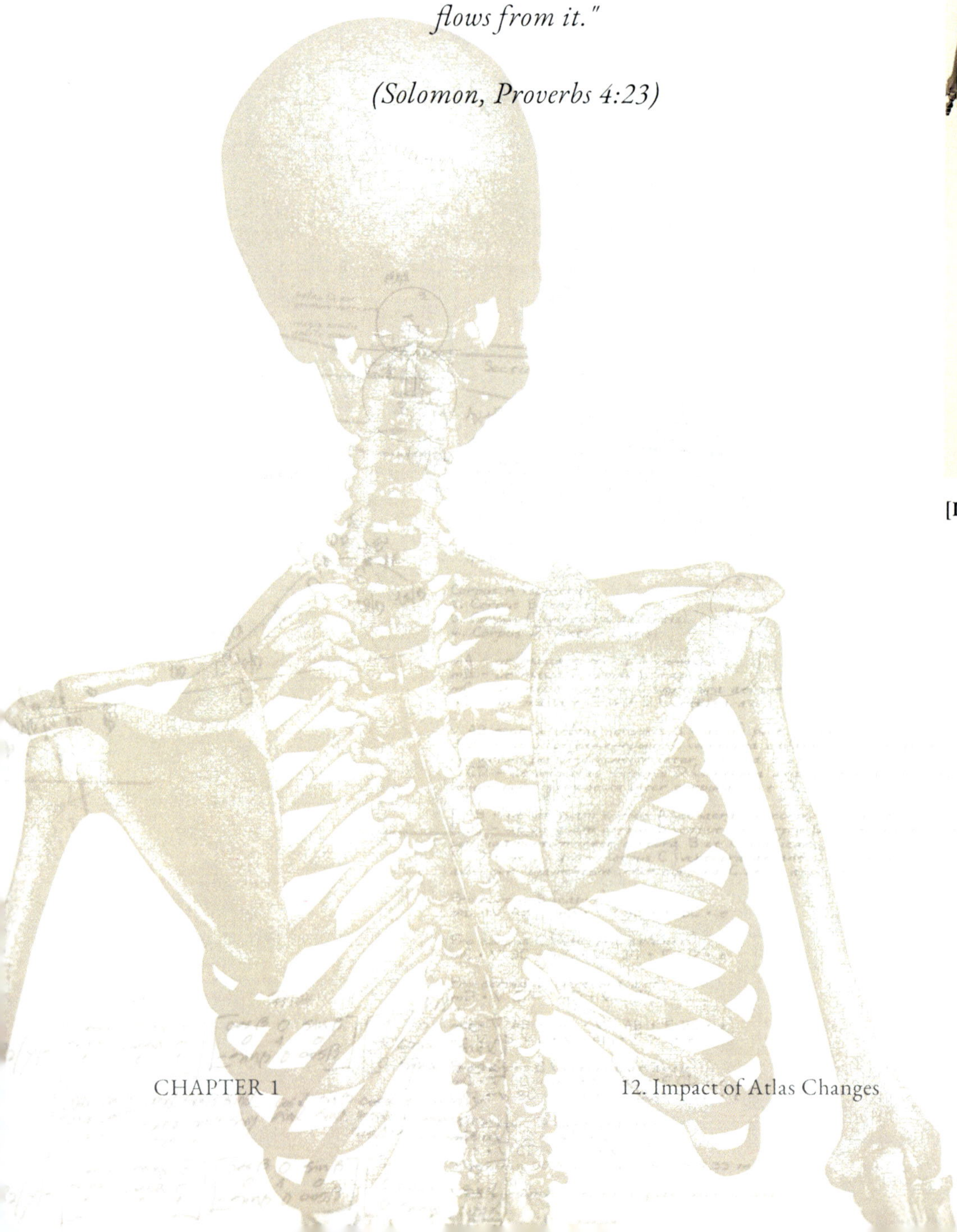

The Atlas: Mobility and Health

The atlas vertebra, situated at the top of the spinal column, plays a crucial role in supporting the skull and facilitating the movements of the head and neck [Image 1]. Its unique structure allows for a wide range of motion, including nodding, rotating, and tilting the head. This mobility is essential for various daily activities, such as driving, working at a computer, or engaging in sports and recreational activities.

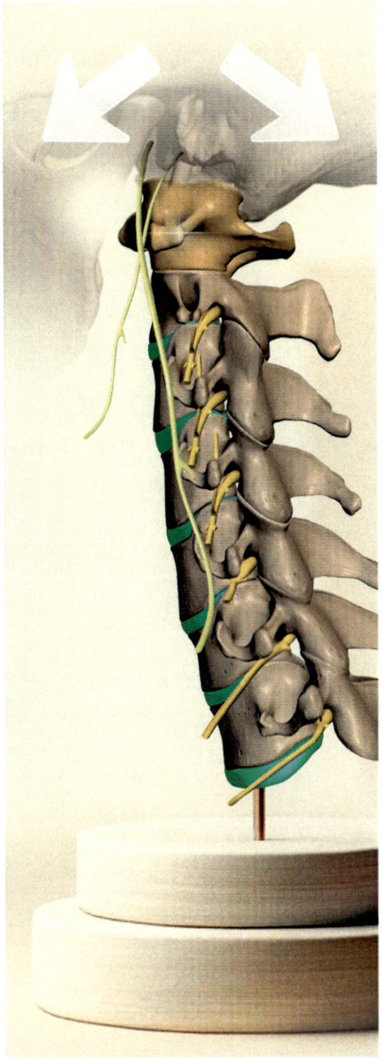

[Image 1] Atlas motion and stability

Moreover, the atlas serves as a vital link between the head and the rest of the body, as it connects the skull to the spinal column. Any compromise in the integrity of the atlas can disrupt this connection, leading to imbalances in posture and movement patterns. Consequently, maintaining the structural integrity of the atlas is essential for preserving overall body mobility and functionality.

Furthermore, the atlas vertebra is closely associated with the nervous system, particularly the brainstem and upper spinal cord. Any misalignment or structural abnormalities in the atlas can potentially impinge on nerve function, affecting sensory perception, motor control, and overall bodily function. Therefore, ensuring the proper alignment and function of the atlas is crucial for optimal nervous system health and body mobility.

In addition to its role in mobility and nervous system function, the atlas is crucial for regulating blood flow to the brain. The vertebral arteries pass through the cervical vertebrae, including the atlas.

"Where the spirit does not work with the hand, there is no art."

(Leonardo da Vinci)

Key Articulations and Functions

The atlas vertebra articulates with the spine at several key points, including the articular surfaces and ligaments that connect the vertebrae. These articulations allow the atlas to move freely and rotate in various directions, which is necessary for normal head and neck rotation [Image 1].

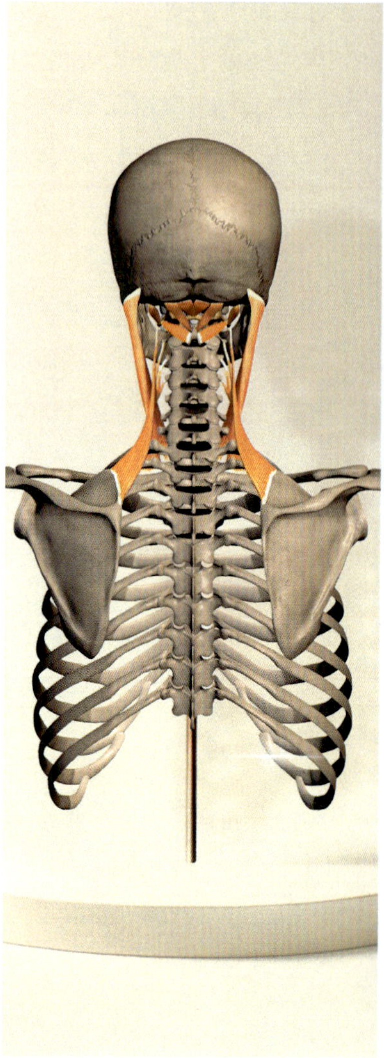

[Image 1] Cervical spine and muscles

A particularly important aspect of the articulation of the atlas vertebra is its connection with other vertebrae in the cervical spine, especially with other cervical vertebrae and the cranial base of the skull. This articulation enables the transfer of the weight of the head along the spine and evenly distributes the load during head and neck movements.

Moreover, the articulation of the atlas with the spine plays a crucial role in maintaining the integrity of the neural structures passing through the cervical spine. Proper articulation allows for optimal flow of information between the brain and the rest of the body, which is essential for sensory-motor function and overall nervous system health.

In addition to facilitating movement and protecting neural structures, the atlas also helps absorb shocks and distribute forces during head and neck movements. This function is essential in reducing strain on the cervical vertebrae and minimizing potential injuries caused by sudden impacts, such as whiplash or other trauma to the neck. The flexibility and stability provided by the atlas ensure that the cervical spine can withstand the daily stresses and sudden movements without compromising structural integrity. Furthermore, the atlas plays a critical role in maintaining overall balance and posture by supporting proper alignment of the head and spine. This alignment not only contributes to physical stability but also helps prevent long-term wear and tear on the musculoskeletal system.

Ligaments of the Atlas

The ligaments of the atlas vertebra play a crucial role in maintaining stability and support for anatomical structures in the cervical spine. This section focuses on studying the various ligaments that connect the atlas vertebra to adjacent structures, including those that stabilize the atlanto-occipital joint.

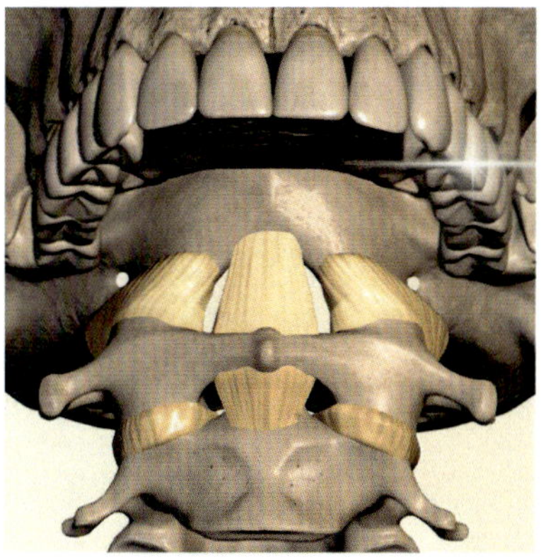

[Image 1] Anterior side

The atlanto-occipital ligaments are particularly significant as they provide stability and support to the head, allowing it to flex forward and backward [Image 1][Image 2]. These ligaments consist of the anterior and posterior arches, as well as the membrane covering the atlanto-occipital space. Their role is to prevent excessive flexion and extension in this joint, which could lead to neck and spine injuries.

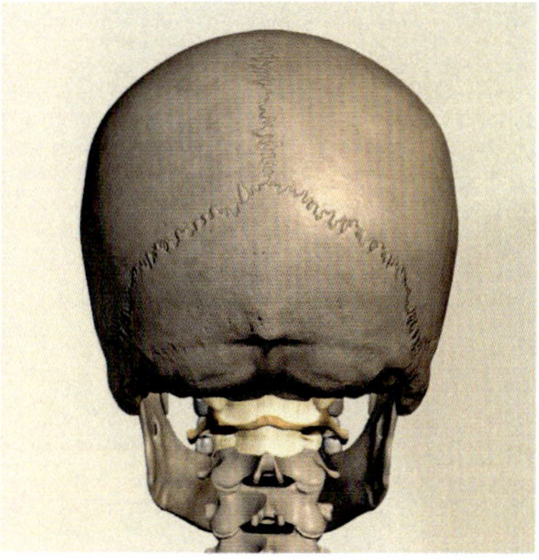

[Image 2] Posterior side

In addition to the atlanto-occipital ligaments, there are other ligaments that contribute to the integrity of the atlas vertebra. This includes the transverse ligament of the atlas, which is part of the cruciform ligament complex [Image 3]. It extends horizontally across the anterior arch of the atlas and serves as a connection between the lateral masses of the atlas. This ligament contributes to the stability of the atlantoaxial joint, a crucial joint that allows for head rotation.

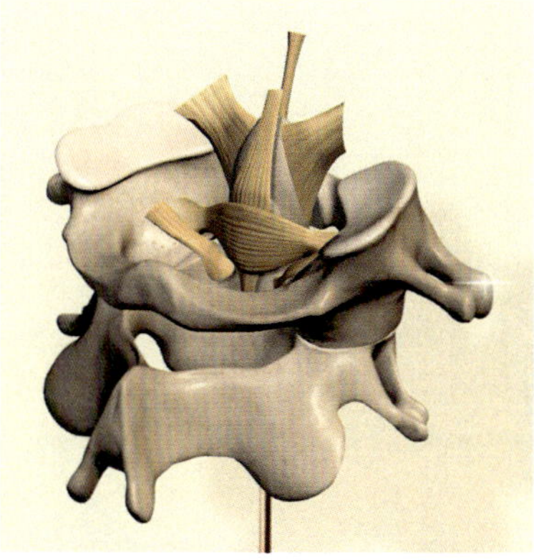

[Image 3] Cruciform ligament

Furthermore, there are interligamentous connections that link the atlas to adjacent vertebrae and surrounding structures. These ligaments play an important role in maintaining balance and stability of the cervical spine, preventing excessive movements and potential injuries.

Understanding these ligaments allows for the diagnosis and treatment of various neck conditions and injuries, as well as the development of effective therapeutic approaches to maintain the health and mobility of the cervical spine.

Anterior Atlanto-Occipital Ligaments

The anterior view of the atlanto-occipital ligaments shows the anterior atlanto-occipital ligament stabilizing the joint between the occipital bone and the atlas. These ligaments allow limited neck movements while maintaining head stability relative to the spine. The anterior perspective clearly illustrates their role as key stabilizers of the atlanto-occipital joint.

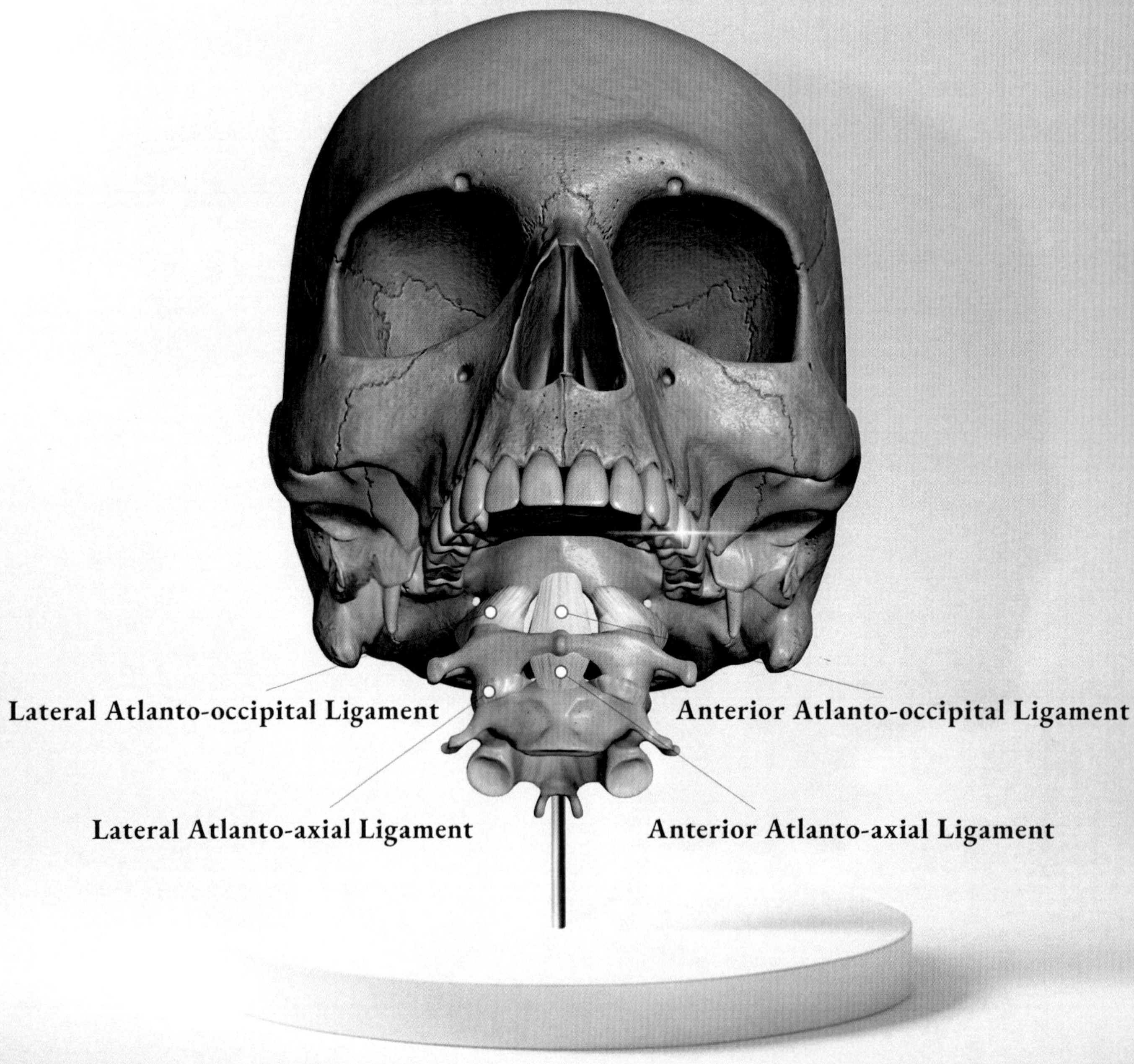

Atlanto-occipital joint

The atlanto-occipital joint is a vital connection between the atlas (C1) and the occipital bone of the skull. It primarily allows for the nodding motion of the head, enabling flexion and extension. This joint is stabilized by ligaments and surrounding muscles, which ensure smooth movement and support the head's balance and stability.

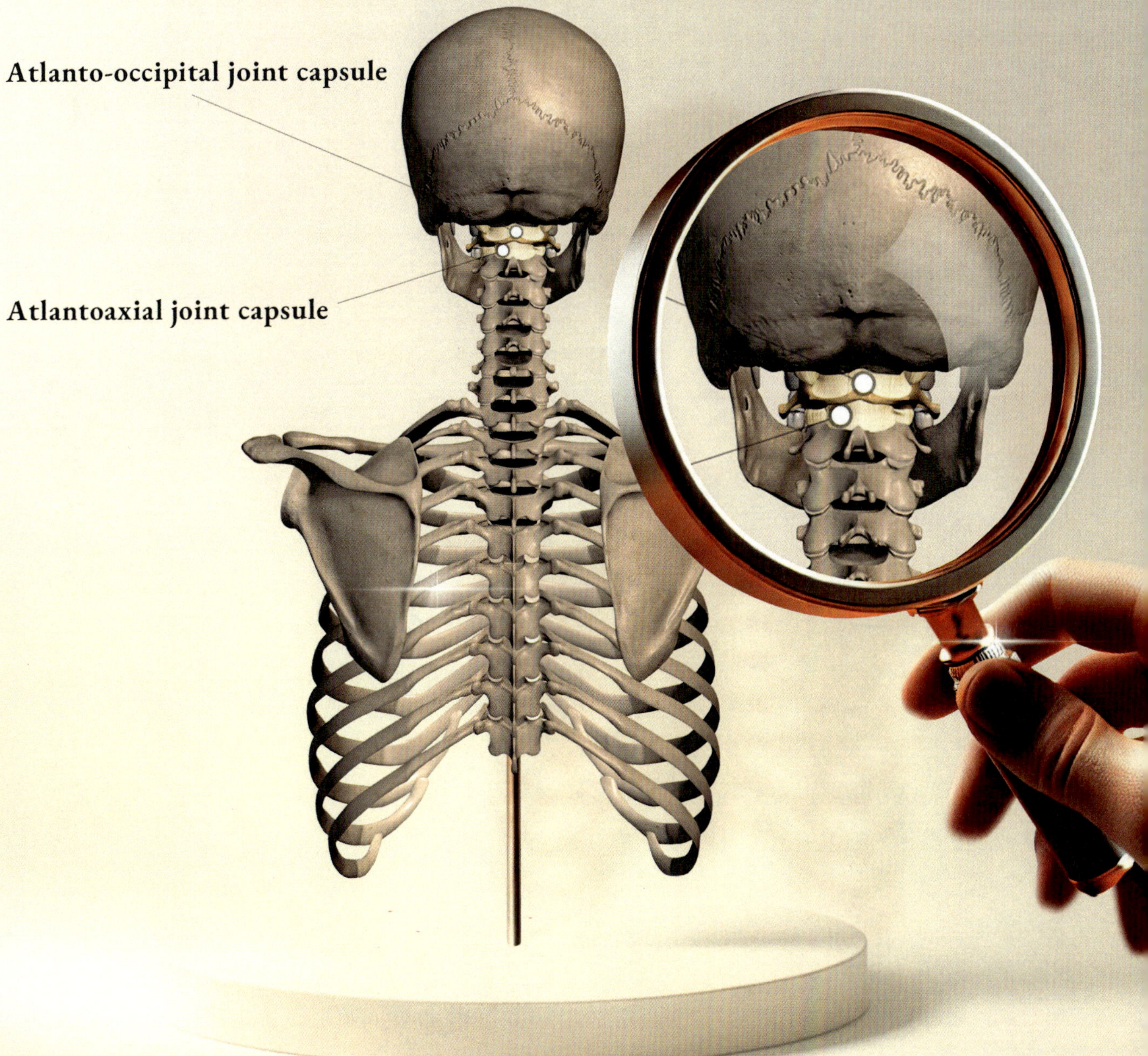

Atlas Ligaments and Their Functions

The ligaments of the atlas vertebra play a crucial role in maintaining stability and support for anatomical structures in the cervical spine. This section focuses on studying the various ligaments that connect the atlas vertebra to adjacent structures, including those that stabilize the atlanto-occipital joint.

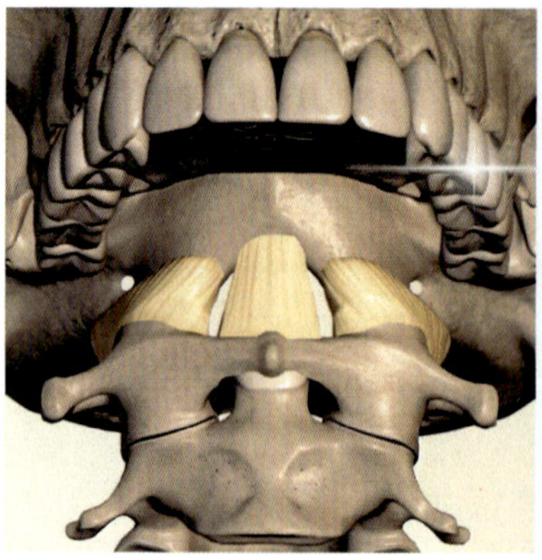
[Image 1] Atlantooccipitalis anterior

1. Atlantooccipitalis anterior ligament

The primary function of the anterior atlanto-occipital ligament is to stabilize the atlanto-occipital joint, which is formed between the base of the skull (occipital bone) and the upper part of the atlas [Image 1]. This ligament prevents excessive backward movement of the head, thereby protecting the spinal cord from damage.

Additionally, the anterior atlanto-occipital ligament assists in supporting the weight of the head and maintaining the optimal position of the neck. Without it, the head would be prone to excessive backward tilting, which could lead to serious spinal cord and nerve injuries in the cervical region.

Furthermore, this ligament contributes to preserving the structure and shape of the atlas, ensuring the integrity of this vertebra and enabling proper functioning of the upper spine.

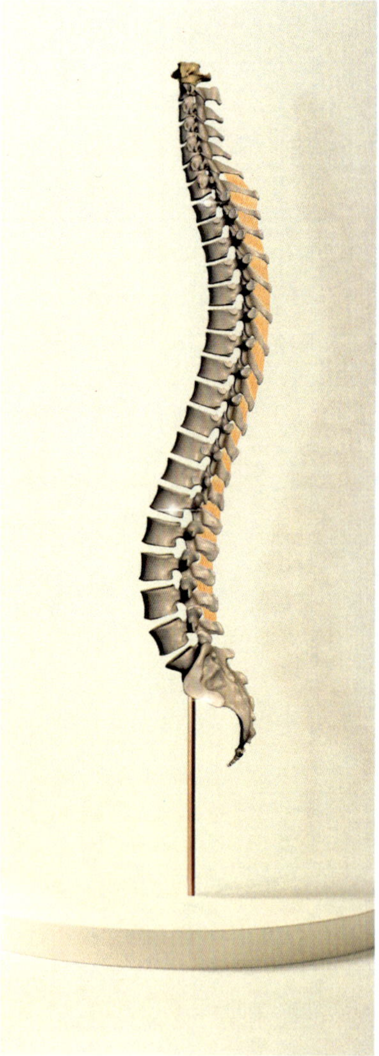
[Image 2] Interspinous ligaments

2. Interspinous ligaments

The primary function of the interspinous ligaments is to stabilize the vertebrae of the spine by connecting their spinous processes along the spinal column [Image 2]. This ligament helps maintain the integrity of the spine, preventing excessive movements that could lead to instability or injury.

Additionally, the interspinal ligament plays a crucial role in supporting the proper alignment of the vertebrae during various body movements, such as bending and twisting. Without this ligament, the vertebrae would be prone to excessive movement, which could result in serious spinal cord and nerve injuries.

Furthermore, the interspinal ligament contributes to preserving the proper curvature of the spinal column, ensuring its stability and flexibility. This allows the spinal column to function correctly, which is essential for daily activities and overall body mobility.

3. Posterior longitudinal

The primary function of the posterior longitudinal ligament is to stabilize the vertebrae of the spine by running along the posterior surface of the vertebral bodies from the base of the skull to the sacrum [Image 1]. This ligament helps maintain the alignment of the vertebrae, preventing excessive forward flexion and protecting the spinal cord from injury.

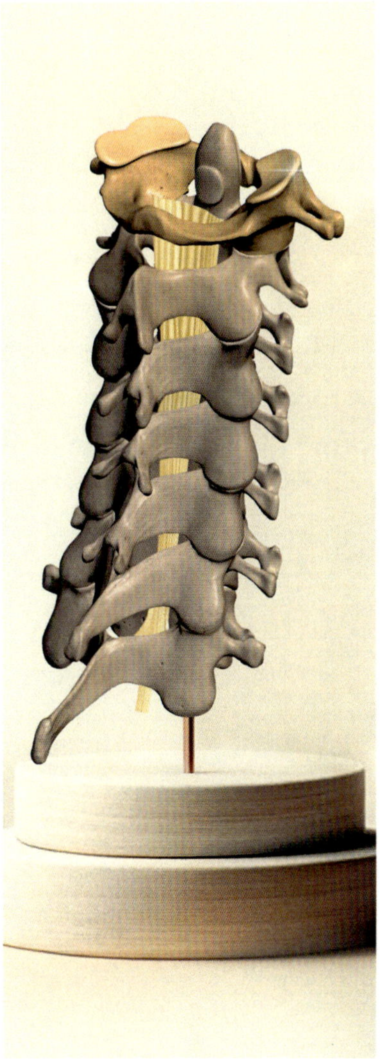

[Image 1] Posterior longitudinal

Additionally, the posterior longitudinal ligament plays a crucial role in supporting the intervertebral discs, helping to distribute the mechanical loads placed on the spine during various movements and activities. Without this ligament, the spine would be more susceptible to disc herniations and other degenerative changes.

Furthermore, the posterior longitudinal ligament contributes to the overall structural integrity of the spinal column, ensuring that the vertebrae and intervertebral discs remain properly aligned. This is essential for maintaining the spine's flexibility and stability, allowing for smooth and pain-free motion while protecting the spinal cord and nerve roots from damage.

4. Towards the anterior tubercle of the atlas

The primary function of the ligament of the apex of the dens is to stabilize the dens (odontoid process) of the second cervical vertebra (axis) and help maintain proper alignment between the atlas and axis [Image 1]. This small but crucial ligament attaches to the tip of the dens and extends to the inner aspect of the base of the occipital bone (foramen magnum).

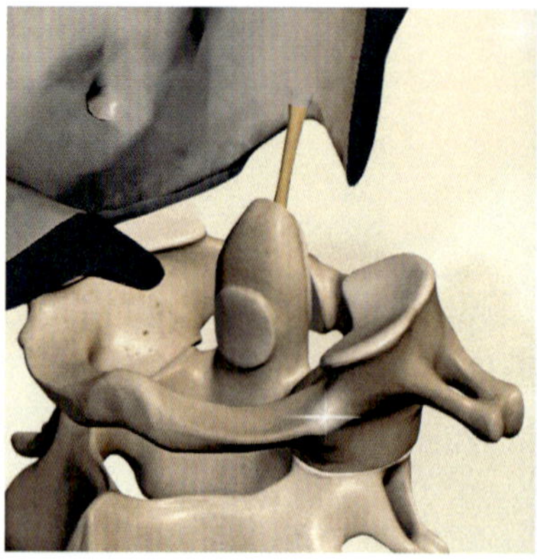

[Image 1] Apical Ligament

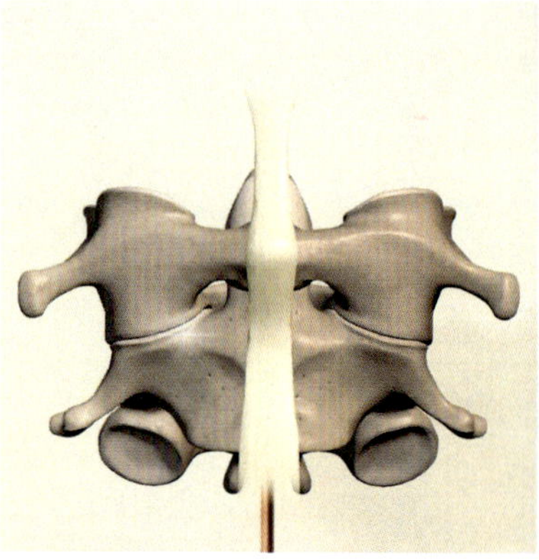

[Image 2] Anterior longitudinal

Additionally, the ligament of the apex of the dens plays a key role in limiting excessive movements of the atlas and axis, preventing dislocation and ensuring the stability of the upper cervical spine. Without this ligament, the head would be prone to excessive rotations and movements, which could lead to serious injuries to the spinal cord and neural structures.

Furthermore, the ligament of the apex of the dens contributes to preserving the anatomical structure and functional integrity of the cervical spine. This allows for normal mobility of the head and neck while protecting the vital neurovascular structures that pass through this region of the spine.

5. Towards the anterior arch of the atlas

The primary function of the anterior longitudinal ligament is to stabilize the vertebral bodies and intervertebral discs along the anterior surface of the spine, extending from the base of the skull down to the sacrum [Image 2]. This ligament helps maintain the alignment of the spine and prevents excessive extension (backward bending) that could lead to instability or injury.

Additionally, the anterior longitudinal ligament plays a crucial role in supporting the vertebral bodies and intervertebral discs, helping to distribute mechanical loads and protect the spine during various movements and activities. Without this ligament, the spine would be more vulnerable to hyperextension injuries and other degenerative changes.

Furthermore, the anterior longitudinal ligament contributes to the overall structural integrity of the spinal column, ensuring that the vertebrae and intervertebral discs remain properly aligned. This is essential for maintaining the spine's stability and flexibility, allowing for smooth and pain-free motion while protecting the spinal cord and nerve roots from damage.

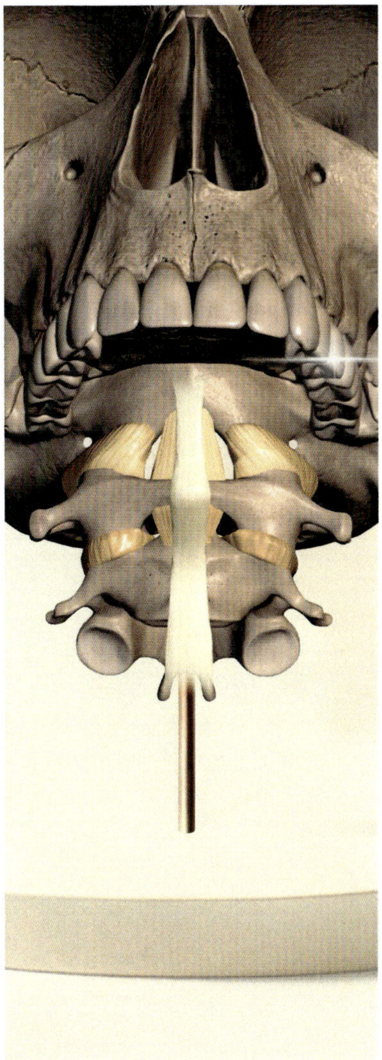

[Image 1] Anterior Spinal Ligaments

6. Towards the anterior surface

The primary function of the anterior articular ligament is to stabilize the joints between the vertebrae, particularly the facet joints, which connect the individual vertebrae of the spine. This ligament spans the anterior aspect of these joints, helping to maintain their proper alignment and prevent excessive movement that could lead to instability or injury.

Additionally, the anterior articular ligament plays a crucial role in supporting the overall structural integrity of the spine, contributing to its ability to bear weight and withstand various mechanical stresses [Image 1]. Without this ligament, the facet joints would be more prone to dislocations and degenerative changes, potentially leading to chronic pain and mobility issues.

Furthermore, the anterior articular ligament helps preserve the natural curvature of the spine, ensuring that the vertebrae move in a coordinated and controlled manner. This is essential for maintaining the flexibility and stability of the spine, allowing for smooth and pain-free motion while protecting the spinal cord and nerve roots from damage.

7. Towards the posterior surface

The primary function of the nuchal ligament is to stabilize the cervical vertebrae and support the head, extending from the occipital bone to the seventh cervical vertebra [Image 1]. This ligament is especially important for maintaining the proper position of the head and neck, preventing excessive forward flexion.

Additionally, the nuchal ligament plays a crucial role in reducing the load on the neck muscles by providing passive support to the head. Without this ligament, the neck muscles would be more prone to fatigue and injury due to constant strain.

Furthermore, the nuchal ligament contributes to the structural stability and flexibility of the cervical spine. This allows for normal mobility of the head and neck, which is essential for daily activities and overall body movement, while simultaneously protecting the spinal cord and nerves in the cervical region from damage.

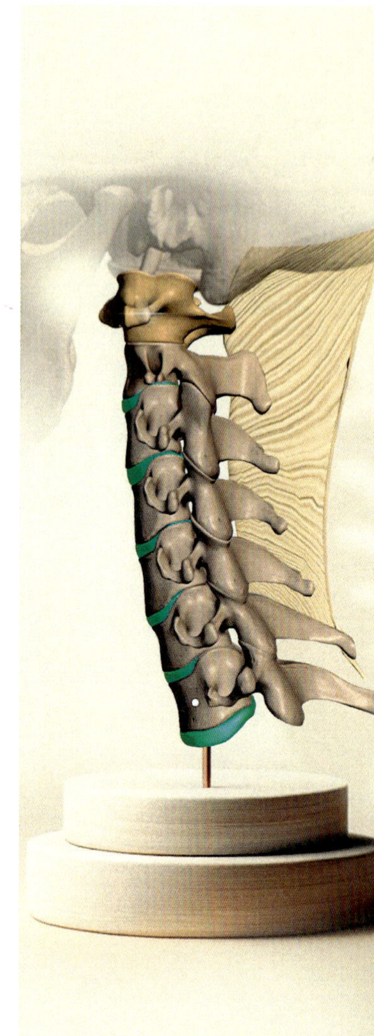

[Image 1] Nuchal ligament

8. Accessory Atlanto-Axial Ligaments [Image 2]

The primary function of the accessory atlanto-axial ligaments is to stabilize the atlanto-axial joint, which connects the atlas (the first cervical vertebra) with the axis (the second cervical vertebra). These ligaments run between the lateral masses of the atlas and the axis, supporting the main structures of the atlanto-axial joint. By providing additional reinforcement, they help to maintain the proper alignment of the cervical

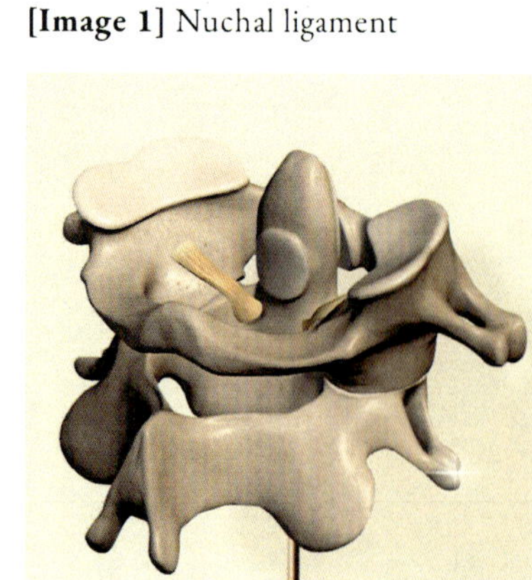

[Image 2] Accessory atlanto-axial

spine and limit excessive or abnormal rotational movements of the head, which could lead to instability or injury.

Additionally, the accessory atlanto-axial ligaments play a key role in distributing mechanical loads across the joint surfaces, ensuring smooth and coordinated movement of the cervical spine. Without these ligaments, the atlanto-axial joint would be more susceptible to dislocations and degenerative changes, potentially leading to serious neurological issues and decreased functionality.

Furthermore, the radial ligament contributes to the overall structural integrity of the radial side of the limb, supporting the muscles and tendons that facilitate movement. This is essential for performing everyday tasks and activities that require fine motor skills and strength, while also protecting the nerves and blood vessels that traverse these regions.

9. Transverse Ligament of the Atlas

The primary function of the transverse ligament of the atlas is to stabilize the atlantoaxial joint, which connects the atlas (the first cervical vertebra) with the axis (the second cervical vertebra) [Image 1]. This ligament extends between the lateral masses of the atlas, securing the dens of the axis and helping to maintain proper alignment while limiting excessive rotational movements of the head.

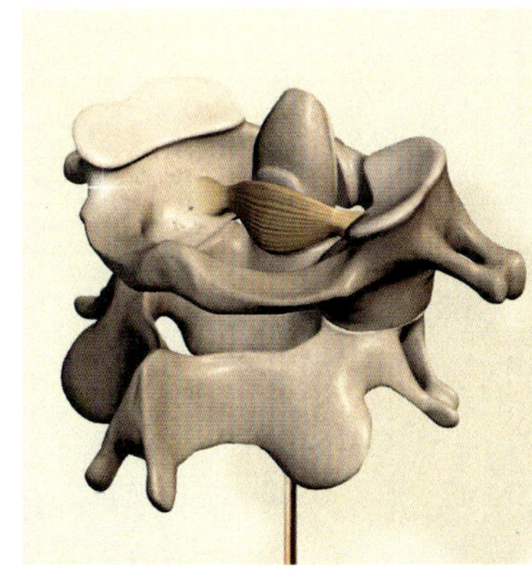
[Image 1] Transverse ligament

Additionally, the transverse ligament of the atlas plays a crucial role in supporting normal cervical spine mobility, allowing the head to move freely while simultaneously protecting the spinal cord from injury. Without this ligament, the cervical vertebrae would be more prone to dislocations and instability, which could lead to serious neurological issues.

Furthermore, the transverse ligament of the atlas contributes to the overall structural integrity of the cervical spine, supporting the muscles and tendons that facilitate head and neck movement. This is essential for daily activities that re-

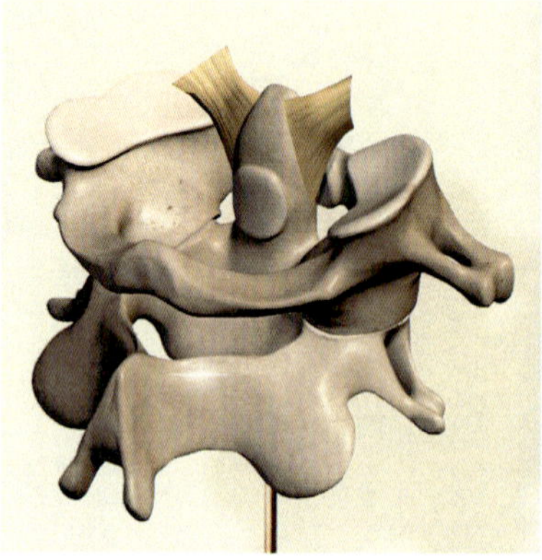
[Image 1] Alar ligaments

10. Alar ligaments

The primary function of the alar ligaments is to stabilize the craniovertebral junction by connecting the sides of the dens (odontoid process) of the axis (the second cervical vertebra) to the medial sides of the occipital condyles of the skull [Image 1]. These ligaments are crucial in limiting the rotation and side-to-side movement of the head, thereby preventing excessive or abnormal motion that could result in injury.

Additionally, the alar ligaments play a key role in maintaining the alignment of the atlas and axis, which is essential for the proper function of the upper cervical spine. Without these ligaments, the head and neck would be more susceptible to hyper-rotation and lateral flexion injuries, potentially leading to severe spinal cord damage and neurological deficits.

Furthermore, the alar ligaments contribute to the overall structural integrity and stability of the cervical spine, particularly during rotational movements of the head. This is vital for ensuring smooth and coordinated head movements, protecting the spinal cord and nerve roots in the cervical region, and supporting the normal range of motion necessary for everyday activities.

11. Interspinal

The primary function of the interspinal ligament of the atlas is to stabilize the cervical vertebrae by connecting the spinous processes of the atlas (the first cervical vertebra) to the axis (the second cervical vertebra). This ligament plays a crucial role in maintaining the integrity and proper alignment of the upper cervical spine, preventing excessive movements that could lead to instability or injury [Image 1].

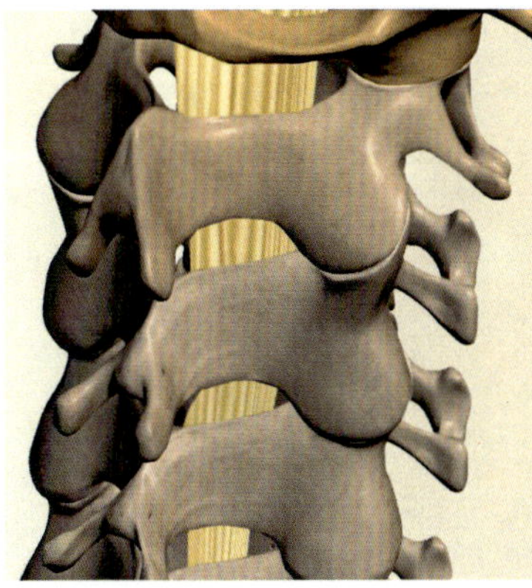

[Image 1] Interspinal ligament

Additionally, the interspinal ligament of the atlas helps facilitate smooth and coordinated movements of the head and neck, particularly during bending and twisting motions. Without this ligament, the cervical vertebrae would be more prone to excessive shifting, which could result in serious spinal cord injuries and damage to the nervous structures.

Furthermore, the interspinal ligament of the atlas contributes to the overall structural stability and flexibility of the cervical spine. This is essential for enabling normal head and neck movements, which are critical for daily activities and overall body mobility, while simultaneously protecting the vital neurovascular structures that pass through this region of the spine.

"What? know ye not that your body is the temple of the Holy Ghost which is in you, which ye have of God, and ye are not your own? For ye are bought with a price: therefore glorify God in your body, and in your spirit, which are God's."

(1 Corinthians 6:19-20)

1. Transverse Ligament of the Atlas

The ligament that extends horizontally around the dens (odontoid process) of the axis. This ligament plays a crucial role in stabilizing the atlanto-axial joint, holding the dens firmly against the anterior arch of the atlas, preventing it from moving backward towards the spinal cord. The Transverse Ligament of the Atlas also helps to allow the rotation of the head while maintaining the alignment of the atlas and axis.

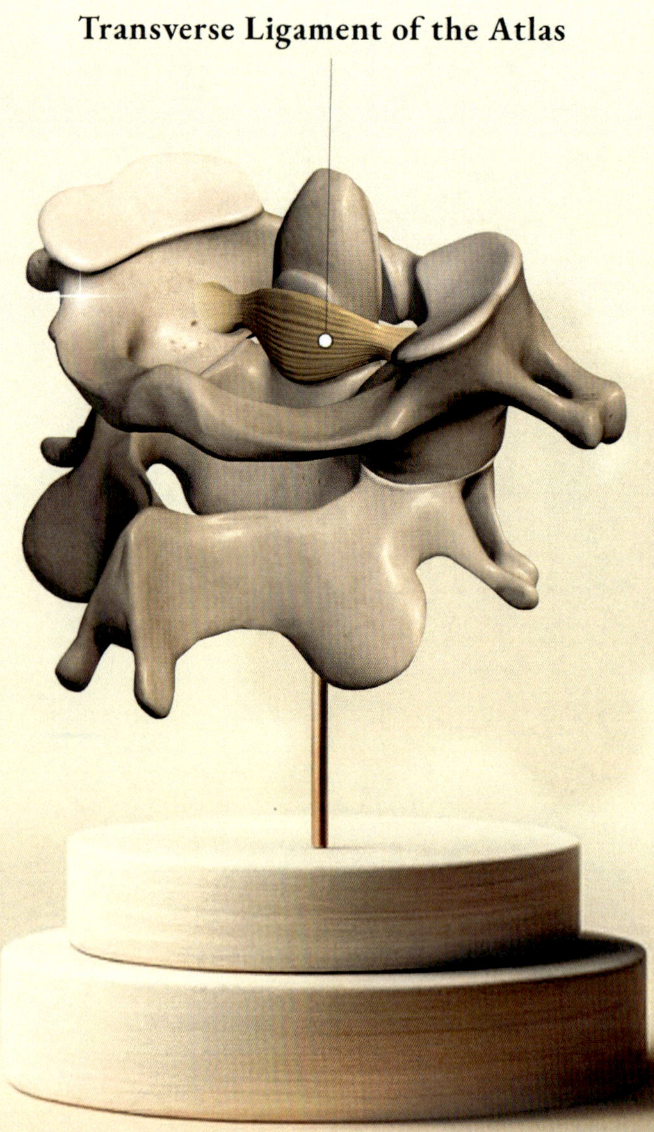

2. Alar Ligaments

The Alar Ligaments are strong, fibrous bands that extend from the sides of the dens (odontoid process) of the axis to the lateral margins of the foramen magnum of the occipital bone. These ligaments play a crucial role in stabilizing the atlanto-axial joint by limiting the amount of rotation and side-to-side movement of the head and atlas relative to the axis. This helps in maintaining the proper alignment and preventing excessive movement that could lead to injury.

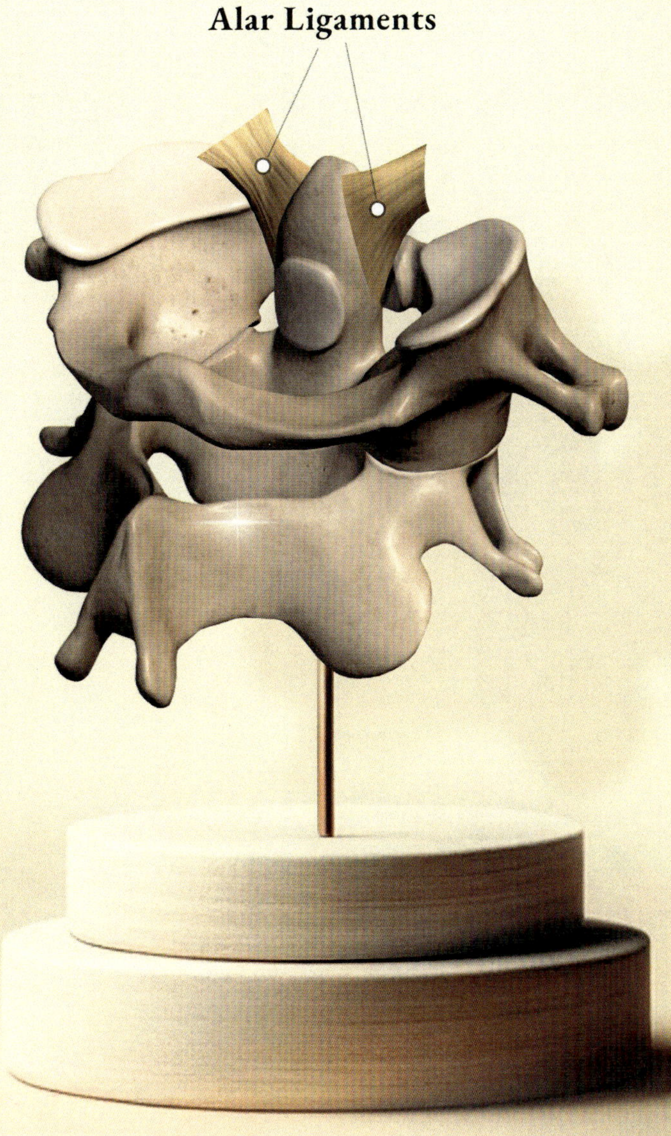

3. Apical Ligament

The Apical Ligament is a slender, fibrous band that extends from the tip of the dens (odontoid process) of the axis to the anterior margin of the foramen magnum of the occipital bone. This ligament plays a significant role in stabilizing the atlanto-occipital joint by providing vertical support and helping to anchor the dens in place. By doing so, it assists in maintaining the alignment of the cervical vertebrae and prevents excessive anterior-posterior movement, thereby contributing to the overall stability of the craniovertebral junction.

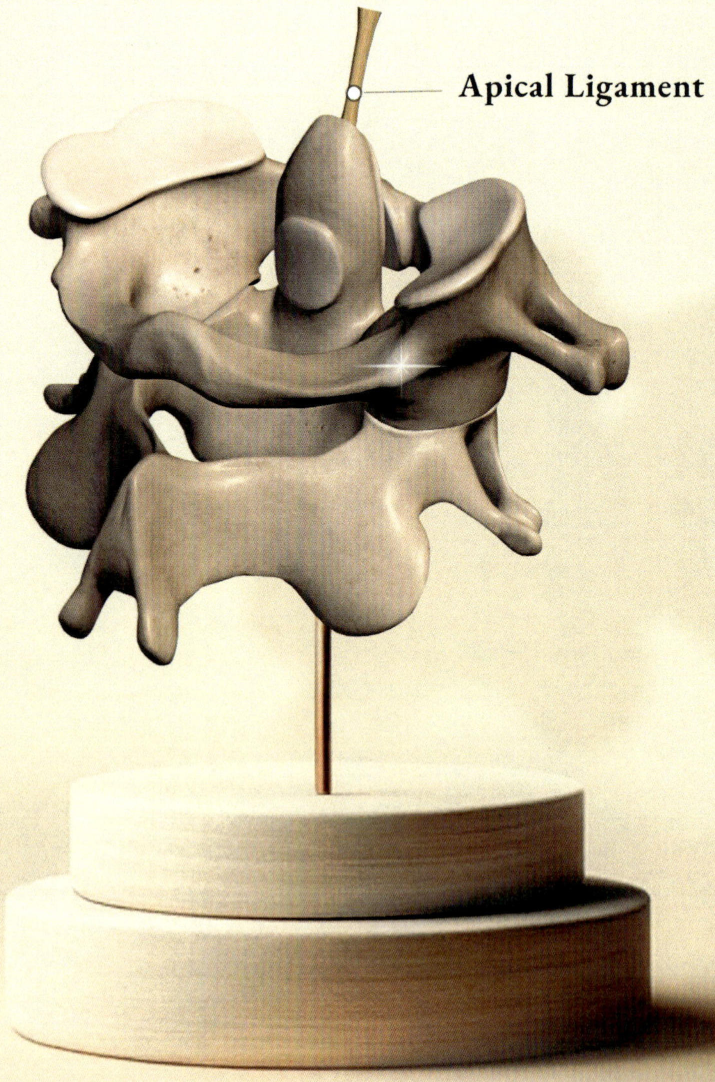

4. Cruciate Ligament

The Cruciate Ligament of the atlas is a key stabilizing structure within the cervical spine. It consists of the transverse ligament of the atlas and two vertical bands, known as the longitudinal fascicles. The transverse ligament extends horizontally around the dens of the axis, anchoring it to the anterior arch of the atlas, while the longitudinal fascicles run vertically, connecting the body of the axis to the basilar part of the occipital bone. This configuration plays a critical role in maintaining the alignment and stability of the atlanto-axial and atlanto-occipital joints, preventing excessive movement that could potentially damage the spinal cord.

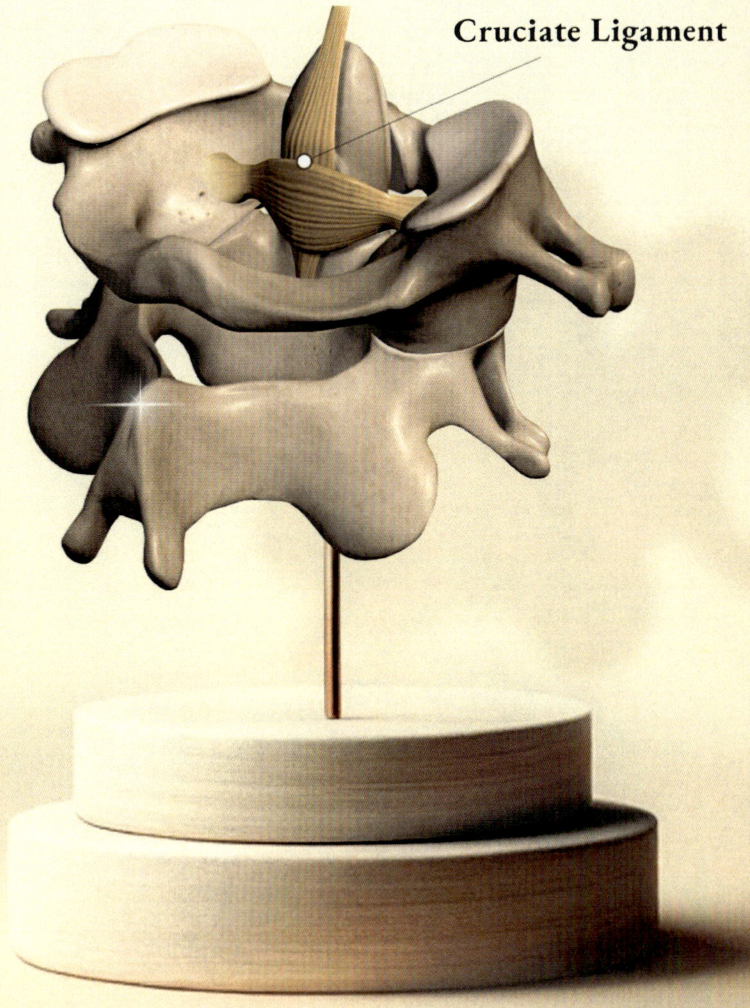

5. Accessory atlanto axial ligaments

The Accessory Atlanto-Axial Ligaments are strong, fibrous bands that extend from the base of the dens (odontoid process) of the axis to the lateral masses of the atlas. These ligaments play an essential role in stabilizing the atlanto-axial joint by providing additional support to the dens, preventing excessive rotational and lateral movements of the atlas relative to the axis. This helps in maintaining proper alignment and stability of the cervical spine, reducing the risk of injury and ensuring smooth and coordinated head movements.

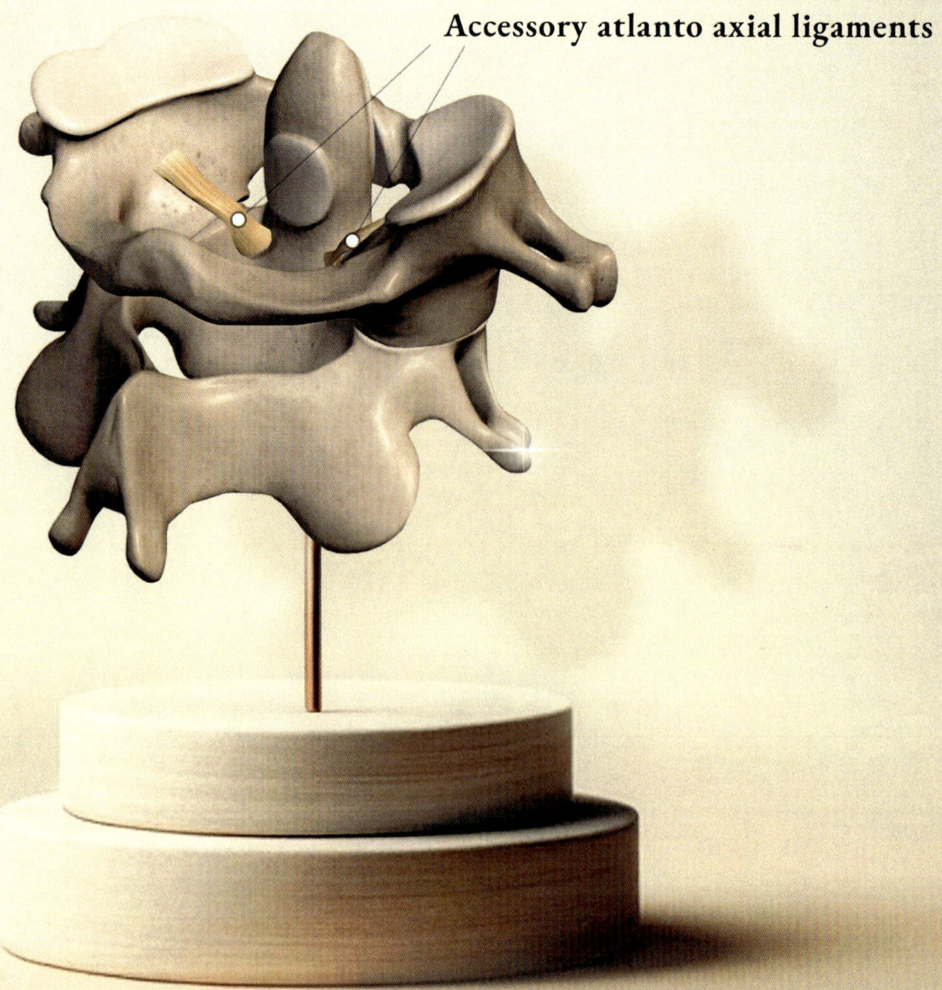

Cervical Vertebrae - *Structure*

The cervical vertebrae are the seven vertebrae (C1-C7) that make up the neck portion of the spinal column. They play a crucial role in supporting the head, allowing for its movement, and protecting the spinal cord. Each vertebra has unique characteristics that enable specific functions.

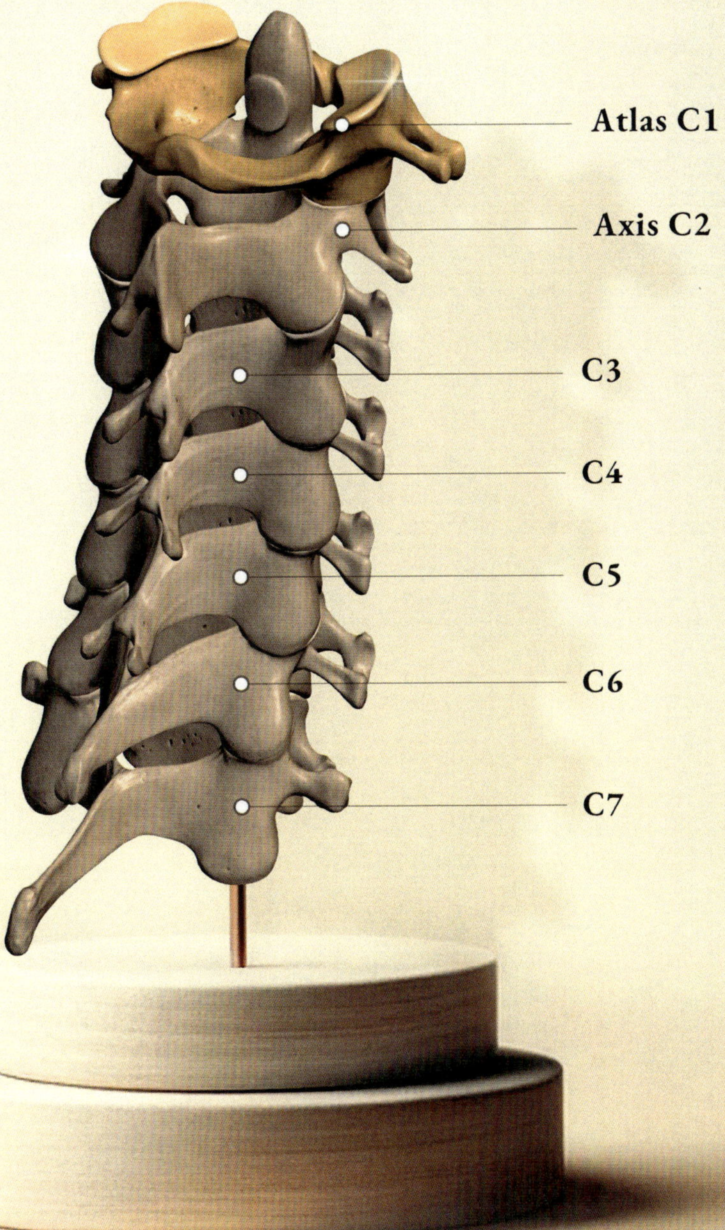

Muscle Structures of the Atlas

An anatomical analysis reveals diverse muscle structures associated with the atlas vertebra [Image 1]. Among them are neck muscles such as the sternocleidomastoid, scalene, and splenius, which have direct or indirect connections to the atlas. These muscles not only provide support and stability to the atlas but also allow for various neck movements, including flexion, rotation, and lateral bending.

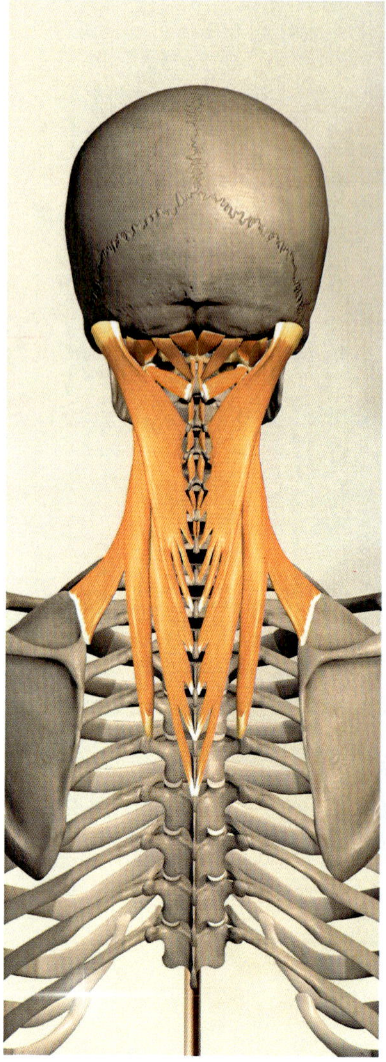

[Image 1] Atlas-Related Muscles

In addition to neck muscles, muscles of the shoulder girdle, such as the levator scapulae and trapezius, contribute to maintaining the stability of the atlas vertebra. These muscles are connected to the cervical spine and can indirectly influence atlas mobility through their connections with neck musculature.

The role of muscles around the atlas vertebra is multifaceted. They not only support this part of the spine and provide stability but also contribute to the range of motion of the neck.

Prolonged muscle tension or imbalance in these structures can lead to atlas dysfunction, potentially causing postural issues or restricted movement. For example, excessive tension in the sternocleidomastoid muscle can pull the atlas out of its proper position, resulting in uneven pressure on the cervical vertebrae. Therefore, maintaining muscle balance and flexibility is essential to ensure the proper functioning of the atlas and the spine as a whole. In addition, poor posture or repetitive strain from activities such as prolonged sitting or improper lifting can further exacerbate muscle imbalances, leading to chronic tension around the atlas. Regular stretching and strengthening exercises targeting the neck and shoulder muscles are crucial for preventing these imbalances and supporting atlas stability.

Muscles Associated with the Atlas

1. Neck Muscles Associated with the Atlas

The primary function of the neck muscles associated with the atlas (the first cervical vertebra) is to facilitate the movement and stabilization of the head and upper cervical spine. Key muscles include the suboccipital muscles, which consist of the rectus capitis posterior major, rectus capitis posterior minor, obliquus capitis superior, and obliquus capitis inferior. These muscles are crucial for fine motor control and proprioception, allowing precise movements of the head.

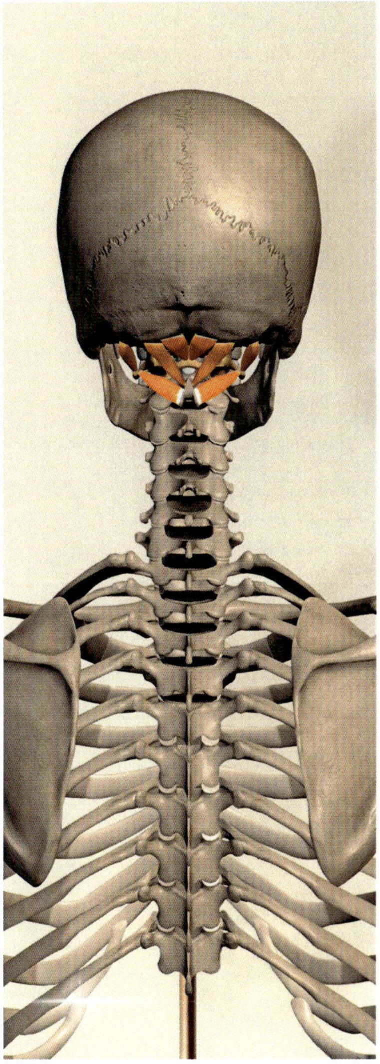

[Image 1] Suboccipital muscles

Additionally, these neck muscles play a vital role in maintaining posture and supporting the weight of the head [Image 1]. They assist in movements such as extension, rotation, and lateral flexion of the head and neck. Without the proper function of these muscles, an individual would experience difficulties in maintaining head stability and performing everyday activities that require head and neck movement.

Furthermore, the neck muscles associated with the atlas help protect the cervical spine and its neurovascular structures. By providing dynamic stabilization, they prevent excessive movements that could lead to injuries or strain. This is essential for ensuring the overall health and functionality of the upper cervical region, contributing to the body's balance and coordination.

2. Splenius Cervicis Associated with the Atlas

The primary function of the splenius cervicis muscle associated with the atlas (the first cervical vertebra) is to extend and rotate the cervical spine, particularly focusing on the lower cervical vertebrae but influencing the upper cervical region as well. This muscle originates from the spinous processes of the upper thoracic vertebrae and inserts into the transverse processes of the upper cervical vertebrae, including the atlas [Image 1].

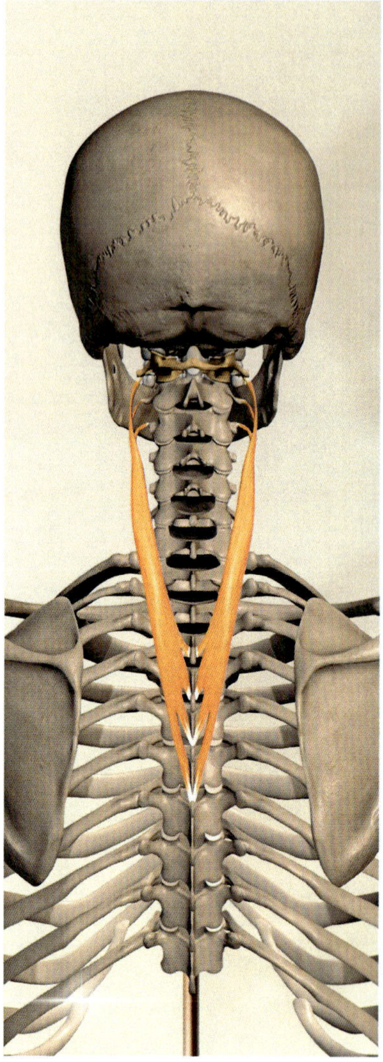

[Image 1] Splenius Cervicis and Atlas

Additionally, the splenius cervicis plays a crucial role in maintaining posture and stabilizing the neck during various movements. It works synergistically with other muscles to facilitate head rotation and lateral flexion. Without the proper function of the splenius cervicis, movements of the head and neck would be less controlled and less stable, leading to difficulties in performing tasks that require precise neck movements.

Furthermore, the splenius cervicis muscle helps protect the cervical spine by distributing mechanical loads and providing support during head and neck movements. This is essential for reducing the risk of neck strain and injury, ensuring the overall health and functionality of the cervical spine, and supporting daily activities that involve head and neck mobility.

3. Sternocleidomastoid Muscle Associated with the Atlas

The primary function of the sternocleidomastoid muscle associated with the atlas (the first cervical vertebra) is to facilitate rotation and flexion of the head and neck. This muscle originates from the manubrium of the sternum and the clavicle, and inserts into the mastoid process of the temporal bone of the skull. While it does not directly attach to the atlas, its actions significantly influence the movements and stability of the upper cervical spine, including the atlas.

Additionally, the sternocleidomastoid plays a crucial role

in maintaining posture and assisting with the balance of the head on the cervical spine. It enables movements such as turning the head from side to side, nodding, and tilting the head. Without the proper function of the sternocleidomastoid, an individual would experience difficulties in these movements, leading to impaired head and neck mobility and stability.

Furthermore, the sternocleidomastoid muscle supports the cervical spine by providing dynamic stability and helping to distribute mechanical loads during various activities. This is essential for reducing the risk of neck strain and injury, ensuring the overall health and functionality of the cervical spine, and supporting everyday tasks that involve head and neck movements [Image 1].

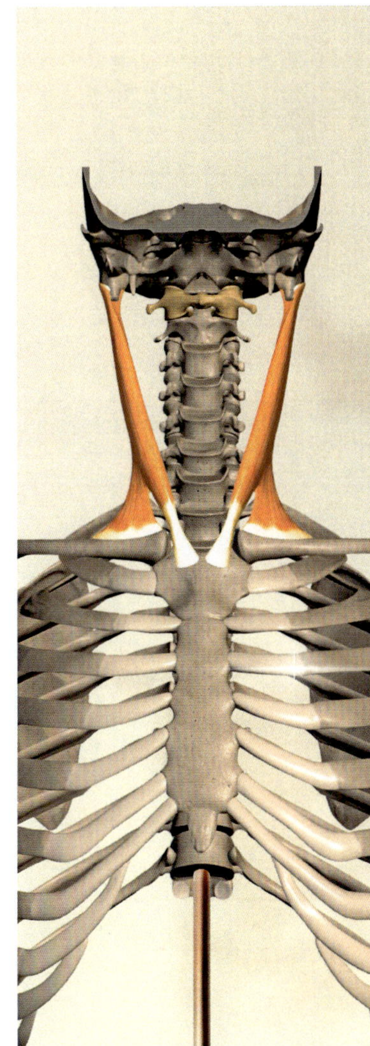

[Image 1] Sternocleidomastoid

4. Scalenes Associated with the atlas

The primary function of the scalene muscles associated with the atlas (the first cervical vertebra) is to facilitate the movement and stabilization of the cervical spine and assist in respiration. The scalene muscles, consisting of the anterior, middle, and posterior scalene, originate from the transverse processes of the cervical vertebrae and insert into the first and second ribs [Image 2]. While they do not directly attach to the atlas, their actions significantly influence the upper cervical spine, including the atlas.

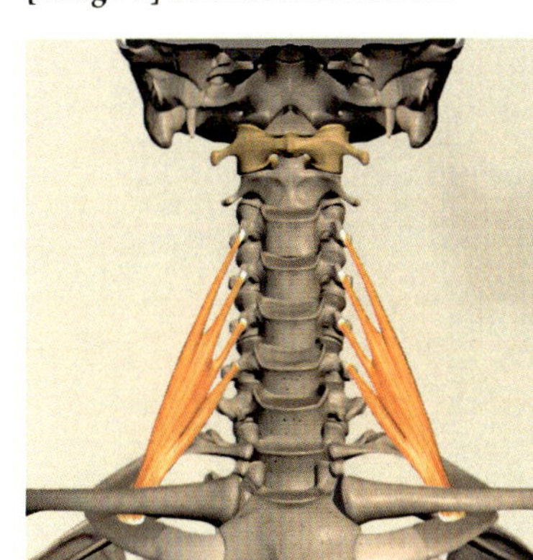

[Image 2] Scalene muscles

Additionally, the scalene muscles play a crucial role in supporting the neck during various movements such as lateral flexion, rotation, and flexion. They also assist in elevating the first and second ribs during deep inhalation, contributing to respiratory function. Without the proper function of the scalene muscles, an individual would experience difficulties in neck movements and breathing.

Furthermore, the scalene muscles help protect the cervical spine by providing dynamic stability and distributing mechanical loads during head and neck movements [Image 1]. This is essential for reducing the risk of neck strain and injury, ensuring the overall health and functionality of the cervical spine, and supporting daily activities that involve head and neck mobility.

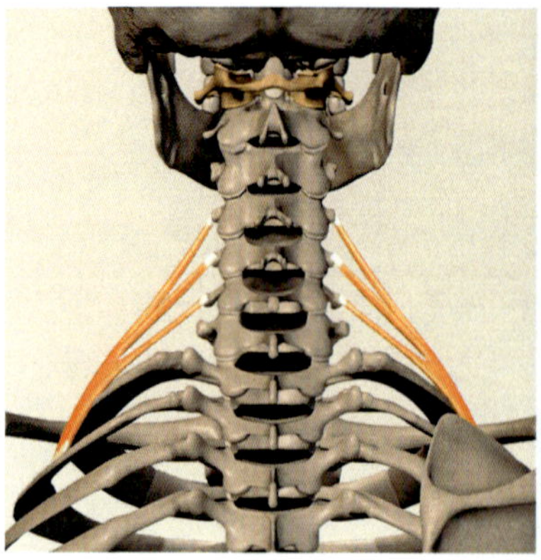

[Image 1] Posterior scalene muscles

5. Levator Scapulae Associated with the Atlas

The primary function of the levator scapulae muscle associated with the atlas (the first cervical vertebra) is to elevate the scapula (shoulder blade) and assist in the movement and stabilization of the cervical spine [Image 2]. This muscle originates from the transverse processes of the first four cervical vertebrae, including the atlas, and inserts into the superior angle of the scapula.

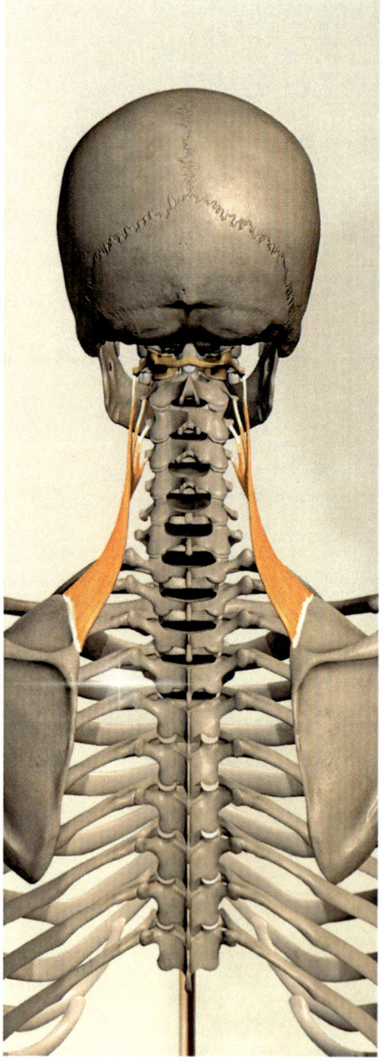

[Image 2] Levator scapulae muscle

Additionally, the levator scapulae plays a crucial role in facilitating neck movements such as lateral flexion and rotation. It also helps maintain proper posture by stabilizing the scapula during upper limb movements. Without the proper function of the levator scapulae, an individual would experience difficulties in shoulder elevation and neck movements, leading to impaired mobility and stability in these areas.

Furthermore, the levator scapulae muscle supports the cervical spine by providing dynamic stability and distributing mechanical loads during head and neck movements. This is essential for reducing the risk of neck strain and injury, ensuring the overall health and functionality of the cervical spine, and supporting daily activities that involve head, neck, and shoulder mobility.

6. Trapezius Muscle Associated with the Atlas

The primary function of the trapezius muscle associated with the atlas (the first cervical vertebra) is to facilitate the movement and stabilization of the shoulder girdle and cervical spine [Image 1]. The upper fibers of the trapezius originate from the occipital bone, the ligamentum nuchae, and the spinous processes of the cervical vertebrae, including the atlas, and insert into the lateral third of the clavicle and the acromion and spine of the scapula.

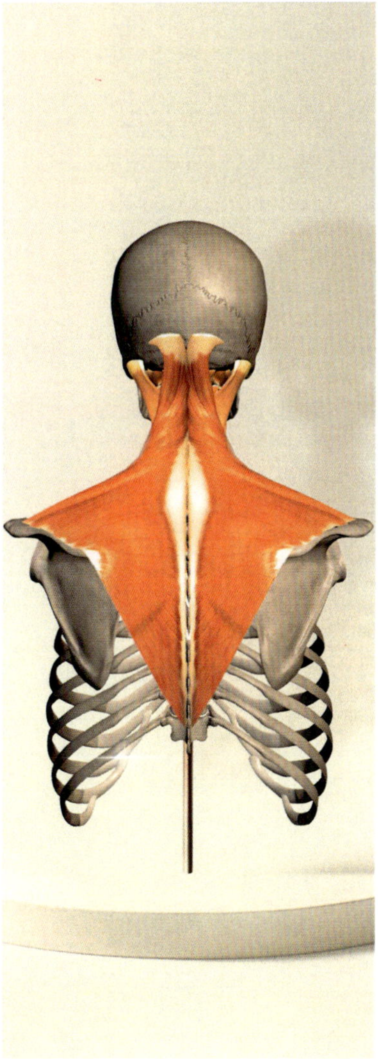

[Image 1] Trapezius muscle

Additionally, the trapezius muscle plays a crucial role in supporting and moving the scapula, including actions such as elevation, retraction, and rotation. It also assists in extending the neck and stabilizing the head. Without the proper function of the trapezius, an individual would experience difficulties in shoulder and neck movements, leading to impaired mobility and stability in these areas.

Furthermore, the trapezius muscle supports the cervical spine by providing dynamic stability and distributing mechanical loads during head, neck, and shoulder movements. This is essential for reducing the risk of neck and shoulder strain and injury, ensuring the overall health and functionality of the upper spine and shoulder girdle, and supporting daily activities that involve head, neck, and shoulder mobility.

7. Shoulder Girdle Muscles Associated with the Atlas

The primary function of the shoulder girdle muscles associated with the atlas (the first cervical vertebra) is to facilitate the movement and stabilization of the shoulder and cervical spine. Key muscles in the shoulder girdle include the trapezius, levator scapulae, and rhomboids. These muscles, although primarily acting on the shoulder blade (scapula), have attachments or functional connections to the cervical spine, including the atlas.

Additionally, the shoulder girdle muscles play crucial roles in various movements such as elevation, depression, retraction, and rotation of the scapula [Image 1]. They also assist in maintaining posture and providing dynamic stability to the upper body. Without the proper function of these muscles, an individual would experience difficulties in shoulder and neck movements, leading to impaired mobility and stability.

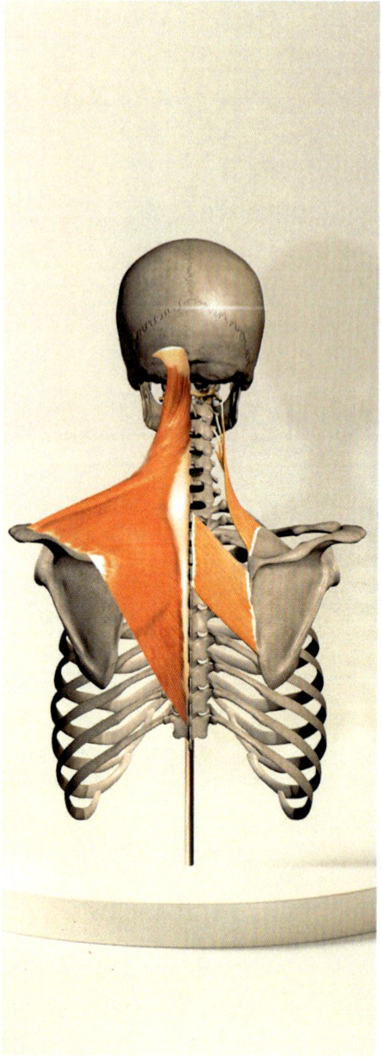

[Image 1] Shoulder girdle muscles

Furthermore, the shoulder girdle muscles support the cervical spine by providing dynamic stability and distributing mechanical loads during head, neck, and shoulder movements. This is essential for reducing the risk of strain and injury, ensuring the overall health and functionality of the upper spine and shoulder girdle, and supporting daily activities that involve head, neck, and shoulder mobility.

8. Levator Scapulae Associated with the Atlas

The primary function of the levator scapulae muscle associated with the atlas (the first cervical vertebra) is to elevate the scapula (shoulder blade) and assist in the movement and stabilization of the cervical spine. This muscle originates from the transverse processes of the first four cervical vertebrae, including the atlas, and inserts into the superior angle of the scapula.

Additionally, the levator scapulae plays a crucial role in facilitating neck movements such as lateral flexion and rotation. It also helps maintain proper posture by stabilizing the scapula during upper limb movements. Without the proper function of the levator scapulae, an individual would experience difficulties in shoulder elevation and neck movements, leading to impaired mobility and stability in these areas.

Furthermore, the levator scapulae muscle supports the cervical spine by providing dynamic stability and distributing mechanical loads during head and neck movements [Image 1]. This is essential for reducing the risk of neck strain and injury, ensuring the overall health and functionality of the cervical spine, and supporting daily activities that involve head, neck, and shoulder mobility.

"Knowing is not enough; we must apply. Being willing is not enough; we must do."

(Leonardo da Vinci)

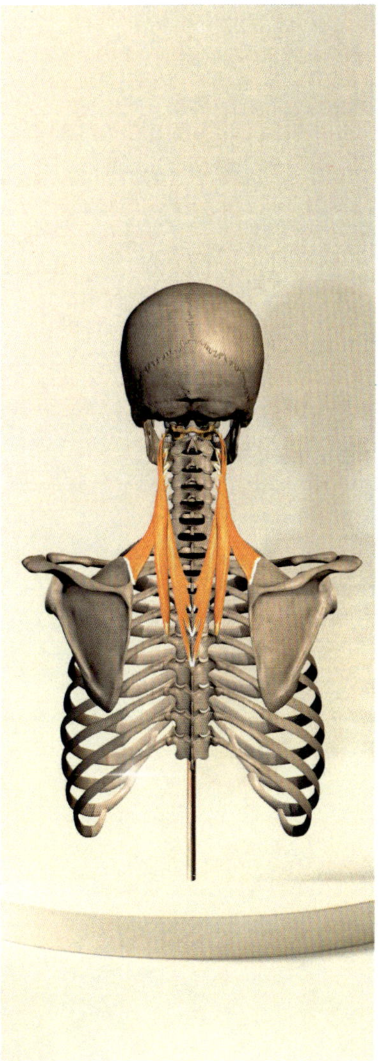

[Image 1] Levator scapulae muscle

Splenius Capitis - *Head Splenius Muscle*

The splenius capitis is a muscle at the back of the neck and upper back. It originates from the lower cervical and upper thoracic vertebrae and inserts at the mastoid process of the temporal bone. Its primary functions are to extend, rotate, and laterally flex the head. The splenius capitis assists in head movements and provides neck stability.

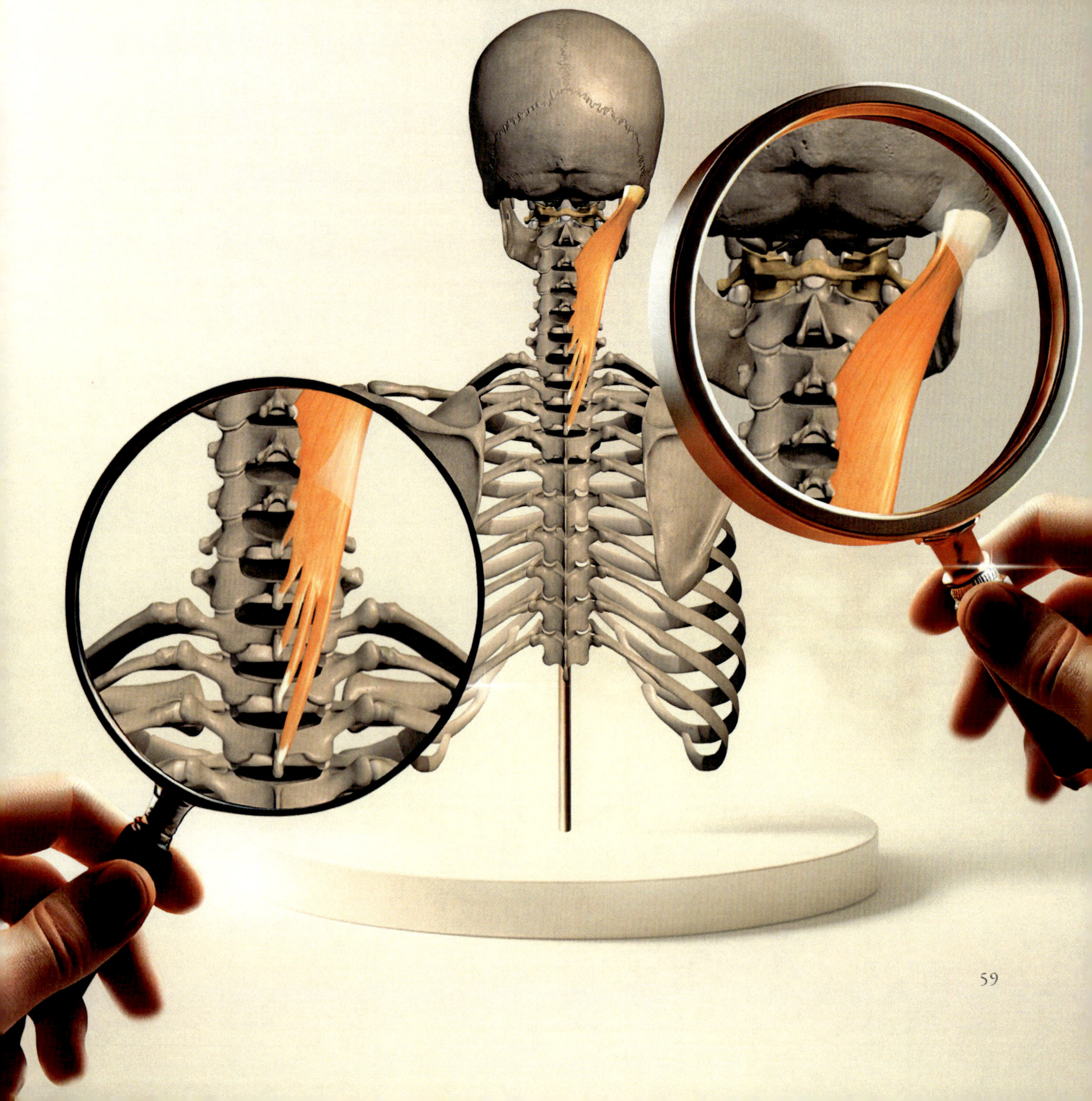

Rectus Capitis Posterior Minor

The rectus capitis posterior minor is a small muscle located at the back of the neck. It originates from the tubercle of the posterior arch of the atlas (C1) and inserts on the inferior nuchal line of the occipital bone. This muscle primarily functions to extend and slightly rotate the head, aiding in the stabilization of the atlanto-occipital joint.

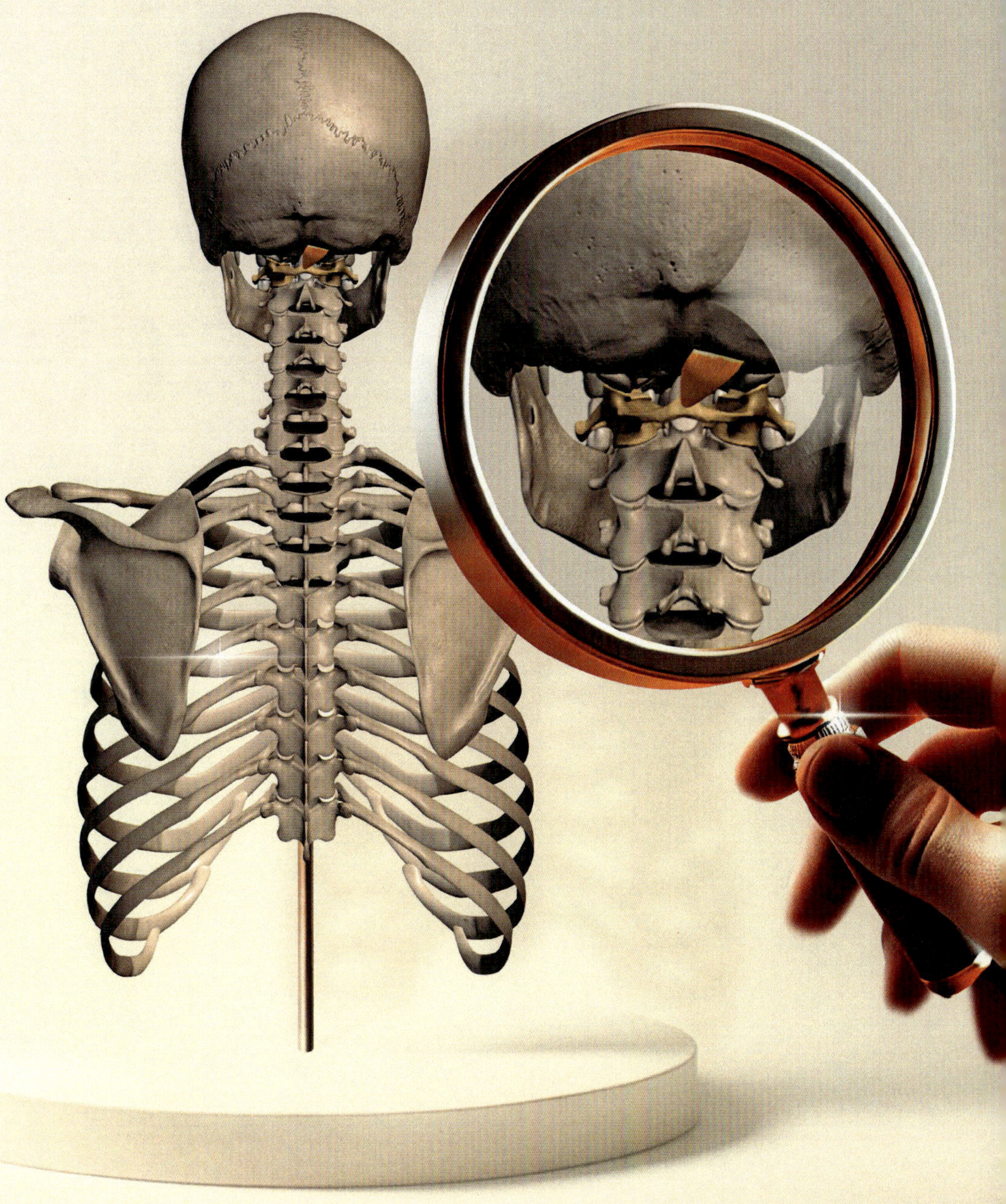

Rectus Capitis Posterior Major - Axis

The rectus capitis posterior major is a muscle located at the back of the neck. It originates from the spinous process of the axis (C2) and inserts on the inferior nuchal line of the occipital bone. This muscle plays a crucial role in extending and rotating the head, thereby providing stability and support to the atlanto-occipital joint.

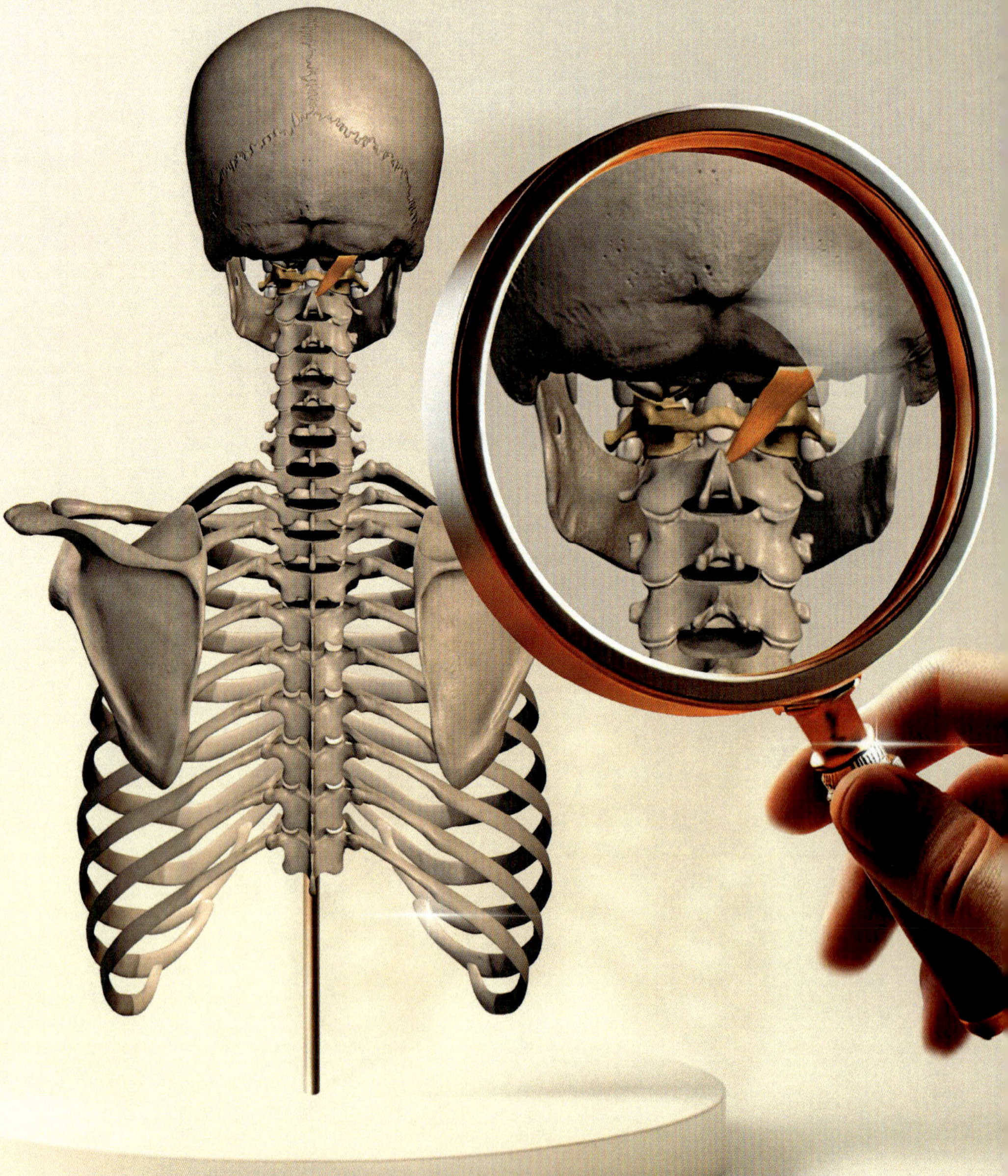

Obliquus Capitis Superior - Atlas

Obliquus capitis superior is a small muscle located at the back of the neck. It originates from the transverse process of the atlas (C1) and inserts on the occipital bone. Its primary functions are to extend and laterally flex the head, aiding in side-to-side movements and maintaining posture. This muscle stabilizes the cervical spine for smooth head movements.

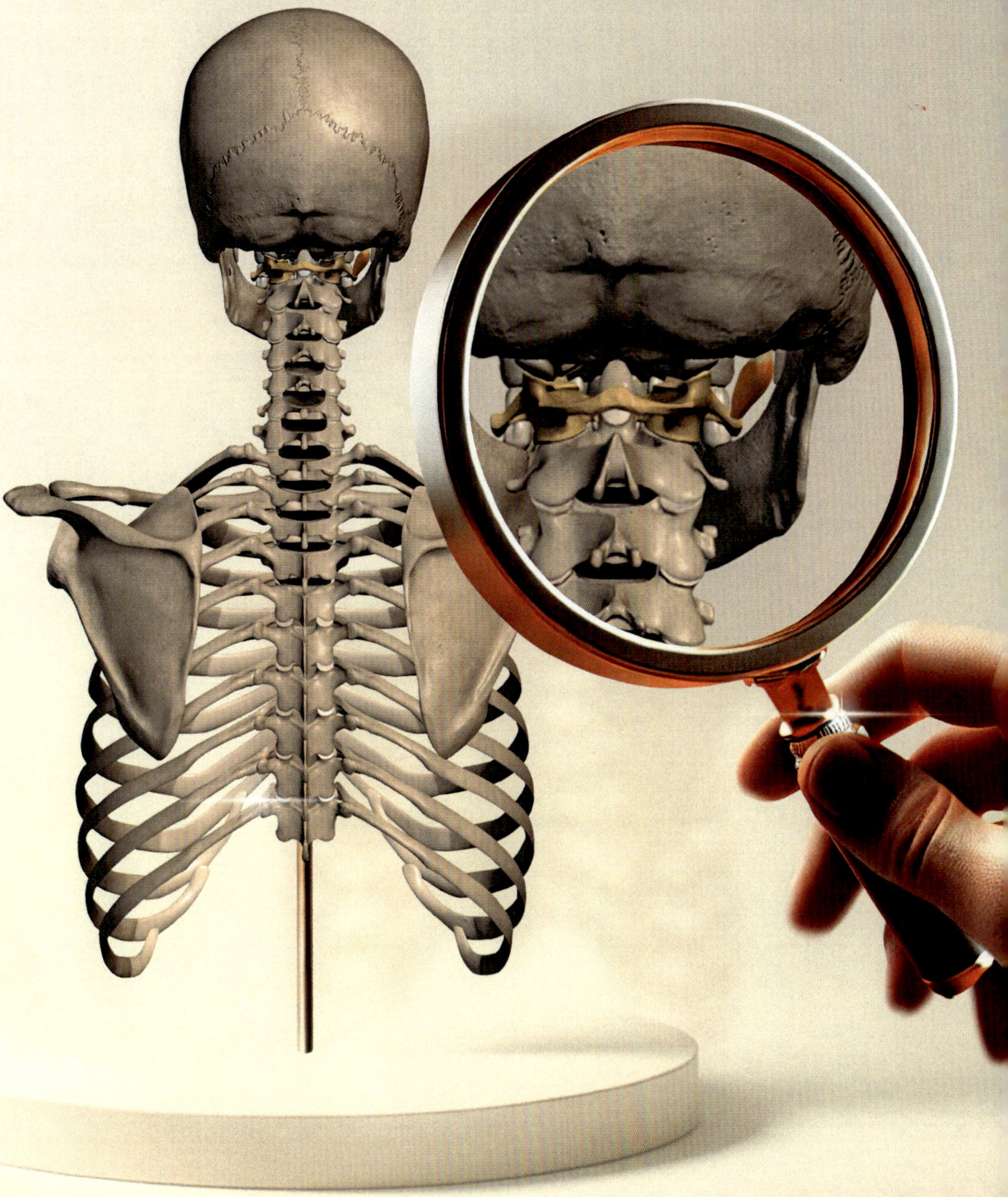

Obliquus Capitis Inferior

Obliquus capitis inferior is a small but significant muscle located at the back of the neck. It originates from the spinous process of the axis (C2) and inserts on the transverse process of the atlas (C1). This muscle primarily functions to rotate the head and atlas on the axis, enabling side-to-side head movements.

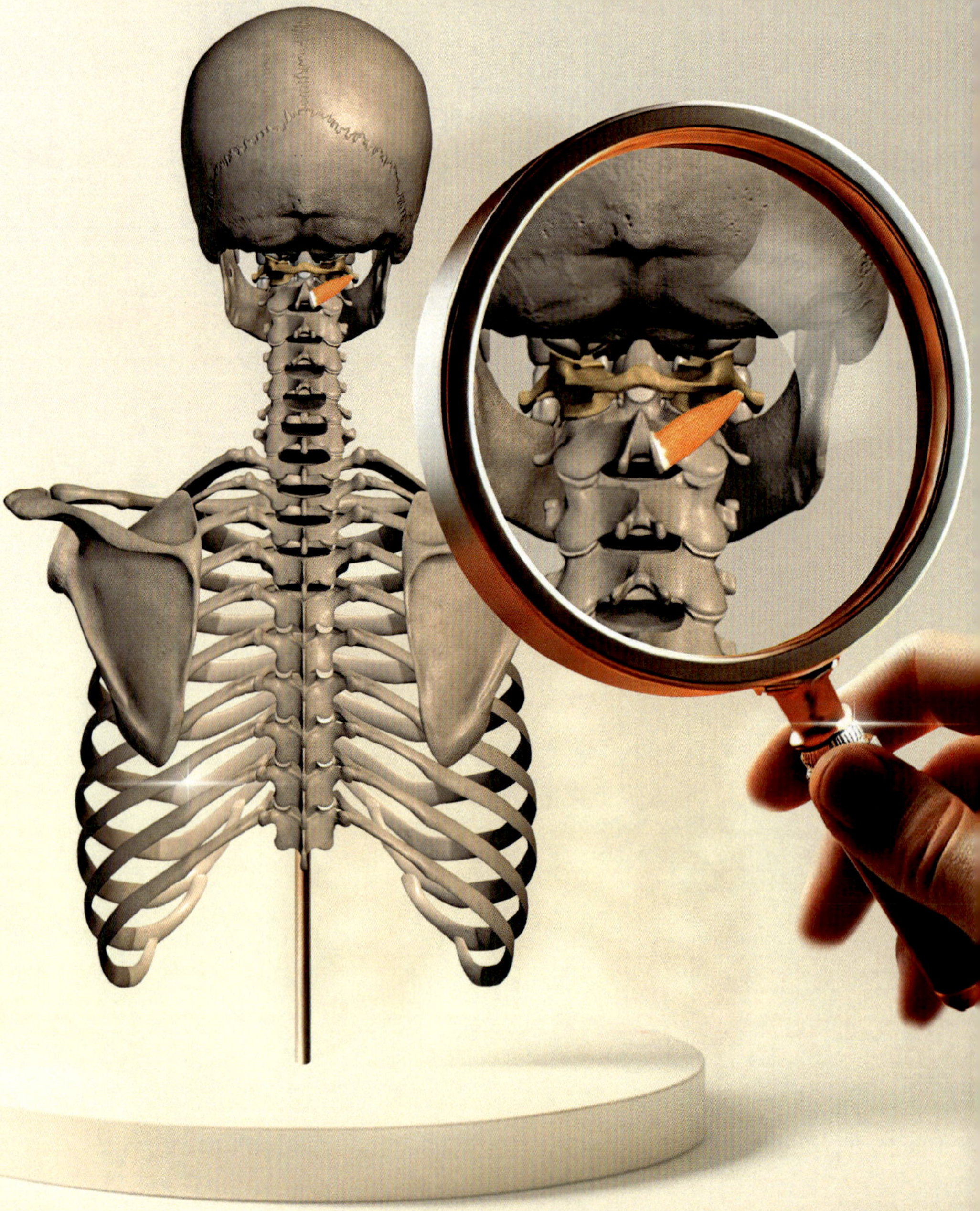

Longissimus Capitis

Longissimus capitis is a muscle located along the back of the neck and head. It originates from the transverse processes of the lower cervical and upper thoracic vertebrae and inserts on the mastoid process of the temporal bone. Its primary functions are to extend, rotate, and laterally flex the head, contributing to head movement and stability.

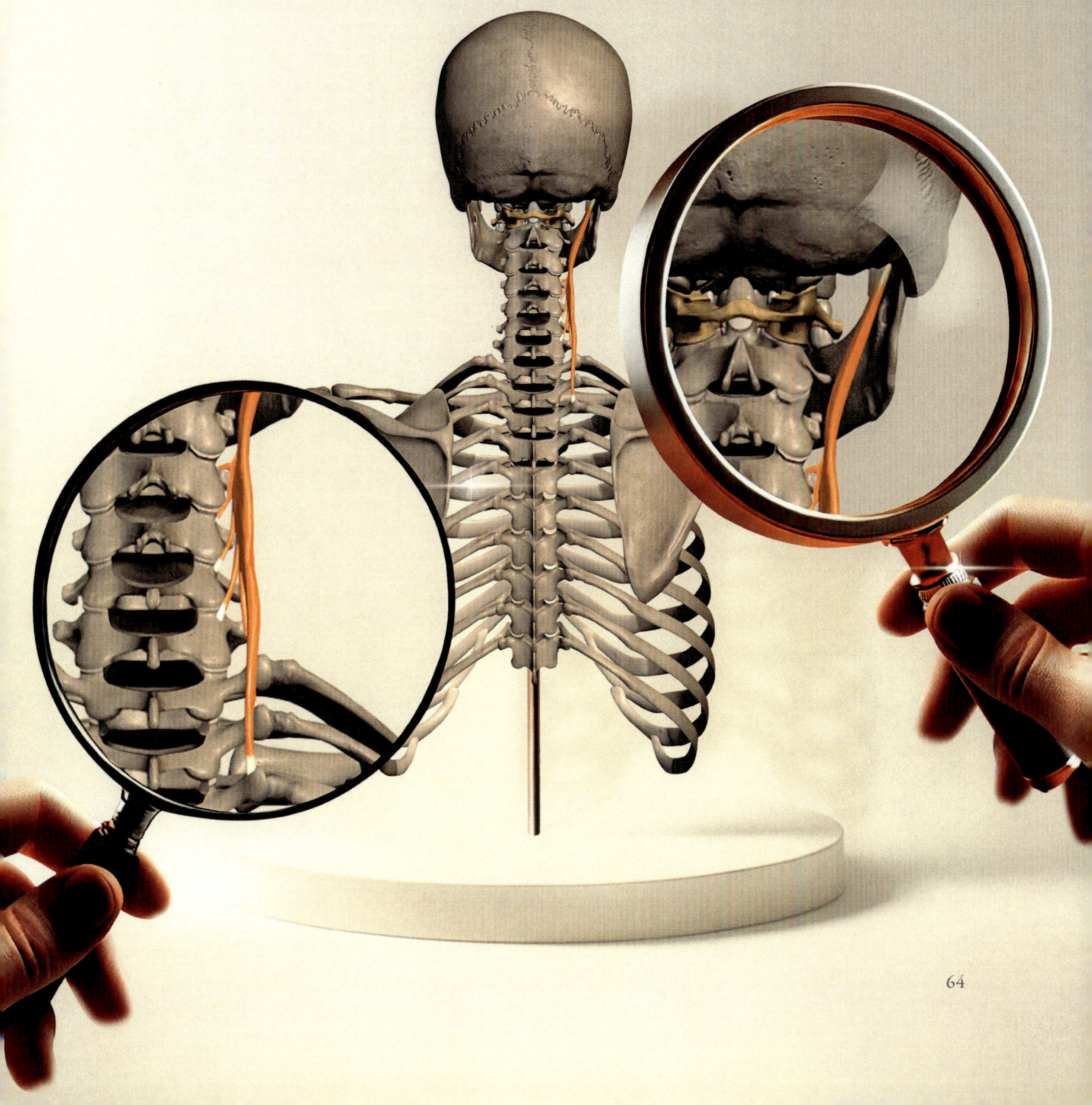

Splenius Cervicis

Splenius cervicis is a muscle located at the back of the neck. It originates from the spinous processes of the upper thoracic vertebrae (T3-T6) and inserts on the transverse processes of the upper cervical vertebrae (C1-C3). Its primary functions are to extend, rotate, and laterally flex the neck, aiding in head and neck movement and stability.

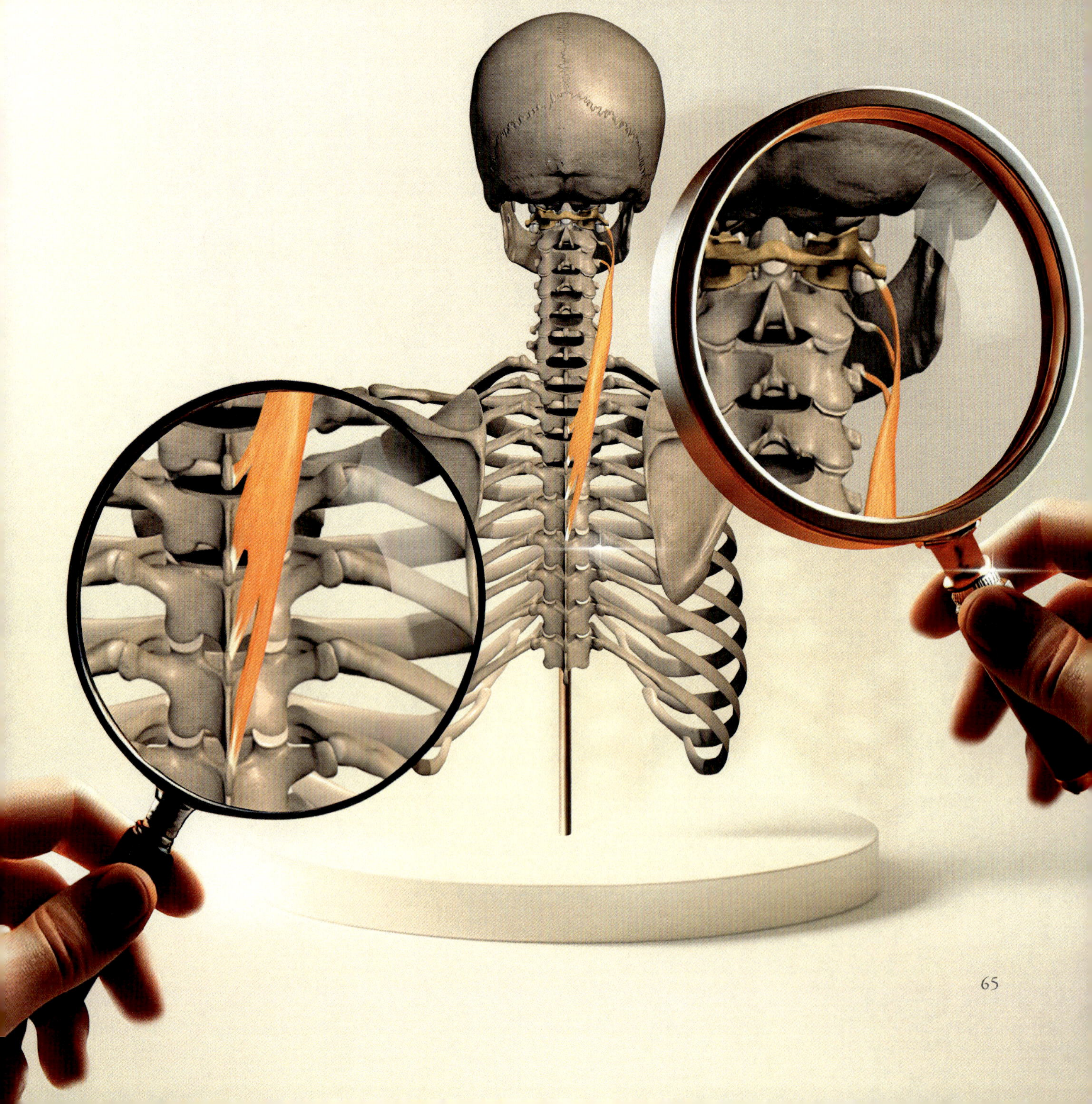

Levator scapulae

The levator scapulae is a long, thin muscle located in the back of the neck. It originates from the transverse processes of the first four to five cervical vertebrae (C1-C4) and extends down to the superior medial border of the scapula. Its primary function is to elevate the scapula, which is particularly useful during shoulder shrugging movements.

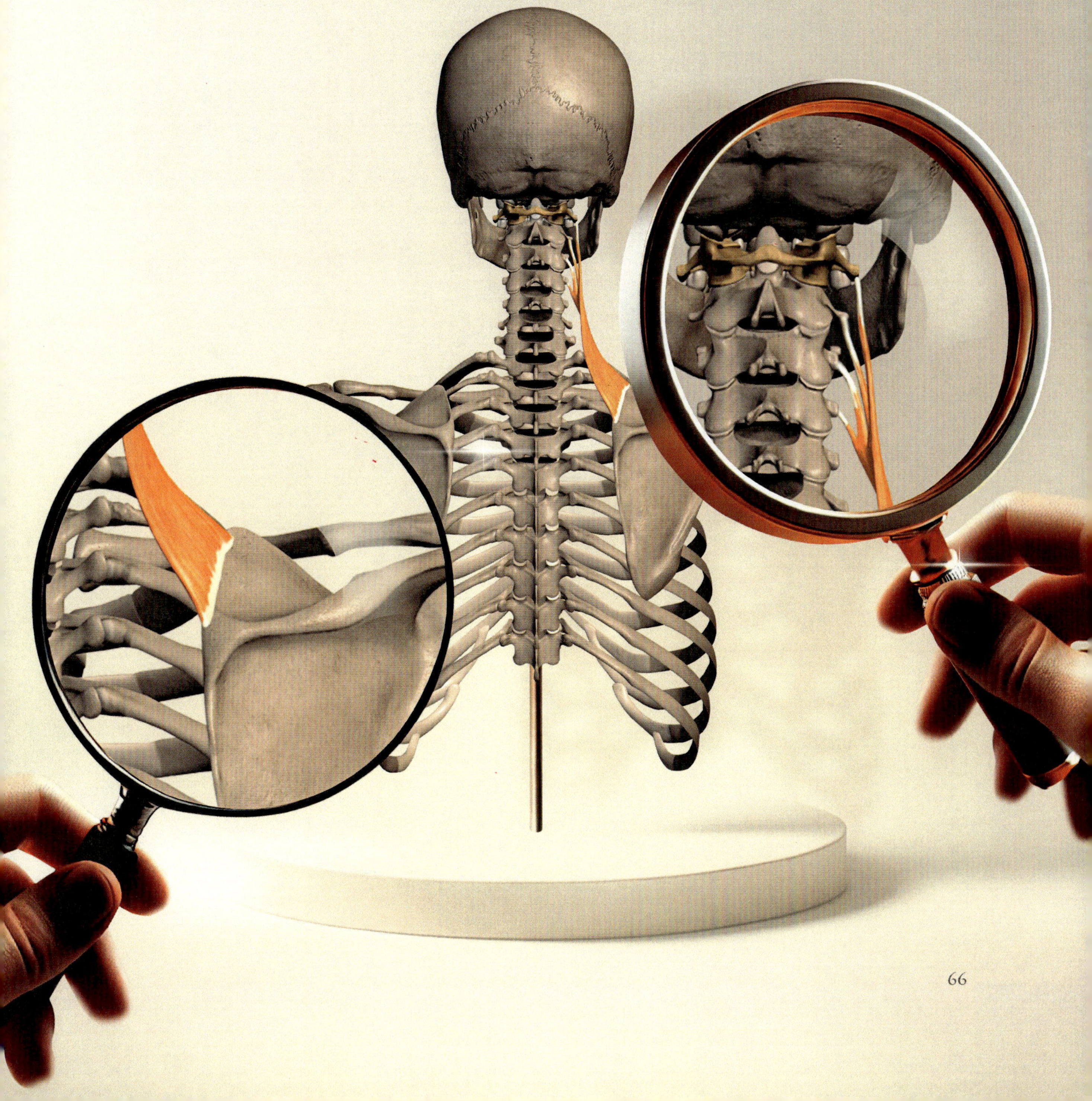

Intertransversarii Anteriores Cervicis

Intertransversarii Anteriores Cervicis are small muscles located between the transverse processes of the cervical vertebrae. They assist in the lateral flexion and stabilization of the neck, helping to maintain proper posture and alignment of the cervical spine. Additionally, they contribute to the fine motor control required for precise neck movements.

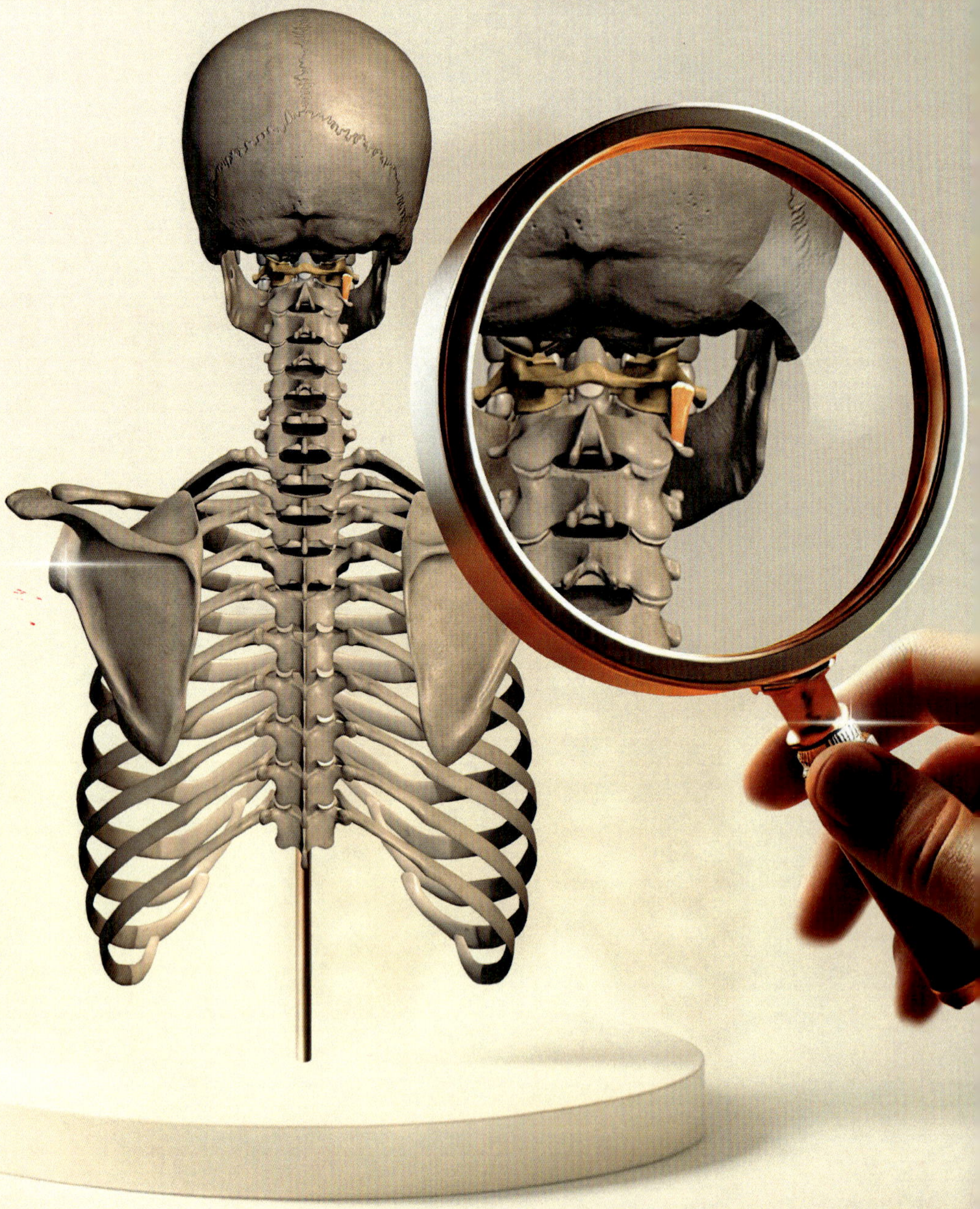

Interspinales Cervicis

The interspinales cervicis muscles are small, paired muscles located between the spinous processes of the cervical vertebrae. They assist in extending and stabilizing the cervical spine, contributing to the neck's overall flexibility and movement. These muscles play a crucial role in maintaining posture and facilitating precise movements of the neck.

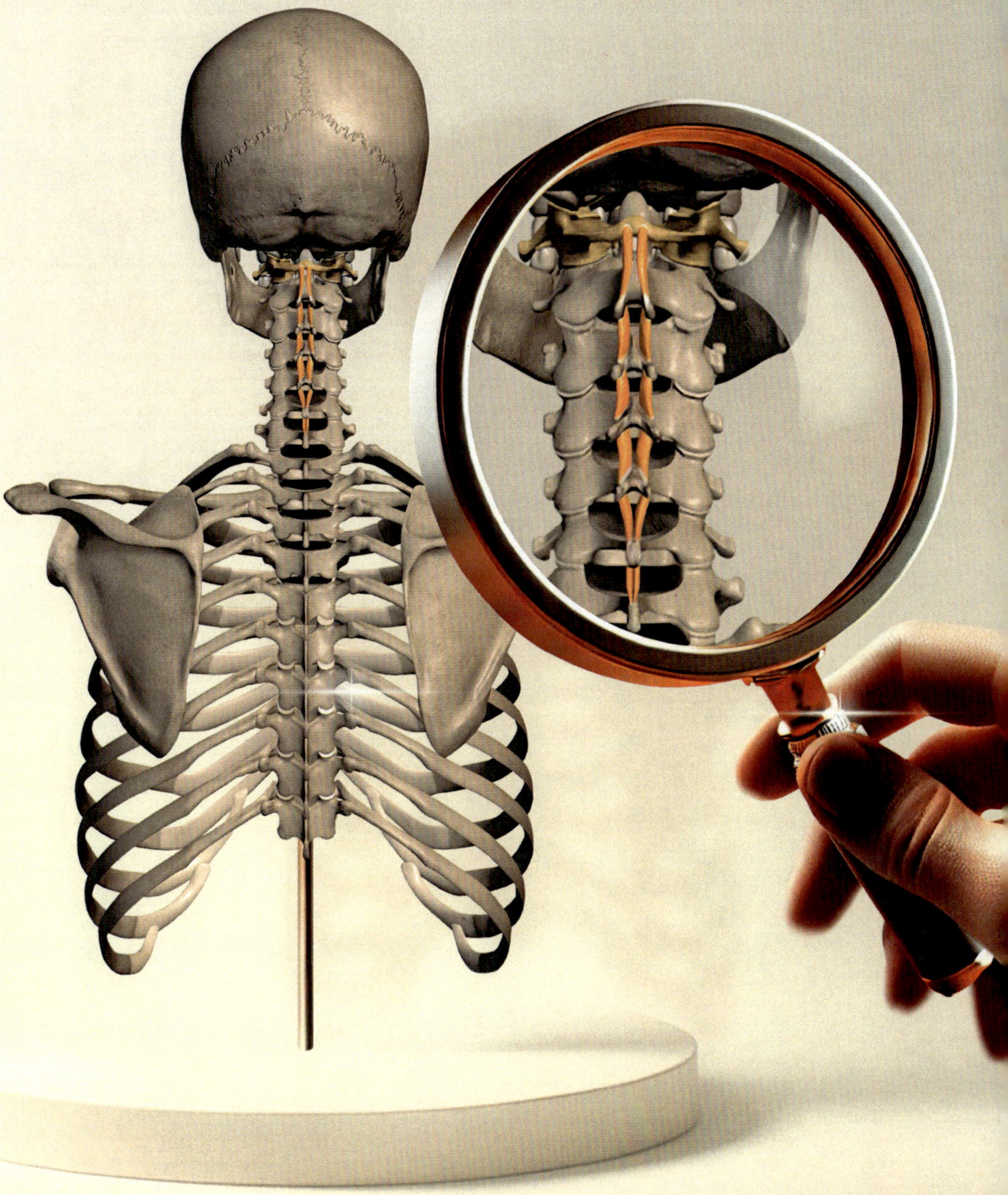

Rectus Capitis Lateralis

Rectus capitis lateralis is a small muscle located at the side of the neck. It originates from the transverse process of the atlas (C1) and inserts on the jugular process of the occipital bone. Its primary function is to assist in lateral flexion of the head, helping to stabilize and support neck movements. Additionally, it plays a role in maintaining proper head alignment.

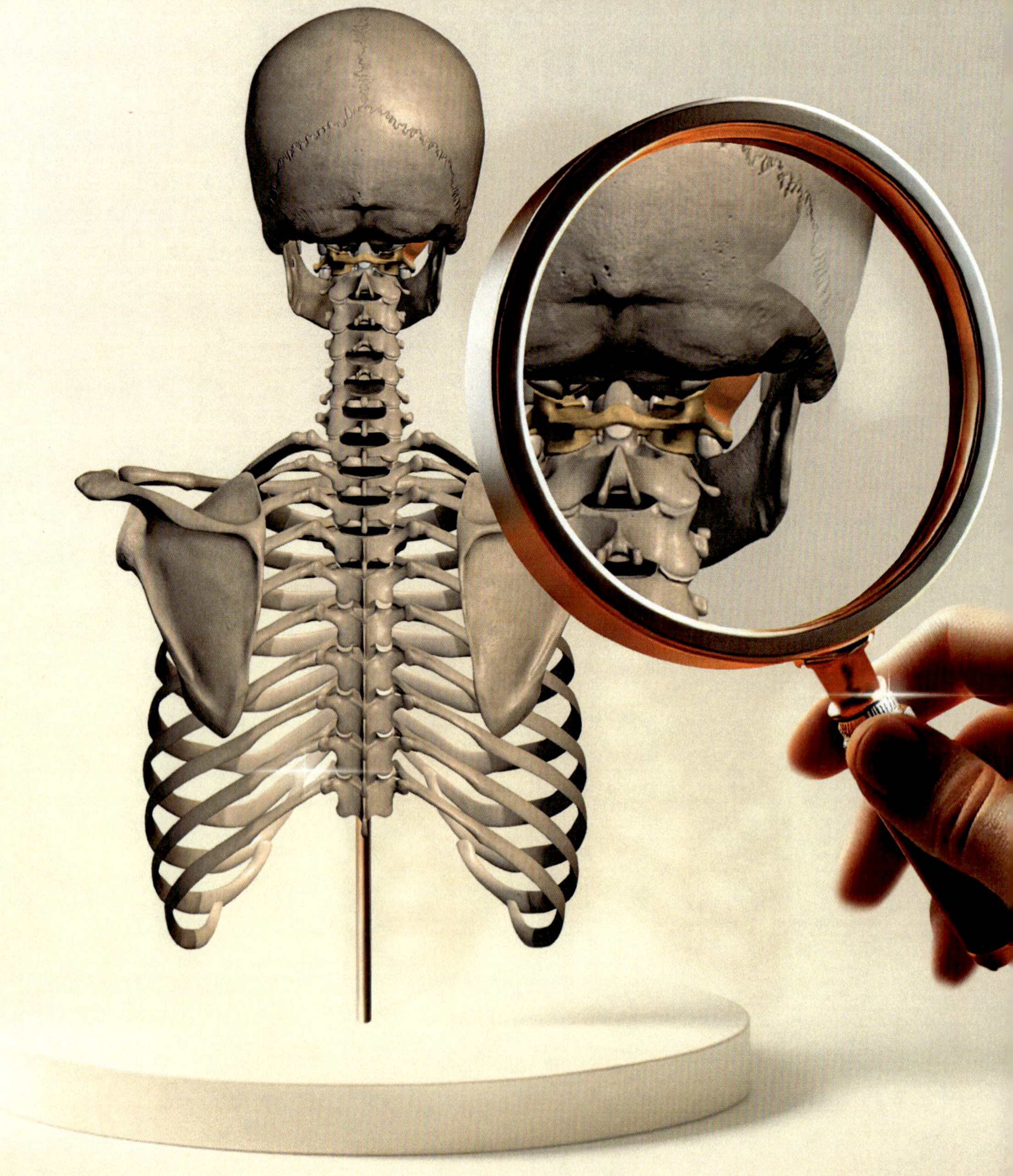

Longissimus Cervicis

Longissimus cervicis is a muscle located along the back of the neck. It originates from the transverse processes of the upper thoracic vertebrae and inserts on the transverse processes of the cervical vertebrae. Its primary functions are to extend, laterally flex, and rotate the neck, providing stability and support for neck movements.

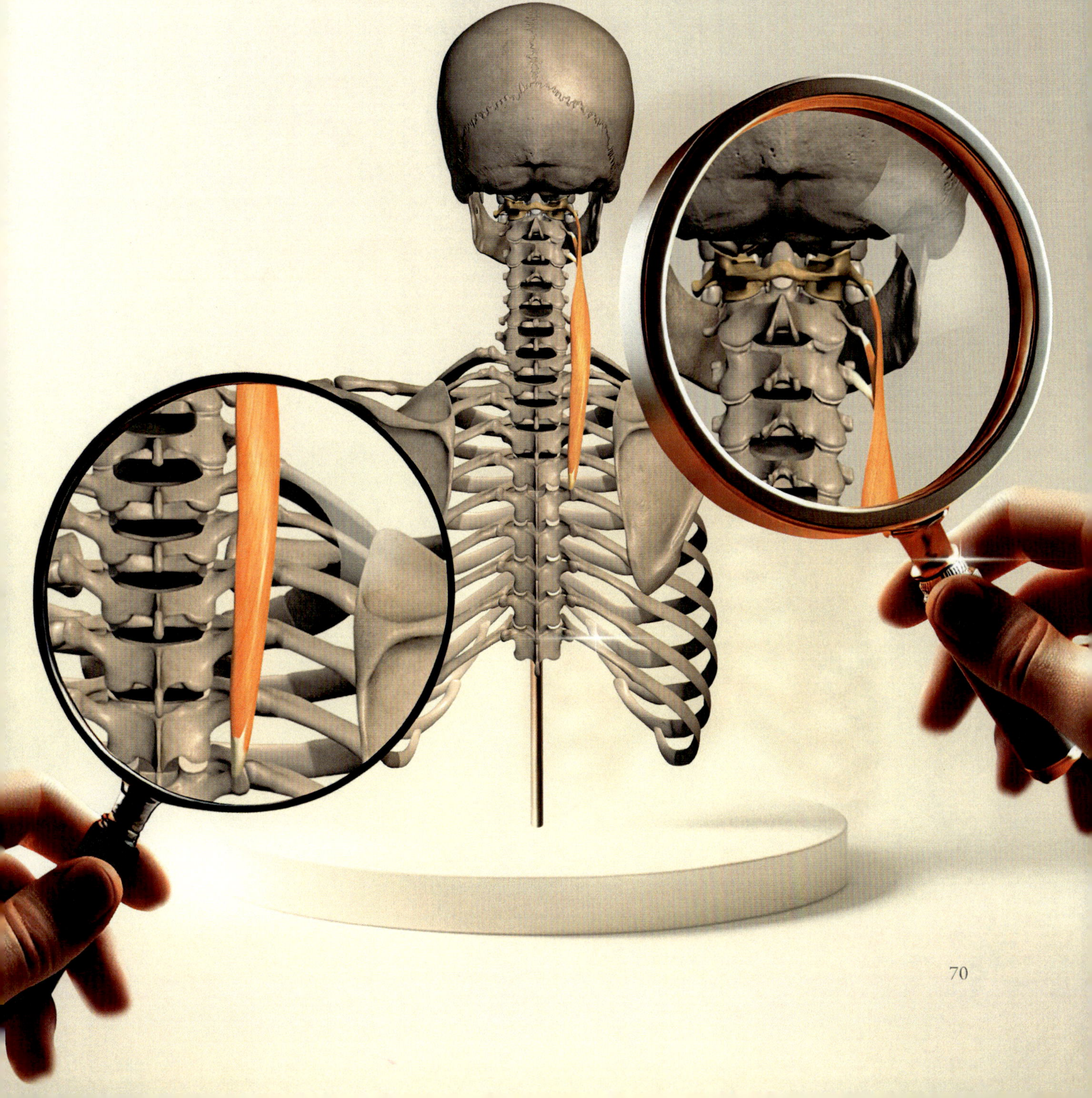

Function of the Posterior Scalene Muscles

The posterior scalene muscles play a crucial role in stabilizing and moving the neck. They assist in lateral flexion, allowing the head to tilt to the side, and contribute to elevating the second rib during inhalation, aiding in the breathing process. Their function is essential for maintaining proper posture and preventing neck strain and injuries.

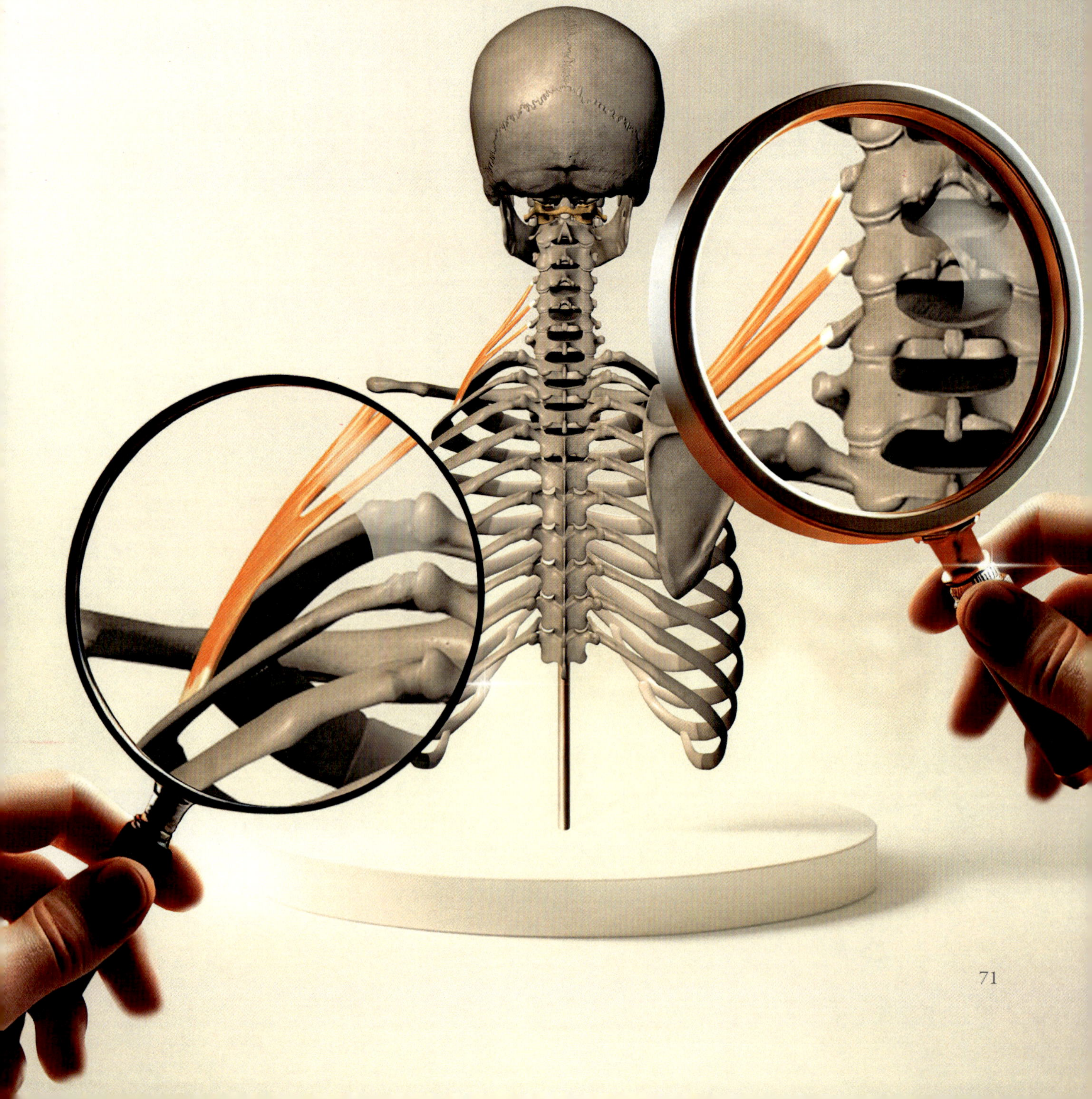

Rectus Capitis Anterior

Rectus capitis anterior is a small muscle located at the front of the neck. It originates from the lateral mass of the atlas (C1) and inserts on the basilar part of the occipital bone. Its primary function is to flex the head, aiding in the stabilization of the atlanto-occipital joint and supporting head movements. Additionally, it helps maintain proper posture.

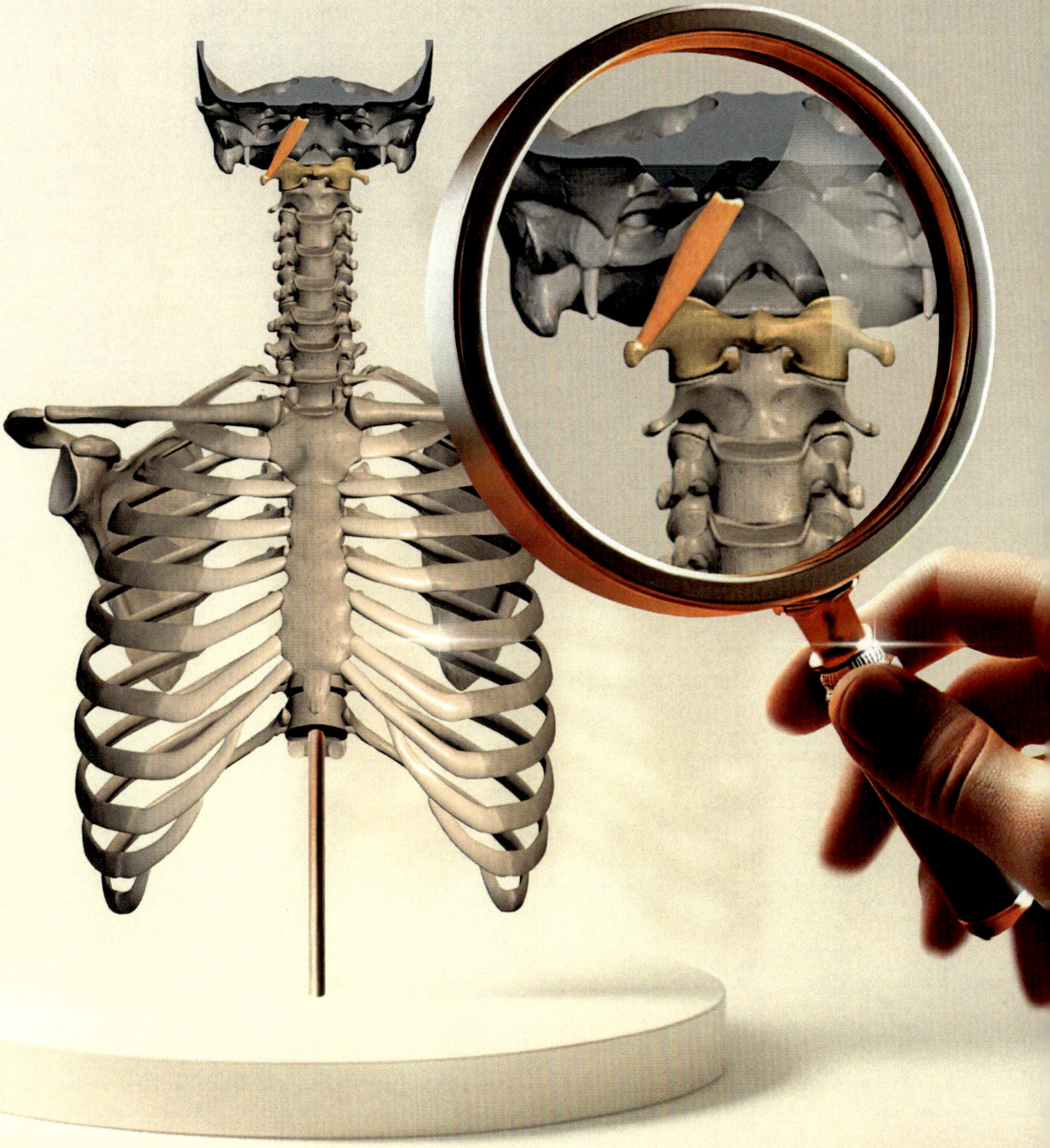

Longus Capitis

Longus capitis is a muscle located at the front of the neck. It originates from the transverse processes of the cervical vertebrae (C3-C6) and inserts on the basilar part of the occipital bone. Its primary functions are to flex the head and neck, aiding in stabilizing and supporting cervical spine movements. Additionally, it helps maintain proper posture.

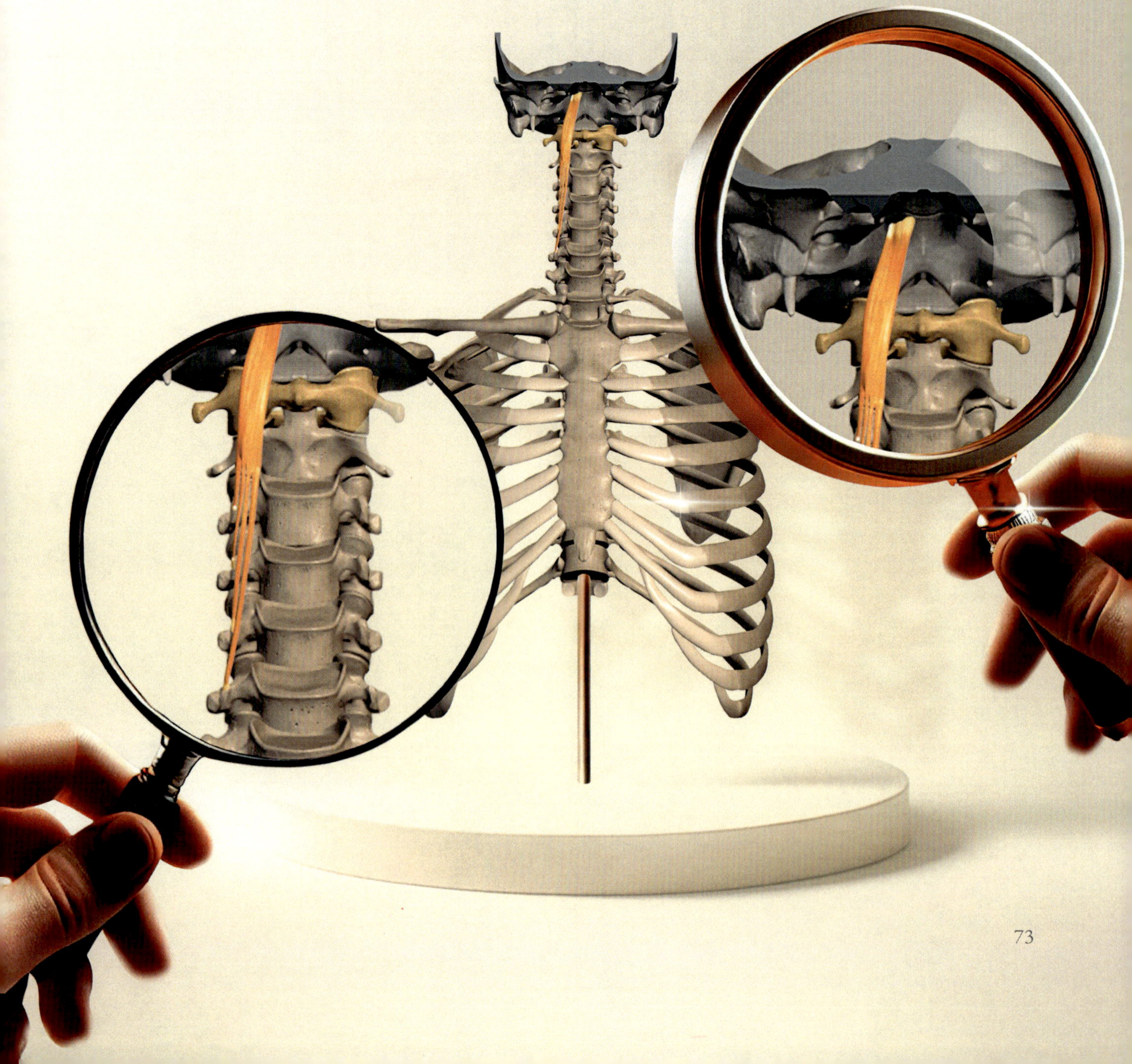

Longus Colli

Longus colli is a muscle located along the front of the cervical spine. It originates from the bodies and transverse processes of the cervical and upper thoracic vertebrae (C1-T3) and inserts on the cervical vertebrae (C2-C6). Its primary functions are to flex and rotate the neck, contributing to the stability and support of cervical spine movements.

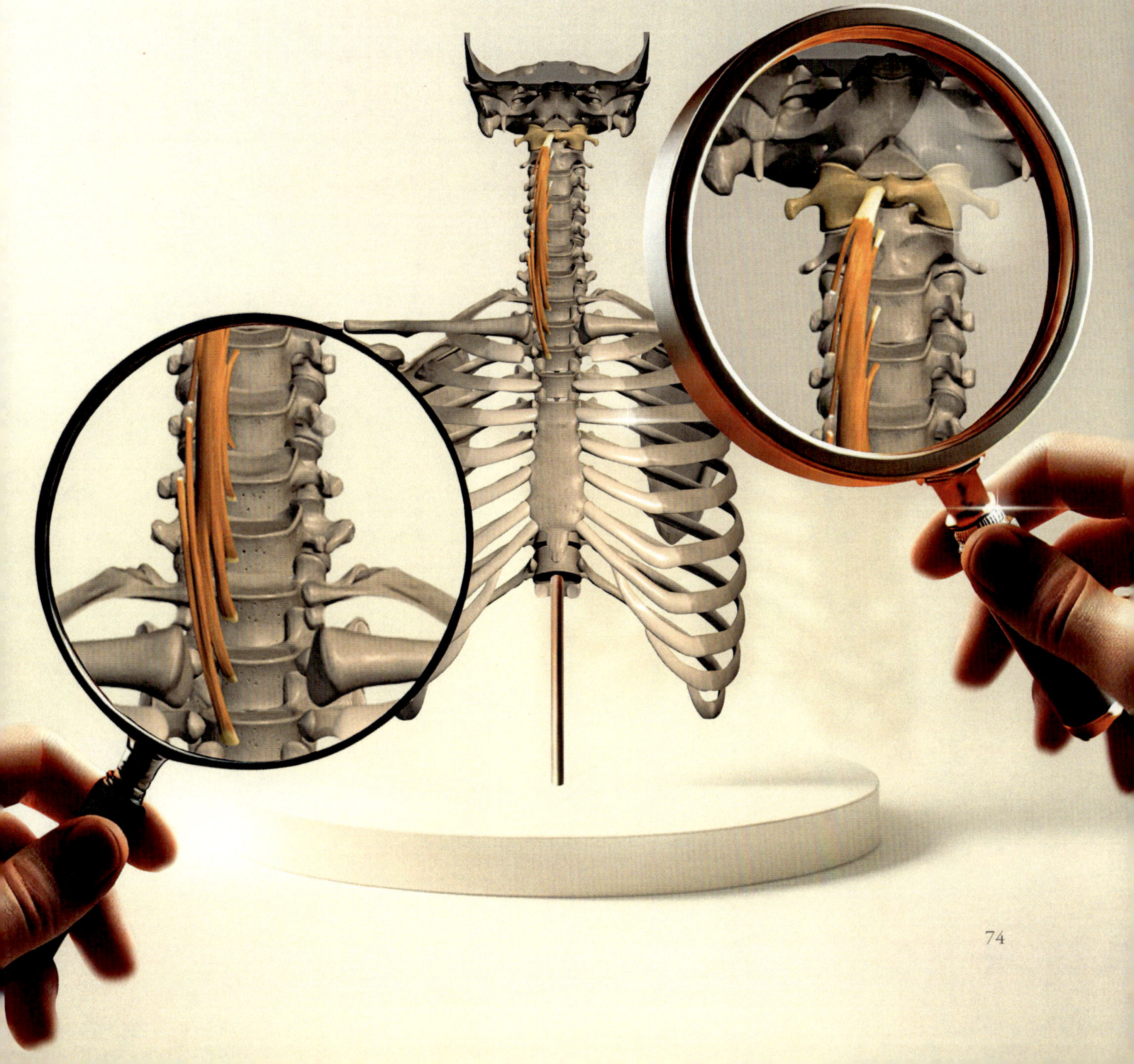

Sternocleidomastoid Muscle

The sternocleidomastoid is a prominent muscle of the neck that originates from the manubrium of the sternum and the clavicle, and inserts into the mastoid process of the temporal bone. Its primary functions include rotating the head to the opposite side and flexing the neck, playing a crucial role in head and neck movements and in maintaining posture.

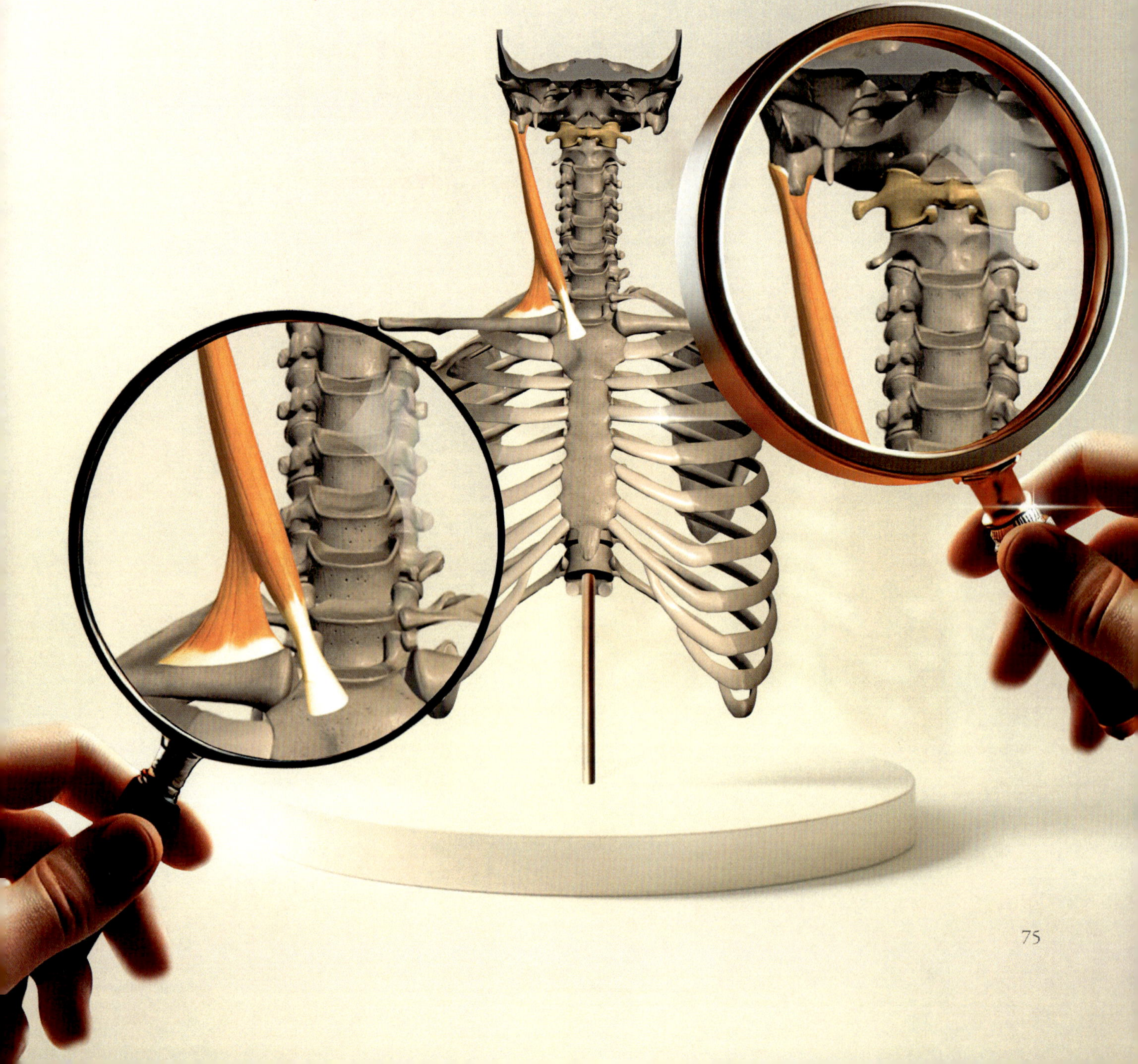

Anterior Scalene Muscle

The anterior scalene muscle is primarily responsible for assisting in the lateral flexion of the neck and elevating the first rib during deep inhalation. It originates from the transverse processes of the cervical vertebrae (C3-C6) and inserts into the first rib. By facilitating these movements, the anterior scalene plays a crucial role in both neck mobility and respiratory function.

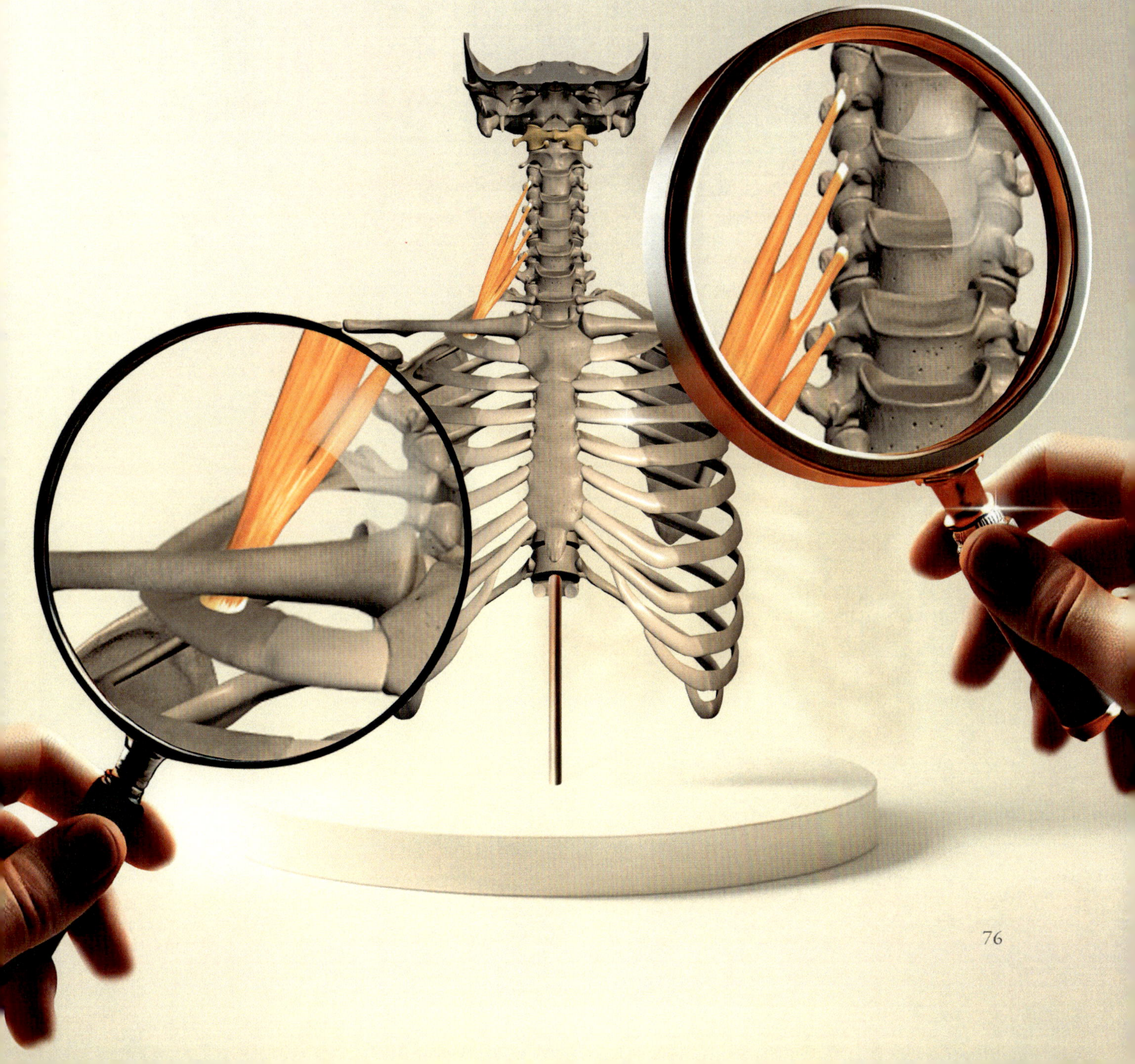

Blood Vessels and the Atlas Vertebra

The blood vessels that pass through and around the atlas vertebra (C1) play a crucial role in supplying blood to the cerebellum, posterior parts of the cerebral hemispheres, and the upper spinal cord. The most important blood vessels in this area are the vertebral arteries, which are part of the vertebrobasilar arterial circulation.

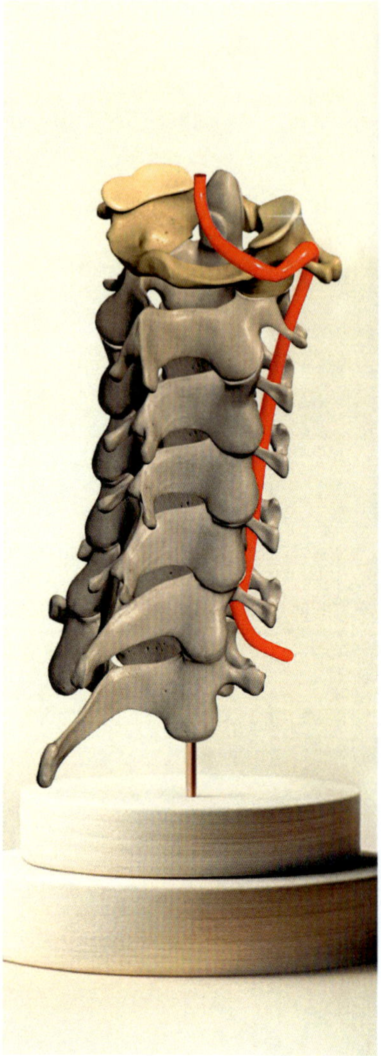

[Image 1] Vertebral artery

Movement or subluxation of the atlas vertebra (C1) can cause significant issues with blood vessels, particularly the vertebral arteries that pass through this part of the neck. Subluxation can lead to compression, stretching, or kinking of these arteries, potentially reducing blood flow and causing various neurological symptoms.

Vertebral Artery

The vertebral artery is a paired blood vessel that branches off from the subclavian artery and ascends through the transverse foramina of the cervical vertebrae. After passing through the transverse foramina from C6 to C1, the vertebral arteries enter the cranium through the foramen magnum, where they merge to form the basilar artery. The vertebral arteries supply blood to the posterior parts of the brain, including the brainstem, cerebellum, and posterior cerebral hemispheres.

This part of its path is known as the "atlanto-occipital" segment of the vertebral artery [Image 1]. This curve allows the artery the flexibility needed to adapt to head movements. The flexibility of this segment is crucial for maintaining uninterrupted blood flow to the brain, despite various head movements and positions.

When the atlas vertebra is displaced from its normal position, it can compress the vertebral arteries, reducing blood flow to the posterior parts of the brain. This reduced blood flow can lead to ischemia, a condition characterized by a lack of oxygen in the brainstem, cerebellum, and posterior cerebral hemispheres. Ischemia can cause various neurological symptoms, including dizziness, headaches, blurred vision, and weakness [Image 1].

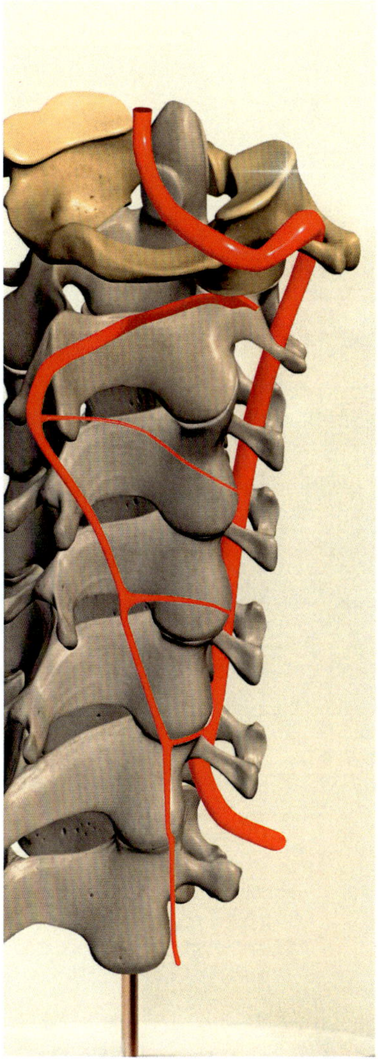

[Image 1] Deep Cervical Artery

In addition to reducing blood flow, displacement of the atlas can cause turbulent blood flow in the vertebral arteries. This turbulence can lead to the formation of a thrombus, a blood clot that can block blood flow and increase the risk of stroke. Thrombosis in the vertebral arteries can have serious consequences, as it can impede blood supply to critical parts of the brain, potentially leading to permanent damage.

Therefore, maintaining the proper position of the atlas is crucial for ensuring adequate blood flow through the vertebral arteries and preventing serious vascular complications. Timely diagnosis and treatment of atlas subluxation can significantly reduce the risk of these complications and improve patients' quality of life.

Because of their anatomical position and path, the vertebral arteries are particularly susceptible to compression or injury during sudden or improper head movements. This can lead to reduced blood flow to the brain, causing dizziness, headaches, or, in severe cases, a stroke. Therefore, maintaining the proper alignment of the atlas is essential for preserving adequate blood flow through the vertebral arteries.

Symptoms of Vertebral Artery Compression

When atlas subluxation, i.e., displacement of the atlas vertebra from its normal position, occurs, it can compress the vertebral arteries, causing numerous health problems. One of the most noticeable symptoms is dizziness, which can occur due to inadequate blood flow to the cerebellum. The cerebellum is crucial for balance and coordination, so reduced blood flow can cause serious stability and movement control issues.

Intense headaches are also a common symptom, often localized at the back of the head or neck. These headaches can result from reduced blood flow, leading to a lack of oxygen in brain tissues. Inadequate blood supply can also cause visual problems. Patients often report blurred vision, double vision, or other visual disturbances, which occur when parts of the brain responsible for vision do not receive enough blood.

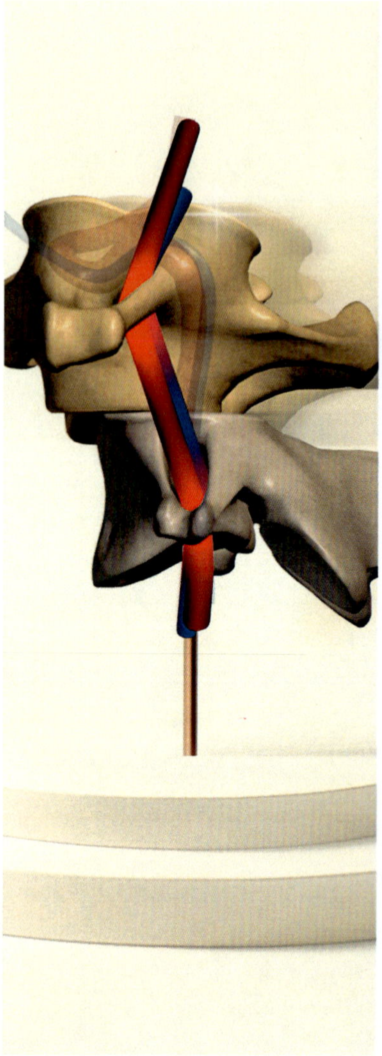

[Image 1] Artery Compression

Dizziness can be accompanied by nausea and vomiting. These symptoms are also a result of a lack of oxygen in the brain, further complicating patients' normal functioning [Image 1]. Additionally, a general feeling of weakness and fatigue can be present due to reduced blood flow and oxygen to the brain. These symptoms often lead to a significant reduction in patients' quality of life, limiting their daily activities and ability to perform usual tasks.

Atlas subluxation and vertebral artery compression present a serious health problem that requires careful diagnosis and appropriate atlas adjustment treatment. Understanding and recognizing these symptoms is important for preventing further complications.

For assessing the condition of the vertebral arteries and blood vessels around the atlas, doctors often use techniques such as magnetic resonance angiography (MRA) or Doppler ultrasound. These methods provide a detailed view of the blood vessels and help identify potential problems like stenosis, compression, or other vascular abnormalities.

Carotid Arteries and the Atlas Vertebra

The carotid arteries are blood vessels that supply the brain with blood. There are two main carotid arteries: the left and right common carotid artery. Each common carotid artery splits into the internal carotid artery (a. carotis interna) and the external carotid artery (a. carotis externa). The internal carotid arteries are particularly important as they directly supply large parts of the brain, including the anterior and middle cerebral arteries, which play a crucial role in cognitive functions and motor control.

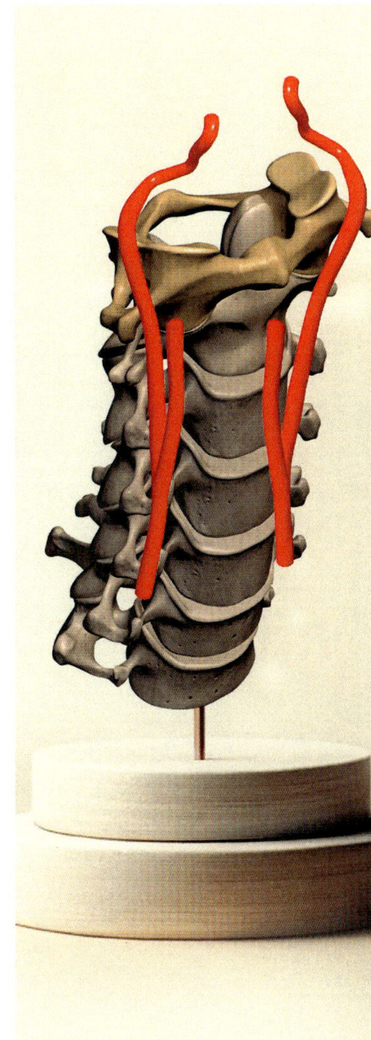

[Image 1] Carotid Artery

The proper position of the atlas vertebra (C1) is vital for maintaining adequate blood flow through the carotid arteries [Image 1]. The atlas vertebra allows for the rotation of the head, but improper alignment or subluxation (atlantoaxial rotation) can lead to compression or impingement of the carotid arteries.

When the atlas vertebra is properly aligned, the carotid arteries remain unobstructed, allowing stable and adequate blood flow to the brain. This is crucial for preventing ischemia, a condition characterized by a lack of oxygen in the brain.

Atlantoaxial rotation can lead to the impingement of one carotid artery. When the carotid artery is impinged, the brain may be deprived of enough oxygen and nutrients. This can lead to symptoms such as dizziness, confusion, weakness, balance and vision problems, and cognitive impairments. In extreme cases, reduced blood flow can cause transient ischemic attacks (TIA) or a stroke.

Therefore, proper alignment of the atlas vertebra is crucial for maintaining unobstructed blood flow through the carotid arteries and preventing serious neurological problems. Regular check-ups and atlas adjustment treatments significantly contribute to maintaining the health and functionality of the carotid arteries, ensuring stable blood supply to the brain.

"In whom we have redemption through his blood, the forgiveness of sins, according to the riches of his grace."

(Ephesians 1:7)

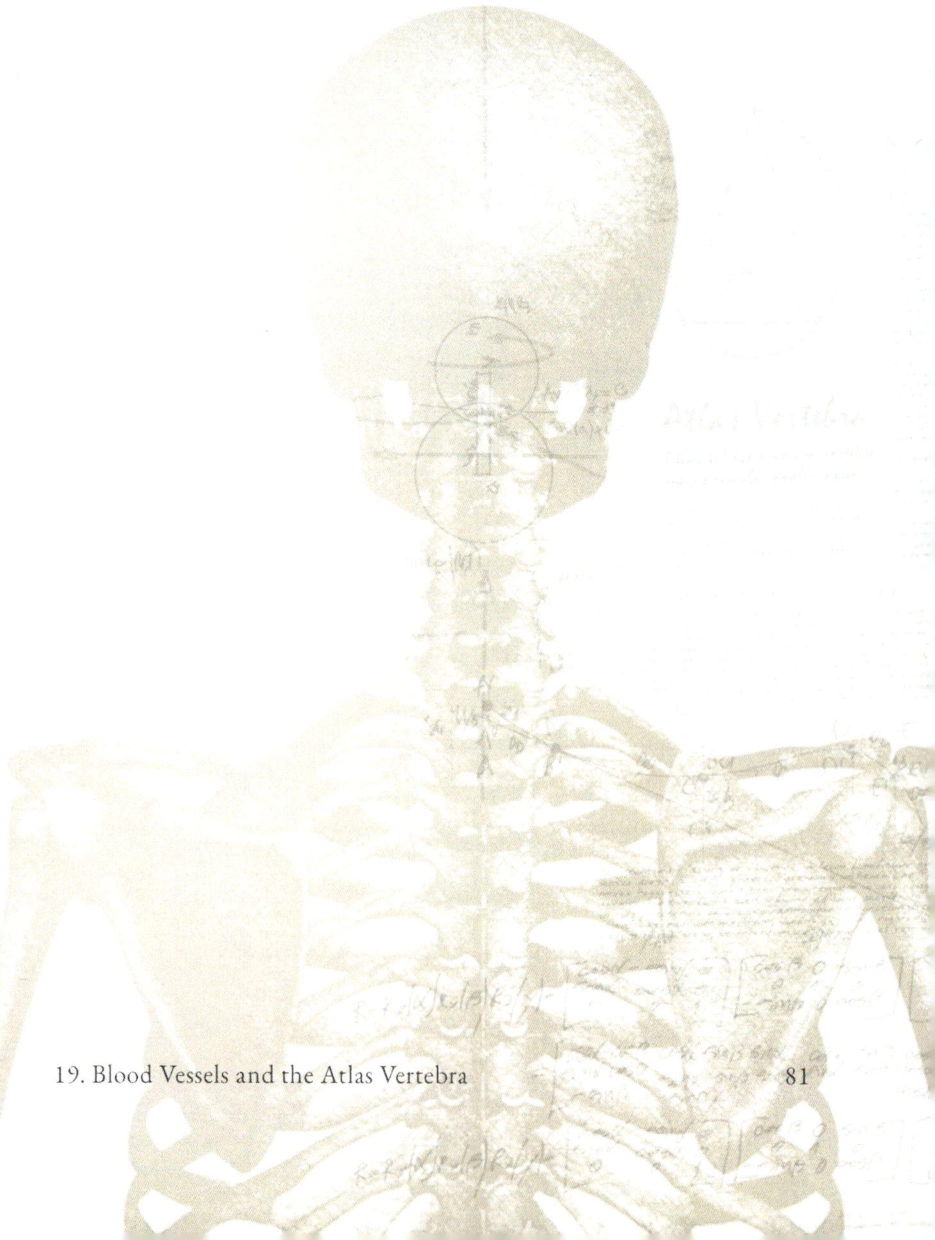

Vertebral Artery - ***Brain Blood Supply***

This artery runs through the transverse foramina of the cervical vertebrae (C6-C1). It supplies blood to the posterior part of the brain, including the cerebellum and brainstem, and helps form the basilar artery. These arteries are crucial for blood circulation in the vertebrobasilar system, essential for brain and central nervous system function.

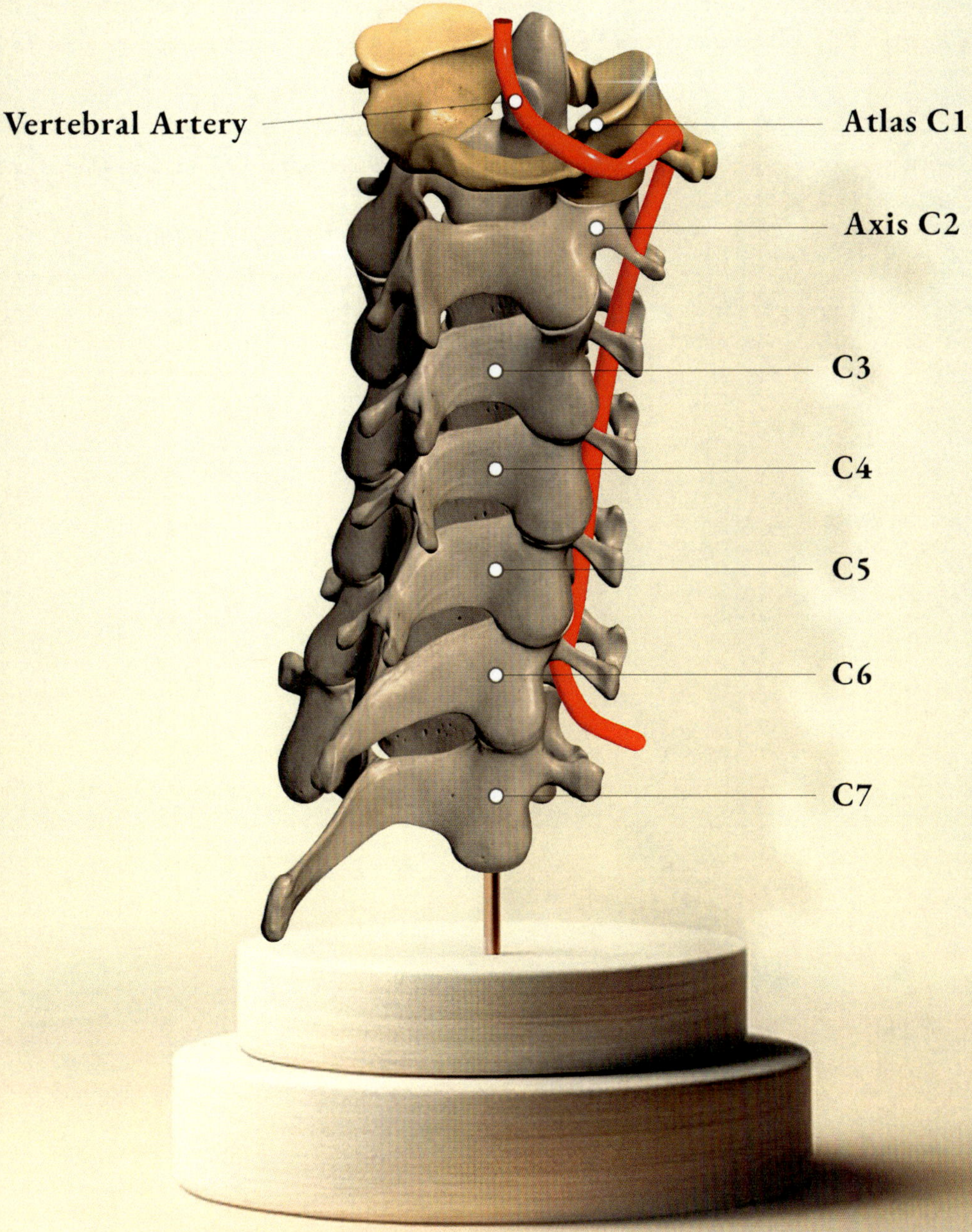

Deep Cervical Artery

The deep cervical artery is a branch of the costocervical trunk, which originates from the subclavian artery. It supplies blood to the deep muscles of the neck, including the semispinalis capitis and semispinalis cervicis muscles, and the spinal cord. This artery also plays a role in providing blood to the vertebrae and the meninges surrounding the spinal cord.

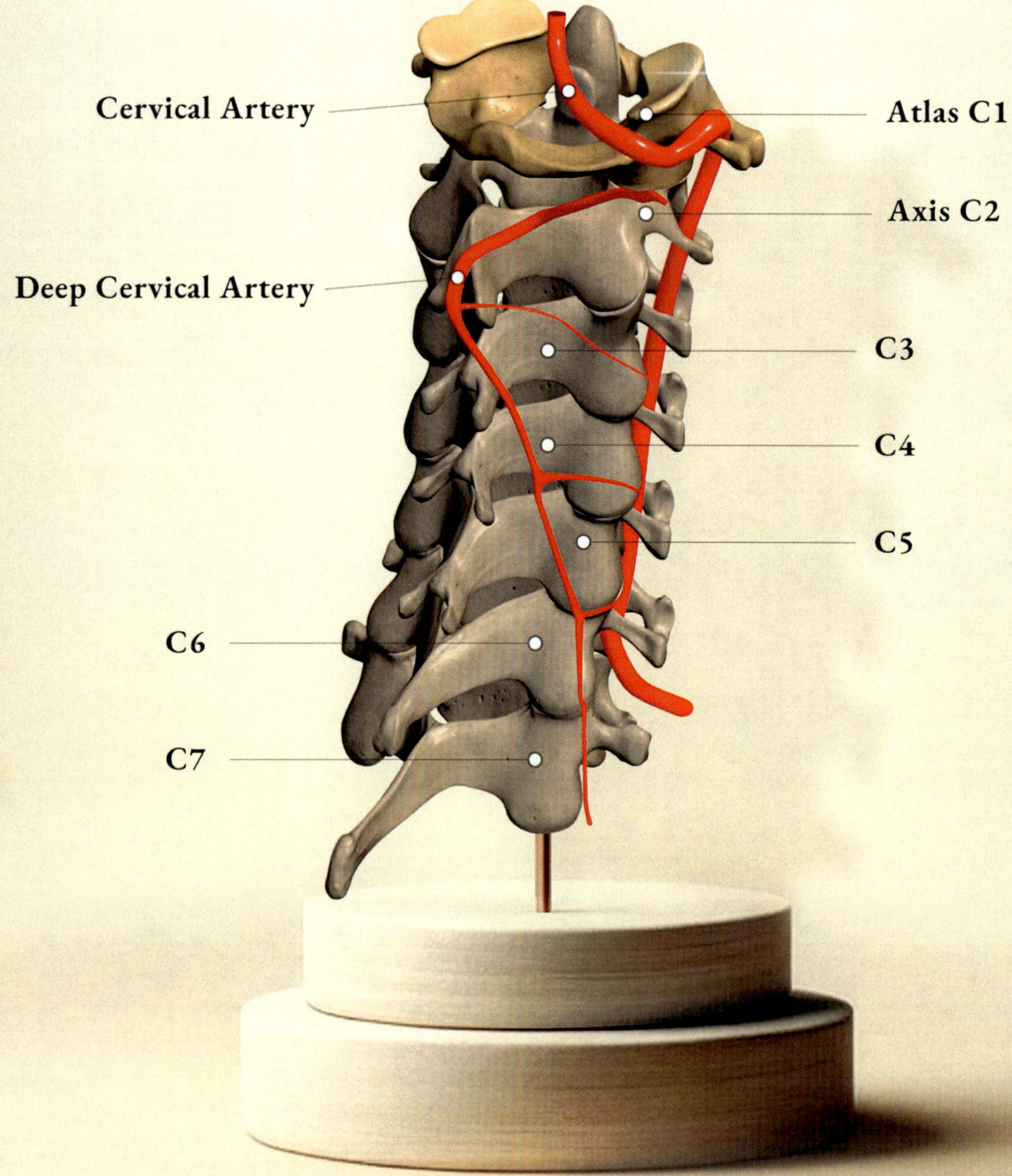

Carotid Arteries - *Vital Blood Supply*

The carotid arteries are major blood vessels that supply oxygenated blood to the brain, neck, and face. There are two carotid arteries: the right and left common carotid arteries. The internal carotid artery passes by the atlas (C1) vertebra. After bifurcation, it ascends towards the brain and enters the skull through the carotid canal in the temporal bone.

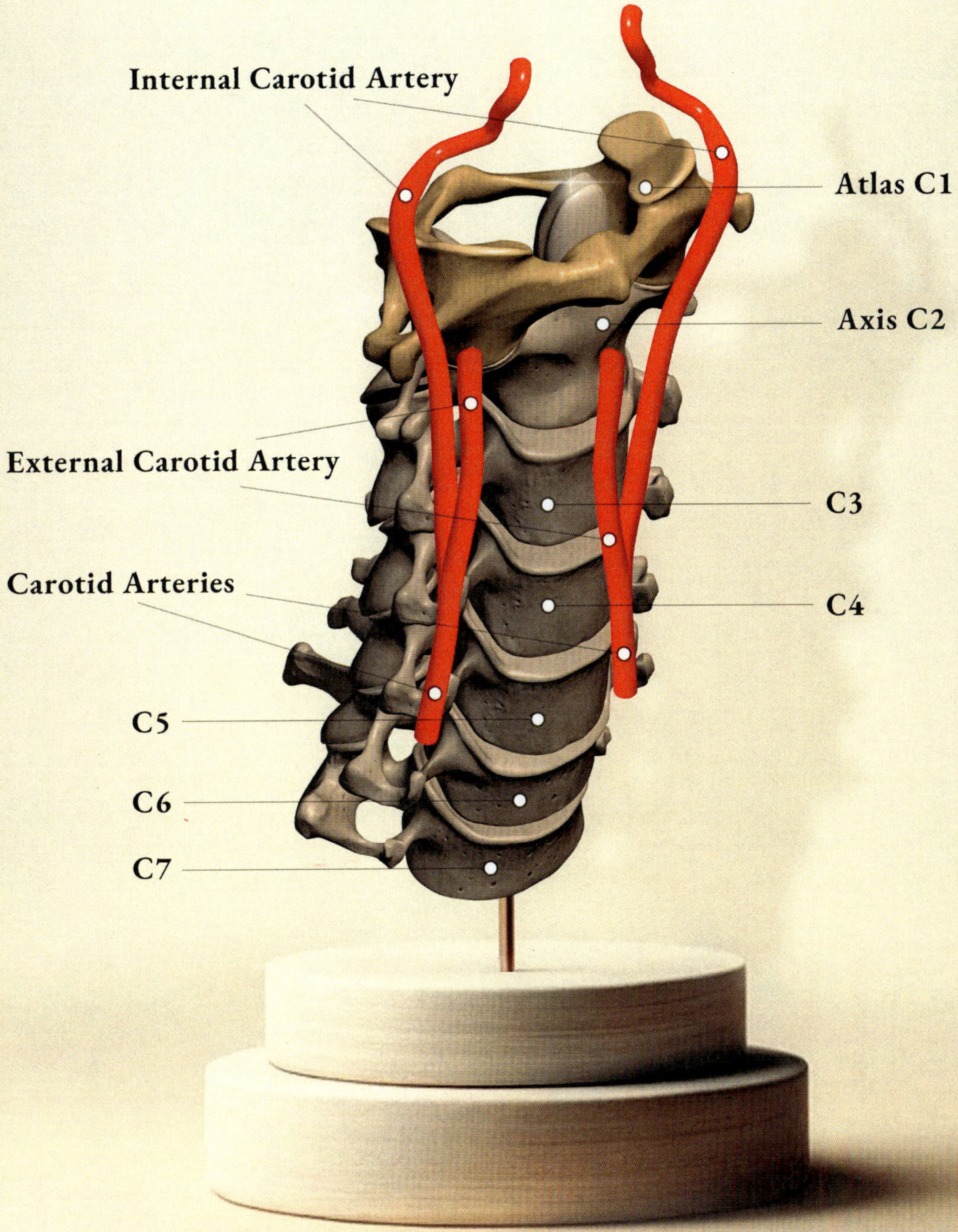

Vertebral Vein

The vertebral vein passes through the transverse foramina of the cervical vertebrae from C1 to C7. This vein follows the path of the vertebral artery and plays a crucial role in draining blood from the cervical structures, including the spinal cord and surrounding muscles. The vertebral vein then empties into the brachiocephalic vein, allowing blood to return to the heart.

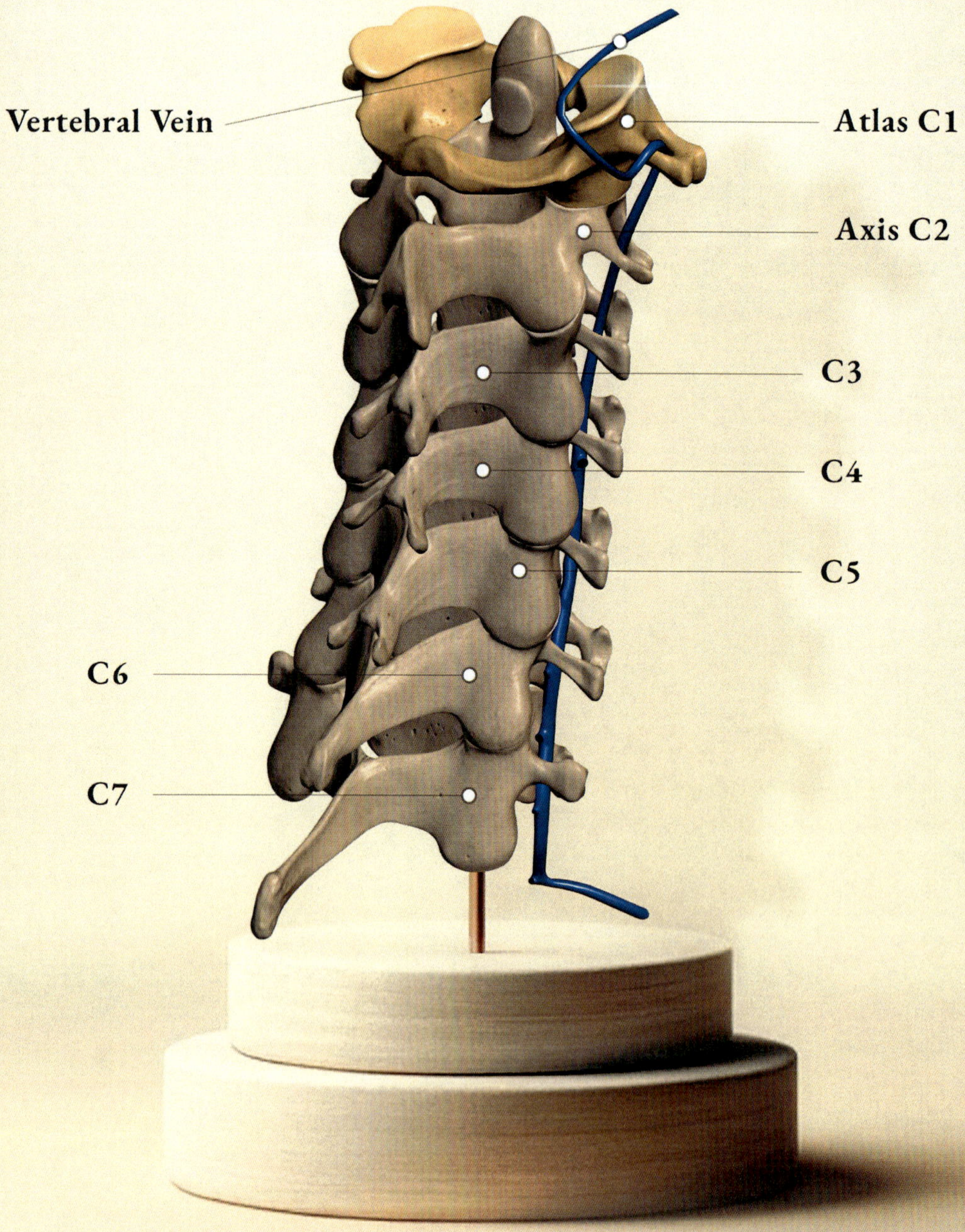

Internal Jugular Vein

The internal jugular vein is the primary vein that drains blood from the brain, face, and neck. It begins at the jugular foramen at the base of the skull, where it collects blood from the dural venous sinuses. The vein descends the neck within the carotid sheath, parallel to the internal carotid artery and the vagus nerve, passing in close proximity to the atlas vertebra.

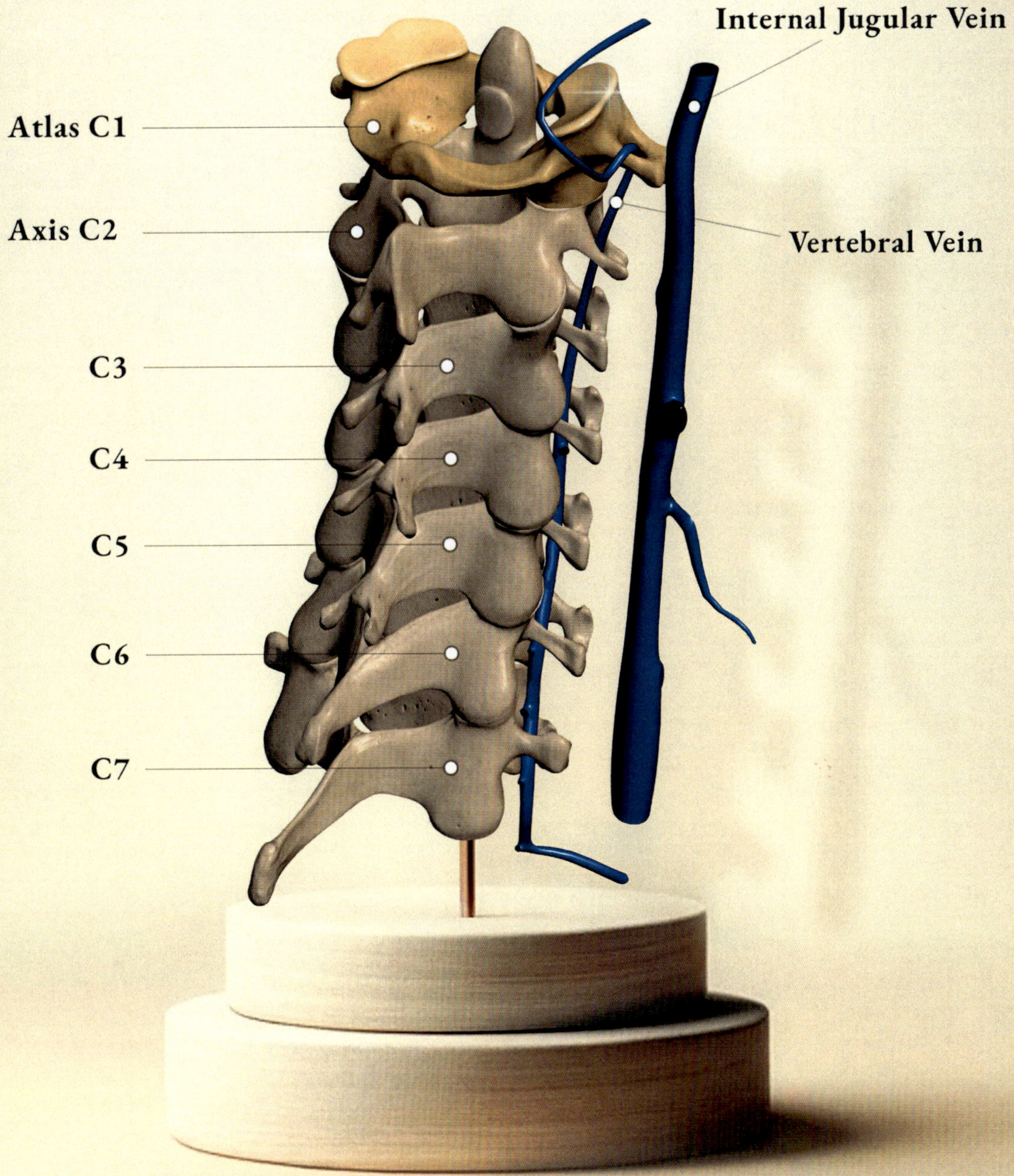

Lymph Nodes in the Area of the Atlas Vertebra

Lymph nodes in the area of the atlas vertebra (C1) are part of the lymphatic system, which is responsible for filtering lymph, removing toxins, waste, and other harmful substances from the body. The proper function of lymph nodes is significant for preventing infections and maintaining health.

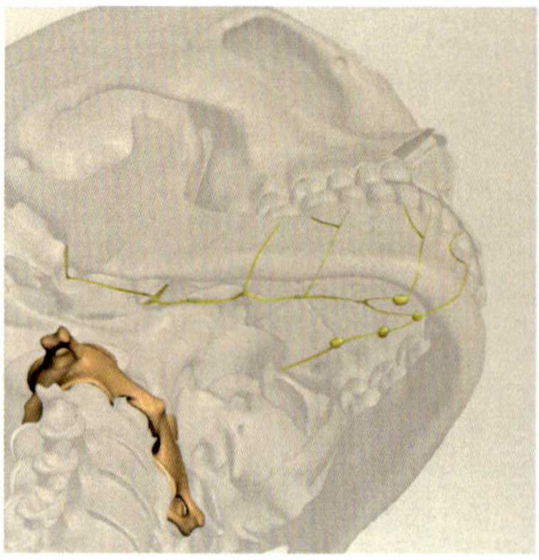

[Image 1] Submental nodes

The cervical region, including the area of the atlas vertebra (C1), contains several important groups of lymph nodes that play a key role in the immune system. These lymph nodes act as filters for lymph, a fluid that circulates through the lymphatic system, removing toxins, waste, and other harmful substances from the body.

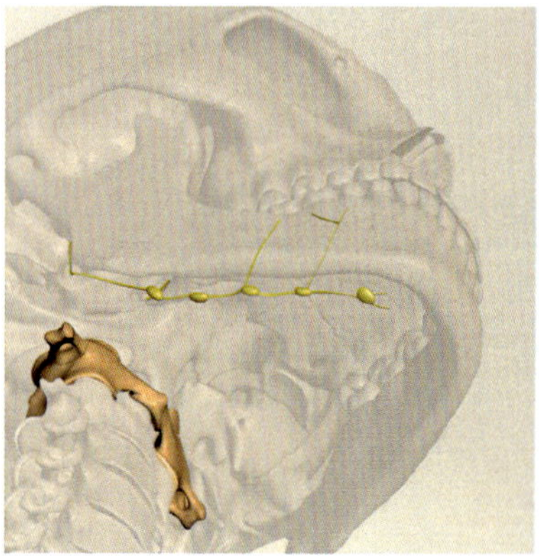

[Image 2] Submandibular nodes

One important group is the submental lymph nodes. These nodes filter lymph from the lower part of the oral cavity and the anterior part of the tongue, providing the first line of defense against infections in this region [Image 1]. The submandibular lymph nodes are located under the lower jaw [Image 2]. Due to their location, the submandibular lymph nodes play a role in protecting against pathogens entering through these parts of the body.

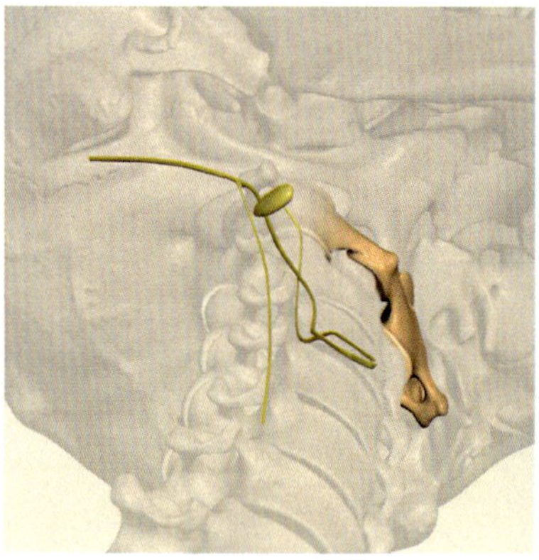

[Image 3] Jugular nodes

Alongside the internal jugular vein are the jugular lymph nodes, which filter lymph from the throat, tonsils, and thyroid gland [Image 3]. These lymph nodes are essential for maintaining the health of the upper respiratory tract and the thyroid gland as they help eliminate bacteria.

The supraclavicular lymph nodes are located above the collarbone and filter lymph from the head, neck, and upper chest. These nodes are particularly important for detecting and combating infections and malignant cells that may spread from these parts of the body.

All these groups of lymph nodes work together to maintain the health and functionality of the immune system. Proper functioning of the lymphatic system in the cervical region is crucial for protecting the body from infections and diseases. Proper alignment of the atlas vertebra can further contribute to the optimal functioning of these lymph nodes if their functionality is compromised. White blood cells in the lymph nodes help fight infections by destroying or trapping pathogens (bacteria) and other harmful substances, preventing their further spread in the body.

Impact of Atlas Subluxation

Atlas subluxation, or displacement of the first cervical vertebra from its normal position, can have significant consequences on the functioning of lymph nodes in the cervical region [Image 1]. This dislocation can cause several serious problems that negatively impact the lymphatic system and overall health.

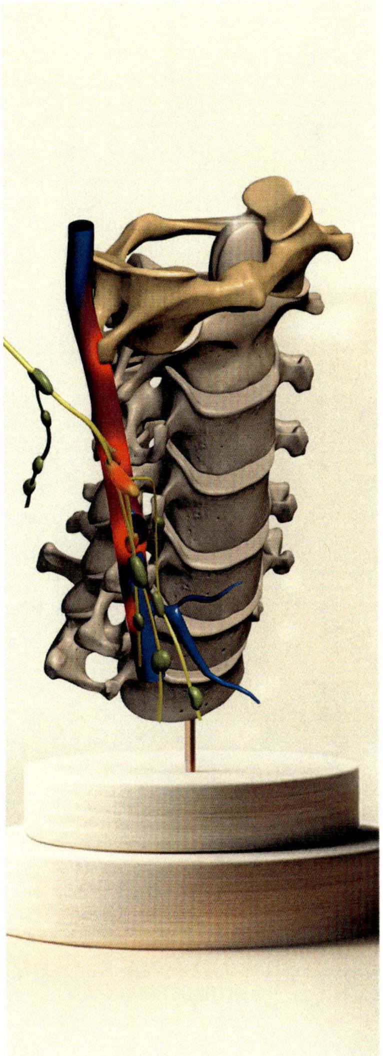

[Image 1] Atlas and lymphatics

When the atlas vertebra is displaced, it can lead to compression of the lymphatic vessels, obstructing the flow of lymph through the cervical region. This compression can result in fluid retention, swelling, and reduced efficiency of the lymphatic system. When lymph cannot circulate freely, the body struggles more to fight infections and less effectively removes toxins, which can negatively impact overall health.

Atlas subluxation can also affect the nerve pathways that regulate the function of lymph nodes. Damaged or irritated nerves can lead to lymph node dysfunction, reducing their ability to effectively filter lymph and respond to infections. When nerve signals are not properly transmitted, lymph nodes cannot adequately perform their role in the immune response, increasing the risk of infections and other health problems.

Displacement of the atlas can cause local inflammatory processes that further burden the lymph nodes. Inflammation can increase the permeability of blood vessels, leading to swelling and reduced functionality of the lymph nodes. Chronic inflammation can weaken the immune system and make it harder for the body to fight off pathogens.

Problems with the lymphatic system in the area of the atlas vertebra can manifest through various symptoms indicating dysfunction of this critical part of the immune system. One of the most common symptoms is swelling. Enlarged or swollen lymph nodes are often a sign of infection or inflammation in the head and neck area. These changes can be visually noticeable and are often accompanied by discomfort.

Pain or tenderness in the lymph nodes can also indicate the presence of infection or other medical issues. When lymph nodes are painful to the touch, it usually means the body is fighting against pathogens or other harmful substances. Reduced efficiency of the lymphatic system can also lead to a general feeling of weakness and fatigue.

When lymph nodes do not function properly, the body struggles more to fight off toxins and infections, resulting in increased feelings of exhaustion. This can significantly impact the quality of life and the ability of a person to cope with daily activities. Additionally, problems with lymph nodes can weaken the immune system, increasing the risk of frequent infections. Proper alignment of the atlas vertebra can significantly contribute to maintaining the health and functionality of the lymphatic system, ensuring an optimal immune response and better resistance to infections.

Jugular Lymphatic Trunk (Right)

The right jugular lymphatic trunk is an essential component of the lymphatic system, responsible for draining lymph from the right side of the head and neck. This trunk collects lymph from the deep cervical lymph nodes and the superficial lymph nodes located in the neck region.

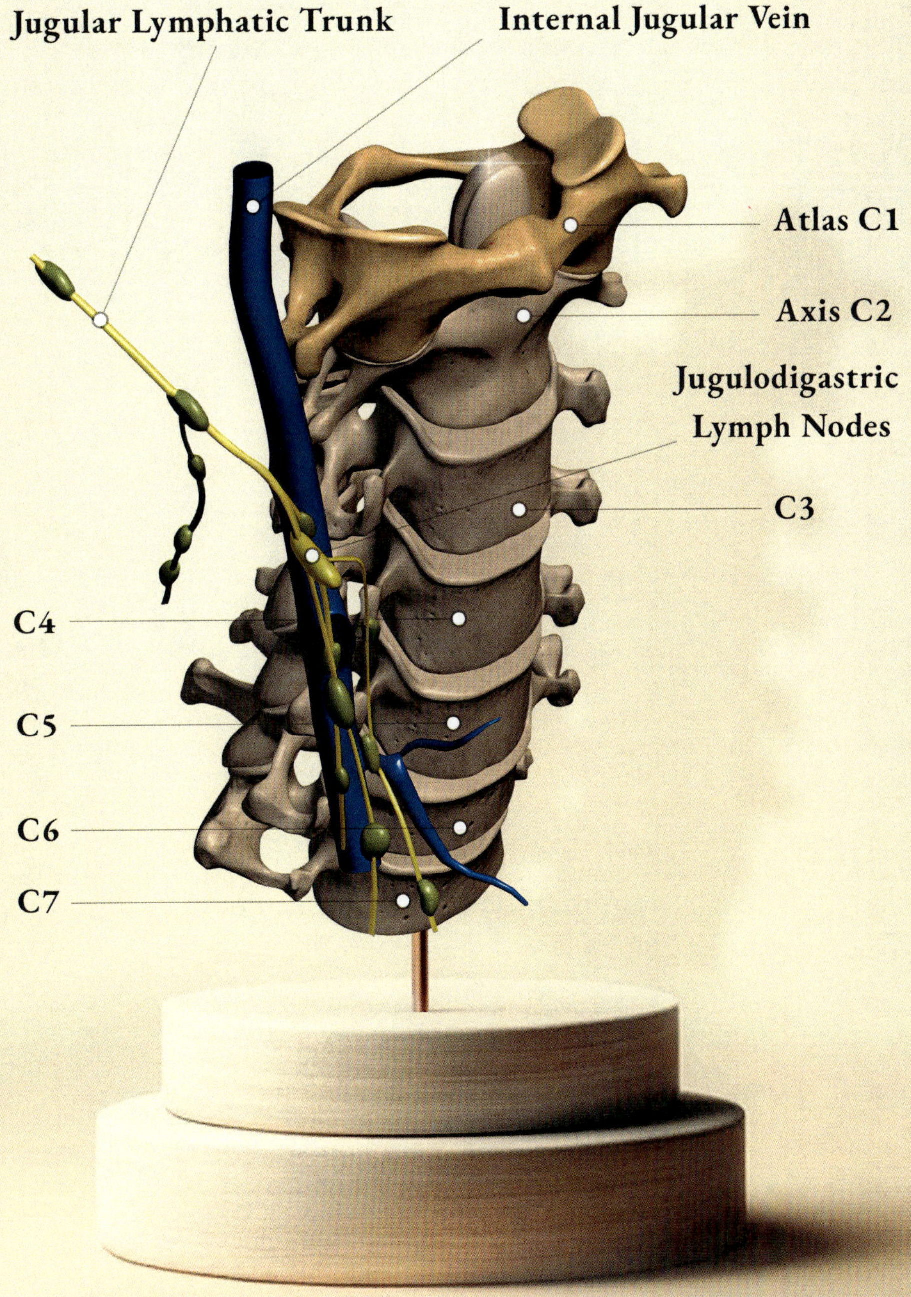

Spinal Nerve C1

The C1 spinal nerve is part of the group of cervical nerves, which are the nerves that exit the cervical (neck) region of the spinal column [Image 1]. The cervical nerves are numbered from C1 to C8 and innervate various parts of the neck, shoulders, arms, and upper torso [Image 2]. The C1 nerve is the first and highest cervical nerve, with a unique role as it is primarily motor with very limited sensory functions.

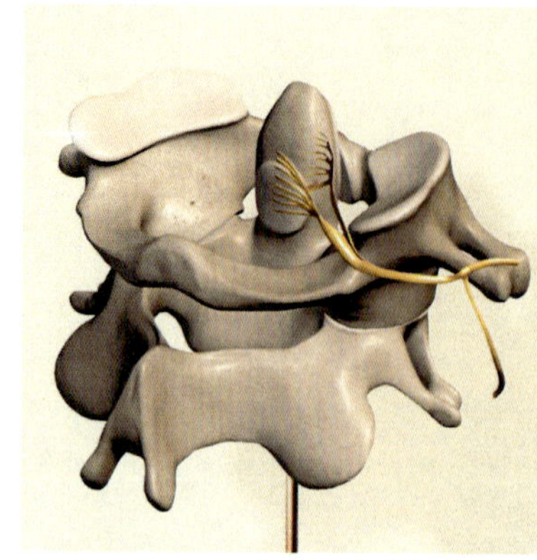
[Image 1] C1 spinal nerve

The C1 spinal nerve exits the spinal canal between the skull and the first cervical vertebra. Spinal nerves, including C1, are part of the peripheral nervous system and exit directly from the spinal cord. In the case of C1, the nerve exits between the occipital bone of the skull and the atlas, then branches out to innervate specific muscle and potentially sensory areas as needed. C1 is unique as it is the first nerve above the atlas and does not have an associated spinal disc, distinguishing it from most other spinal nerves.

The C1 nerve mainly innervates muscles in the cervical region. It branches out to different parts of the head and neck, forming a complex network of nerve pathways that help coordinate and control movements, with branches that help control several key neck muscles, including the suboccipital muscles. These muscles play a crucial role in head movements and stability, allowing for precise and controlled movements.

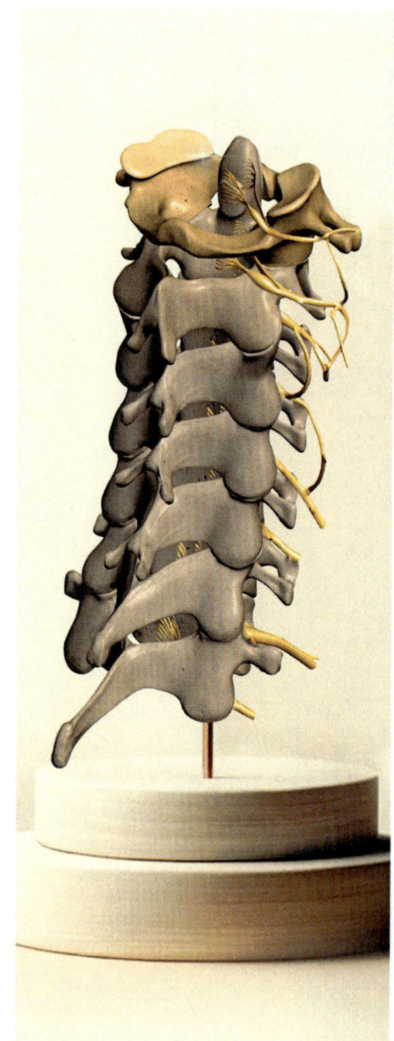
[Image 2] Spinal nerves

In addition to its motor function, the branches of the nerve may play a role in proprioception, which is the body's ability to perceive its position and movements in space. Proprioception is crucial for coordination and balance, allowing the body to effectively adjust to different positions and movements. Thus, the first cervical nerve plays a vital role not only in head and neck movements but also in maintaining the stability and orientation of the entire body.

The C1 nerve can have an indirect impact on some sensory functions through its connected branches that communicate with other nerve pathways, but its primary function is the motor control of specific neck muscles.

One branch of the C1 nerve re-enters the spinal canal as the meningeal branch [Image 1]. This branch can transmit sensory information from the meninges, or brain coverings, in the occipital region. The meningeal branch is significant because it allows for the transmission of sensations important for the protection and function of the central nervous system.

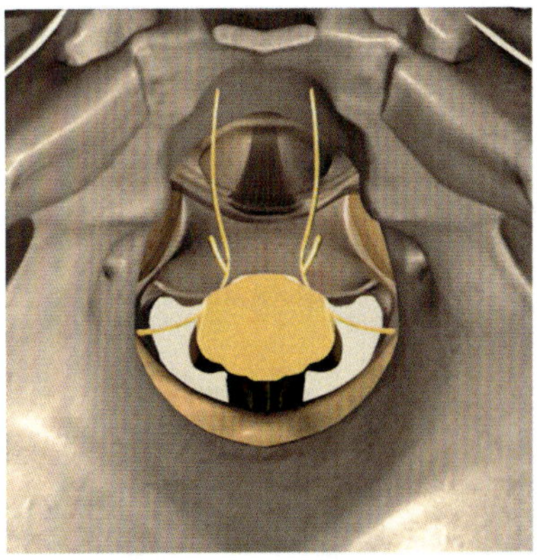
[Image 1] C1 meningeal branch

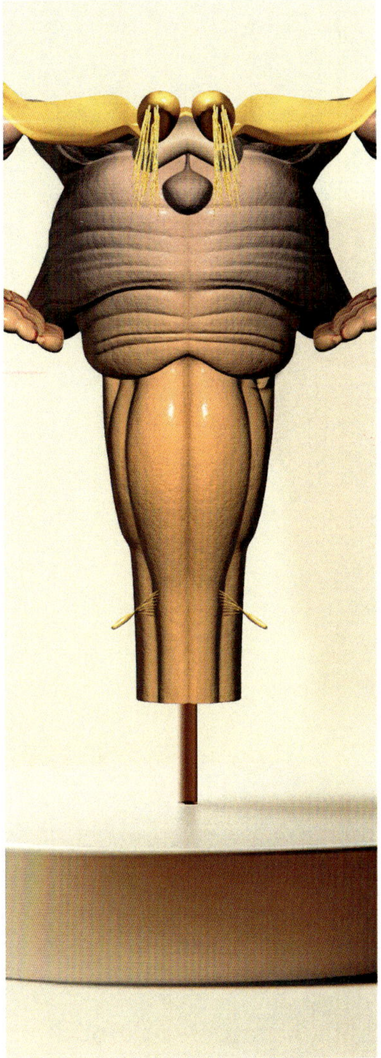
[Image 2] Hypoglossal nerve

The C1 nerve also forms a loop with the XII cranial nerve, known as the hypoglossal nerve [Image 2]. Although the hypoglossal nerve is primarily motor and controls tongue movements, through this connection, C1 may have an indirect role in sensations related to certain parts of the throat and tongue. This collaboration between the nerves enhances coordination and function in the throat.

Besides these specific connections, C1 forms anastomoses with other cervical nerves, such as C2 and sometimes C3. Through these connections, C1 can be involved in sensory pathways related to the skin and deep tissues of the neck. These anastomoses allow for the integration of sensory and motor functions, which is crucial for maintaining balance and coordination in the cervical region of the body.

The role of the C1 spinal nerve in the nervous system is complex and multifaceted. Its motor functions are primary, but the sensory functions it performs through connections with other nerves contribute to the overall functioning and adaptability of the nervous system. Understanding these connections and functions can be crucial for diagnosing and treating various neurological and musculoskeletal disorders.

Through these anastomoses, C1 can act as a sort of relay station for sensory signals. Sensory signals from the skin and deeper structures of the neck can be partially transmitted to C1 and its connected branches. This allows for the integration of sensory information from different sources, contributing to more precise coordination of motor responses. This ability of C1 to integrate sensory information is key for faster and more efficient responses to environmental stimuli.

C1, through its connections, also affects proprioceptive signals, which help in the perception of position, movement, and balance of the head. Proprioception is critical for regulating muscle tone and the position of the head relative to the body, which is necessary for maintaining balance and coordination. Through anastomoses with other cervical nerves, C1 plays a key role in fine-tuning these functions.

Through such anastomoses, sensory information can be integrated more quickly and efficiently into the central nervous system, enabling faster and more precise responses to sensory stimuli from the environment. This increase in sensory efficiency contributes to the overall functionality of the cervical region, allowing better adaptation and reaction to various situations that require coordinated movements and head and neck stability.

When the atlas vertebra, or the first cervical vertebra, compresses or exerts pressure on the C1 spinal nerve, it can cause a range of symptoms primarily associated with pain and restricted mobility. The most common symptom is neck pain, which can be sharp or dull and often worsens with head movements. Additionally, the pain can radiate to the back of the head or the crown, often described as a deep, piercing headache that can significantly diminish the patient's quality of life.

Restricted mobility is another common symptom. There can be a decrease in the range of motion in the neck, especially when trying to rotate or bend the head. This restriction can significantly hinder daily activities and cause additional problems with muscles and joints.

Dizziness and balance problems are symptoms that occur due to the role of the C1 nerve in proprioception. Compression of this nerve can affect the sense of balance, resulting in dizziness or instability. This can be particularly dangerous as it increases the risk of falls and injuries.

Changes in skin sensation on the head or neck can also occur as a result of disruptions in sensory signals. Patients may experience tingling, burning, or numbness in these areas, which can be uncomfortable and alarming.

Muscle weakness is another potential symptom, especially if the compression affects the motor branches of the C1 nerve. Weakness in the muscles innervated by C1 can impact head and neck stability, further complicating mobility and daily functions.

Symptoms can vary depending on the degree of compression and the individual's anatomy. If these symptoms occur, timely diagnosis and treatment of atlas adjustment are crucial for preventing further complications and preserving the patient's quality of life.

Spinal Nerves - *Connect and Control*

Cervical spinal nerves are eight pairs of nerves (C1-C8) that transmit sensory information from the neck, shoulders, and arms to the brain, and motor signals from the brain to these areas. They are crucial for reflexes and movement coordination, connecting the central and peripheral nervous systems.

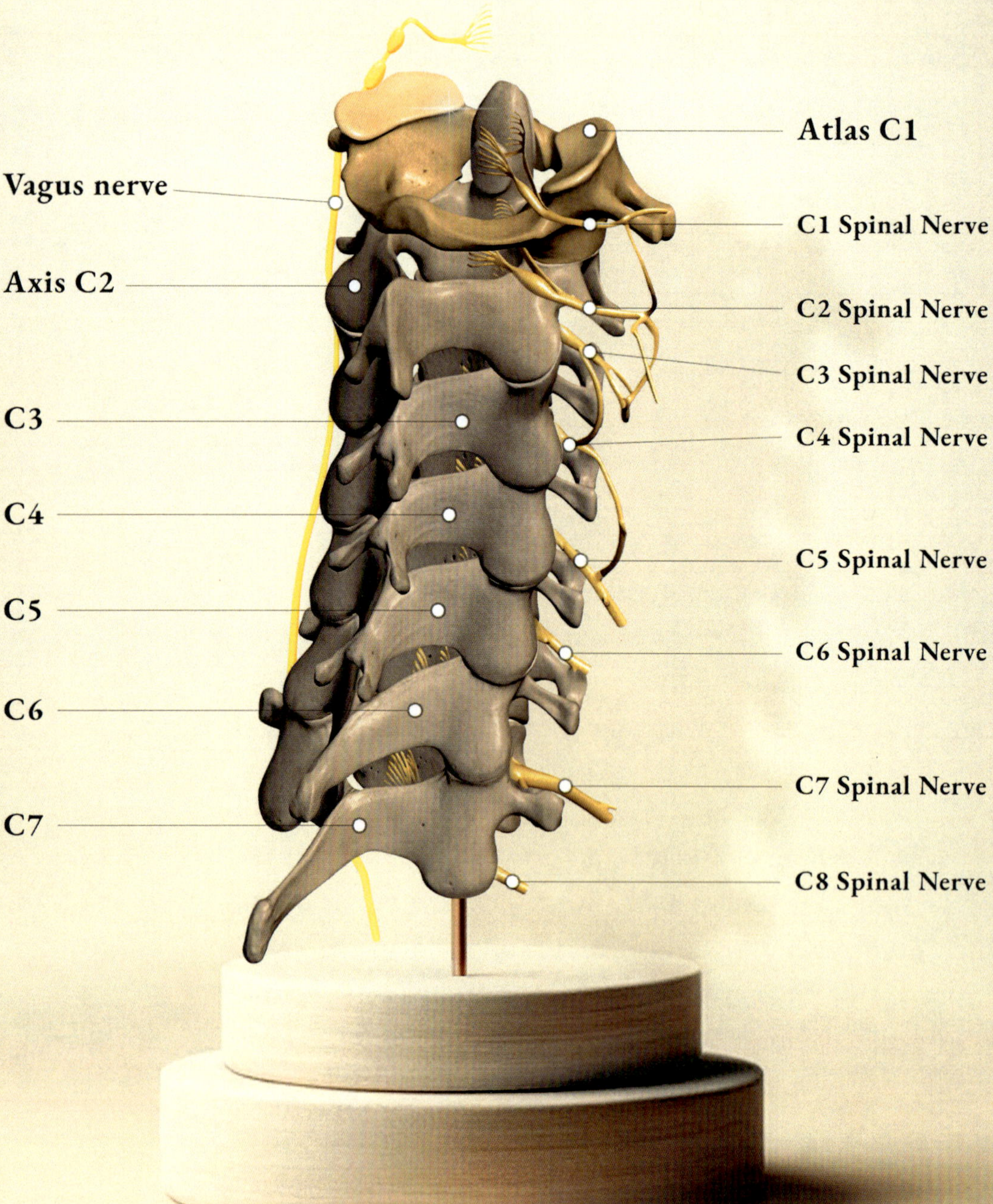

The Medulla Oblongata

Medulla oblongata, also known simply as the medulla, is a critical structure located at the base of the brainstem, connecting the brain to the spinal cord [Image 1]. It serves as a vital pathway for various sensory and motor nerves traveling between the brain and the body. Despite its relatively small size, the medulla plays a crucial role in regulating essential bodily functions such as heart rate, blood pressure, breathing, and swallowing.

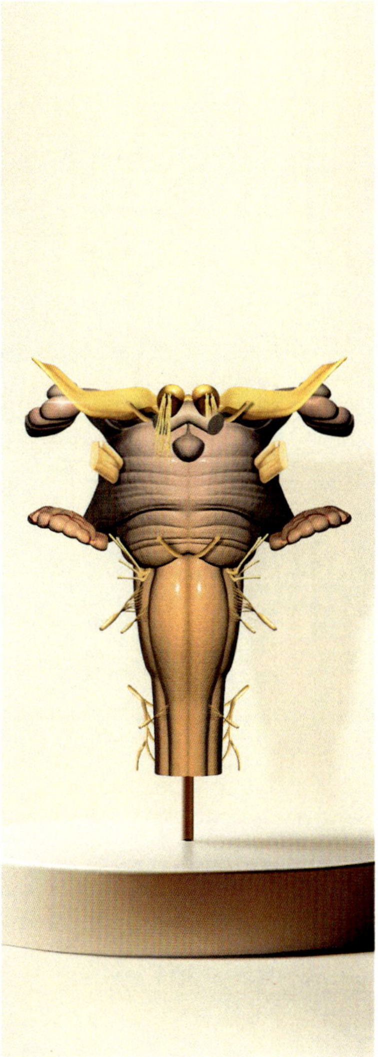

[Image 1] Anterior medulla oblongata

One of the key functions of the medulla is to control autonomic functions, which are involuntary processes essential for maintaining homeostasis in the body. For example, it regulates heart rate and blood pressure by adjusting the activity of the cardiac and vasomotor centers located within its structure. Through its connections with the cardiovascular system, the medulla ensures that blood flow and pressure remain within optimal ranges to support organ function and overall health.

In addition to cardiovascular regulation, the medulla oblongata is involved in respiratory control, coordinating the rhythm and depth of breathing to maintain adequate oxygen levels in the body. It receives sensory input from chemoreceptors that detect changes in blood oxygen and carbon dioxide levels, allowing it to adjust breathing rate and depth accordingly. This intricate control ensures efficient gas exchange in the lungs, essential for sustaining cellular respiration and overall metabolic function.

Furthermore, the medulla is integral to the coordination of swallowing and other reflex actions. It receives sensory input from various cranial nerves, integrating this information to initiate appropriate motor responses such as swallowing, coughing, and sneezing. This reflexive control helps protect the airway and facilitate the ingestion of food and liquids, contributing to overall digestive health and nutrition.

In summary, the medulla oblongata serves as a vital relay center for sensory and motor signals between the brain and the body [Image 1]. Its multifaceted functions encompass autonomic regulation, respiratory control, and coordination of reflex actions, all of which are essential for maintaining homeostasis and ensuring the body's optimal functioning. Studying the medulla provides valuable insights into the intricate neural circuits underlying fundamental physiological processes and their relevance to overall health and well-being.

"And the LORD God formed man of the dust of the ground, and breathed into his nostrils the breath of life; and man became a living soul."

(Genesis 2:7)

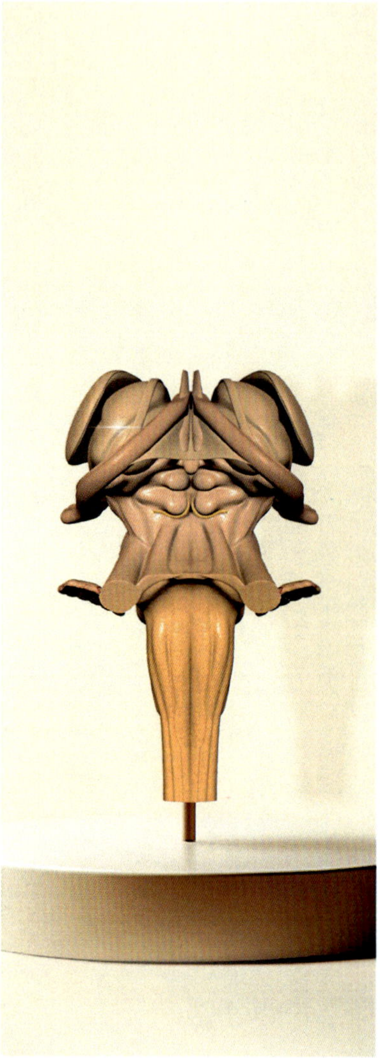

[Image 1] Posterior Medulla Oblongata

Medulla Oblongata - Anterior View

The medulla oblongata, located at the base of the brainstem, is crucial for regulating vital autonomic functions. It controls heart rate, blood pressure, and breathing. Additionally, it coordinates reflexes such as swallowing, coughing, and sneezing. This structure acts as a conduit for nerve signals between the brain and spinal cord, ensuring seamless communication within the central nervous system. Damage to the medulla oblongata can result in severe, life-threatening consequences due to its essential role in maintaining homeostasis.

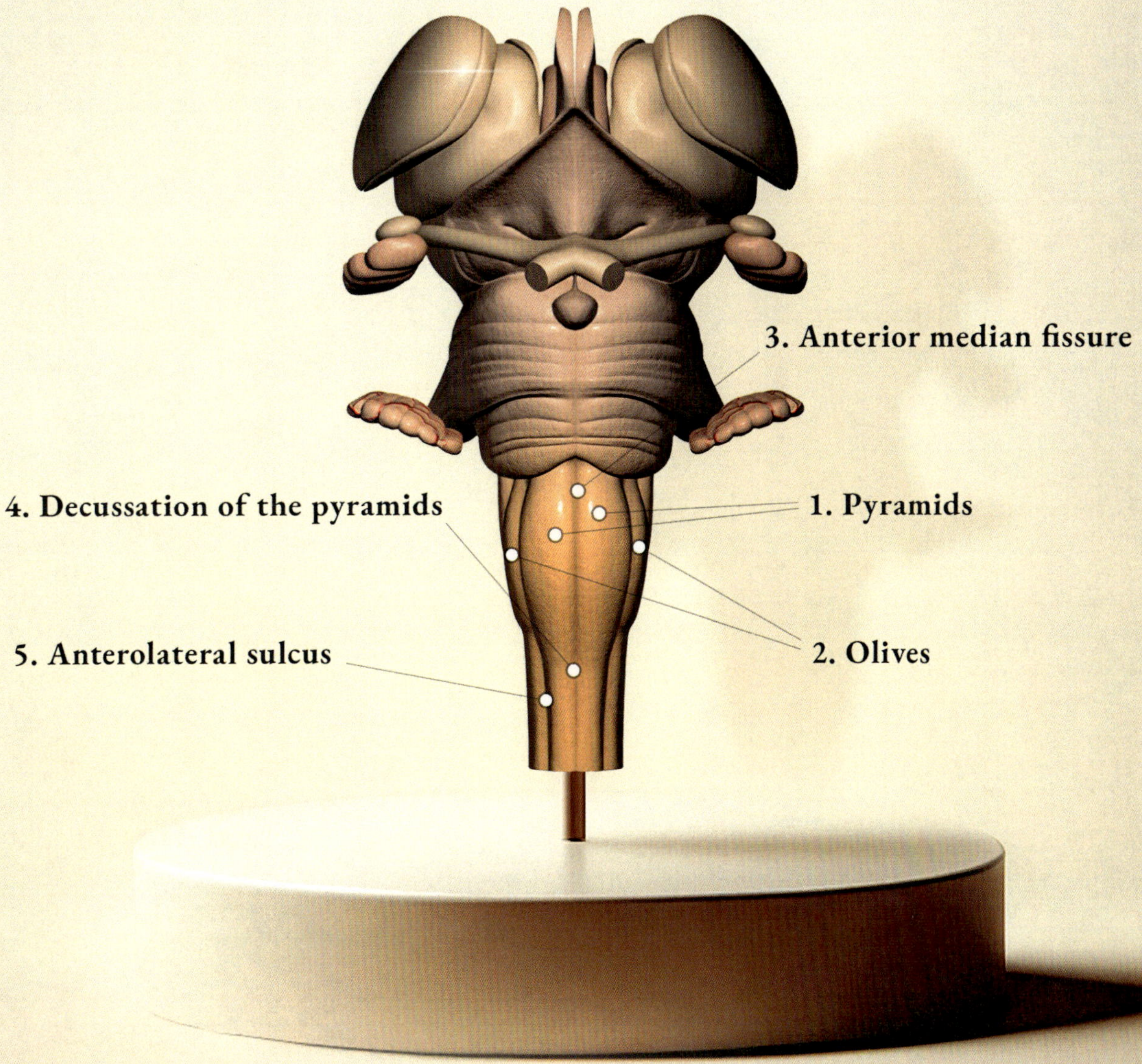

1. Pyramids

The pyramids are paired structures located on the anterior (ventral) side of the medulla oblongata. They contain the corticospinal tracts, which are major motor pathways that transmit signals from the cerebral cortex to the spinal cord, facilitating voluntary motor control. The pyramidal decussation, where the fibers cross to the opposite side, is also found here. This crossing allows for the contralateral control of motor functions, meaning each side of the brain controls the opposite side of the body. Damage to the pyramids can result in motor deficits and loss of voluntary muscle control.

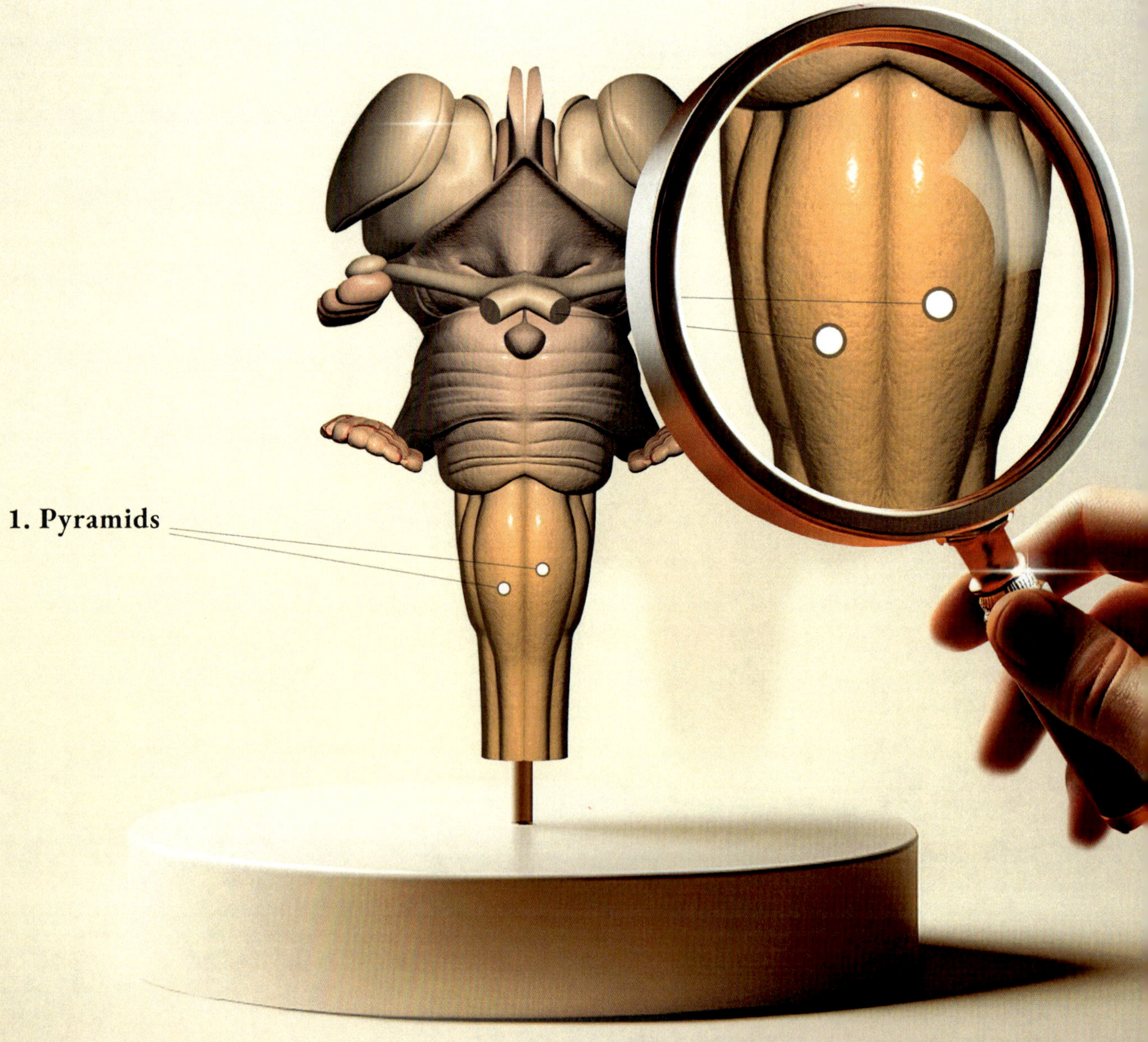

2. Olives

The olives are prominent oval-shaped structures located laterally to the pyramids on the anterior side of the medulla oblongata. They contain the inferior olivary nuclei, which play a crucial role in motor coordination and learning. The olives receive input from various parts of the brain and spinal cord and send output to the cerebellum, helping to refine motor movements. Damage to the olives can result in impaired motor coordination and difficulties with learning new motor skills. Proper functioning of the olives is essential for precise and coordinated motor activities.

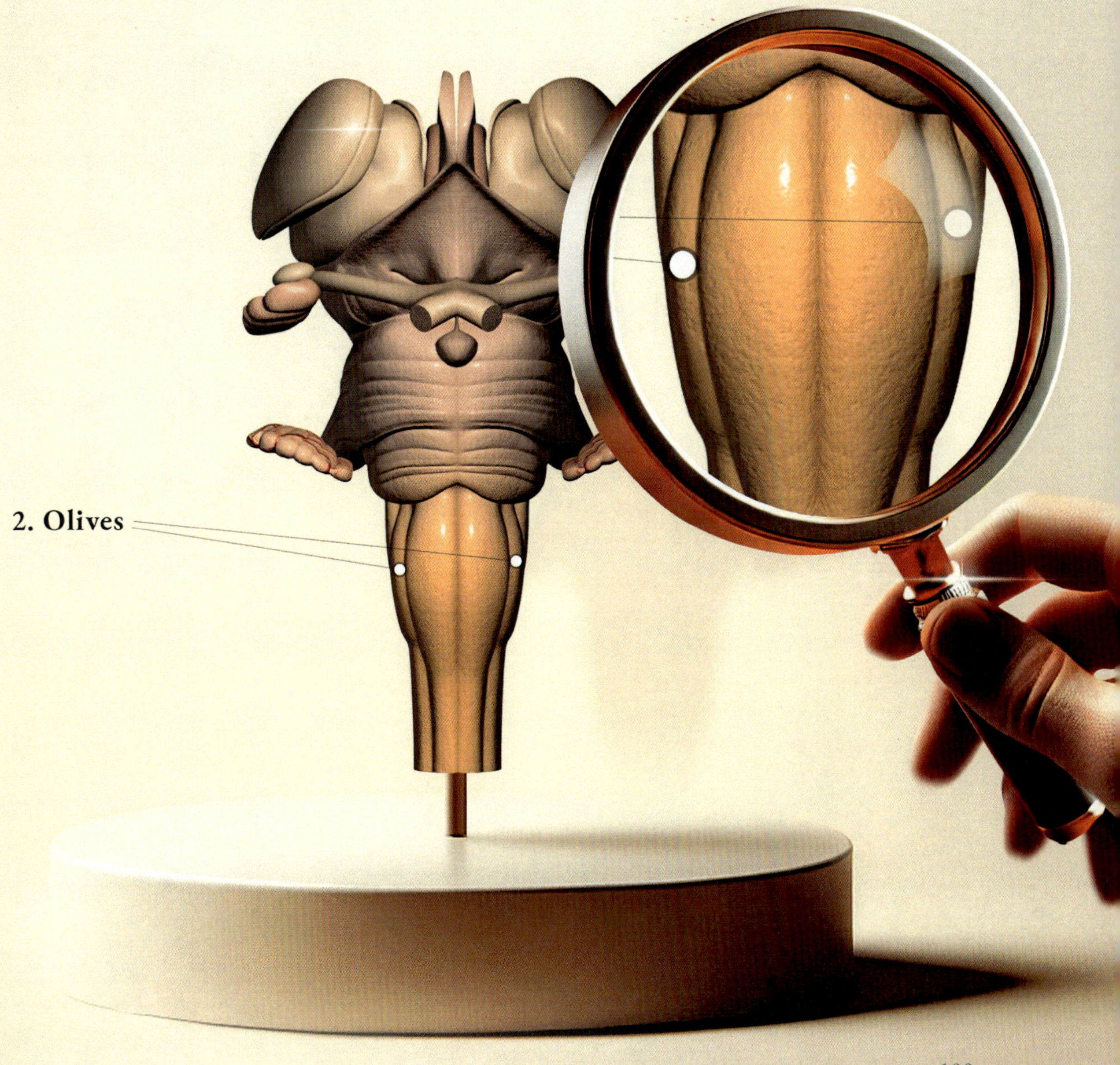

3. Anterior Median Fissure

The anterior median fissure is a deep groove that runs along the midline of the anterior side of the medulla oblongata. This fissure helps to separate the two pyramids and serves as an important anatomical landmark. While it does not have a direct sensory or motor function, the anterior median fissure is significant for the organization and identification of surrounding neural structures. It helps to delineate the left and right sides of the medulla, providing a reference point for neuroanatomical studies and surgical procedures.

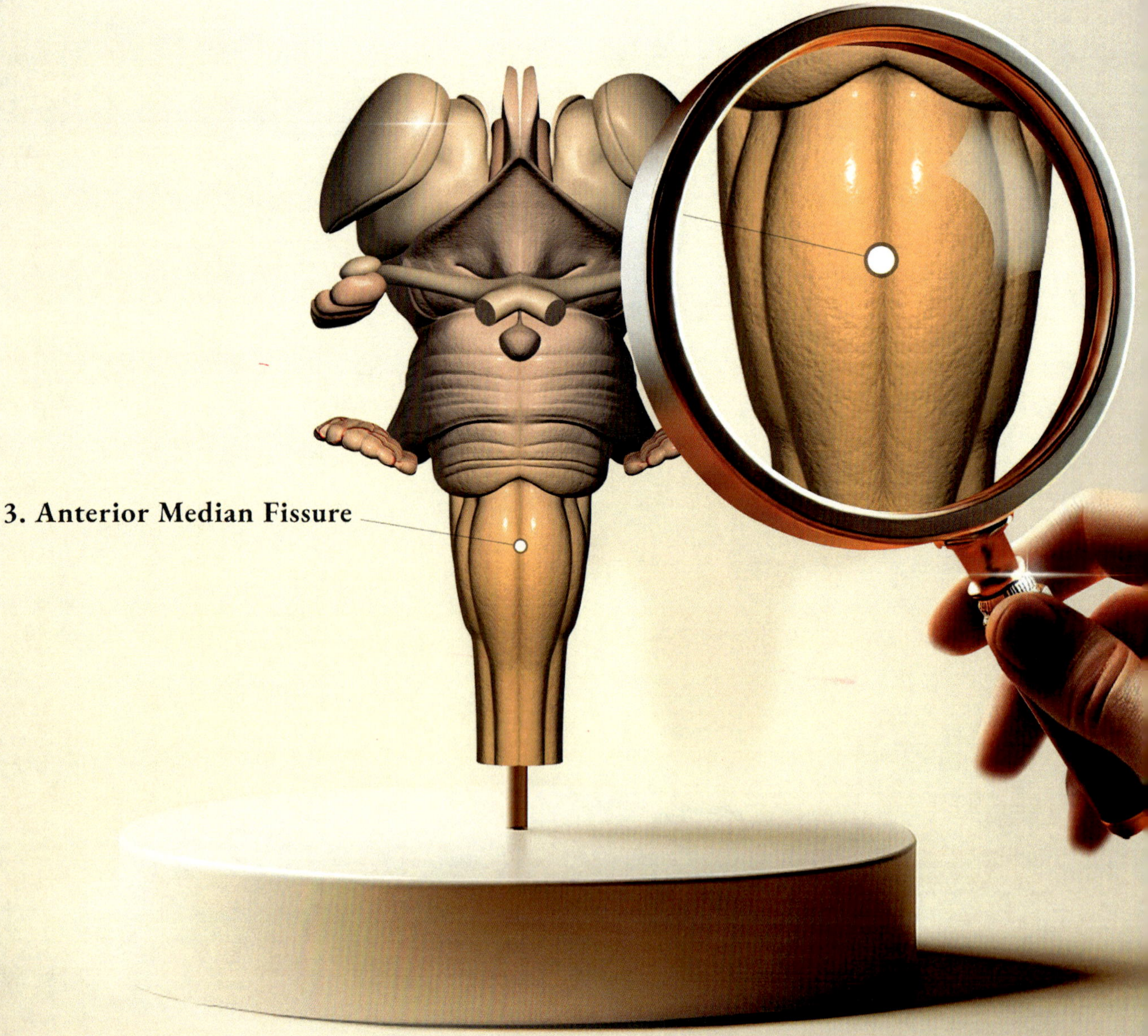

4. Decussation of the Pyramids

The decussation of the pyramids is the point where the majority of the fibers in the corticospinal tracts cross from one side of the medulla oblongata to the other. This crossing occurs at the junction between the medulla and the spinal cord and is essential for the contralateral control of motor functions. The decussation allows each hemisphere of the brain to control the opposite side of the body. Damage to the decussation of the pyramids can result in significant motor deficits and loss of voluntary muscle control on the contralateral side of the body.

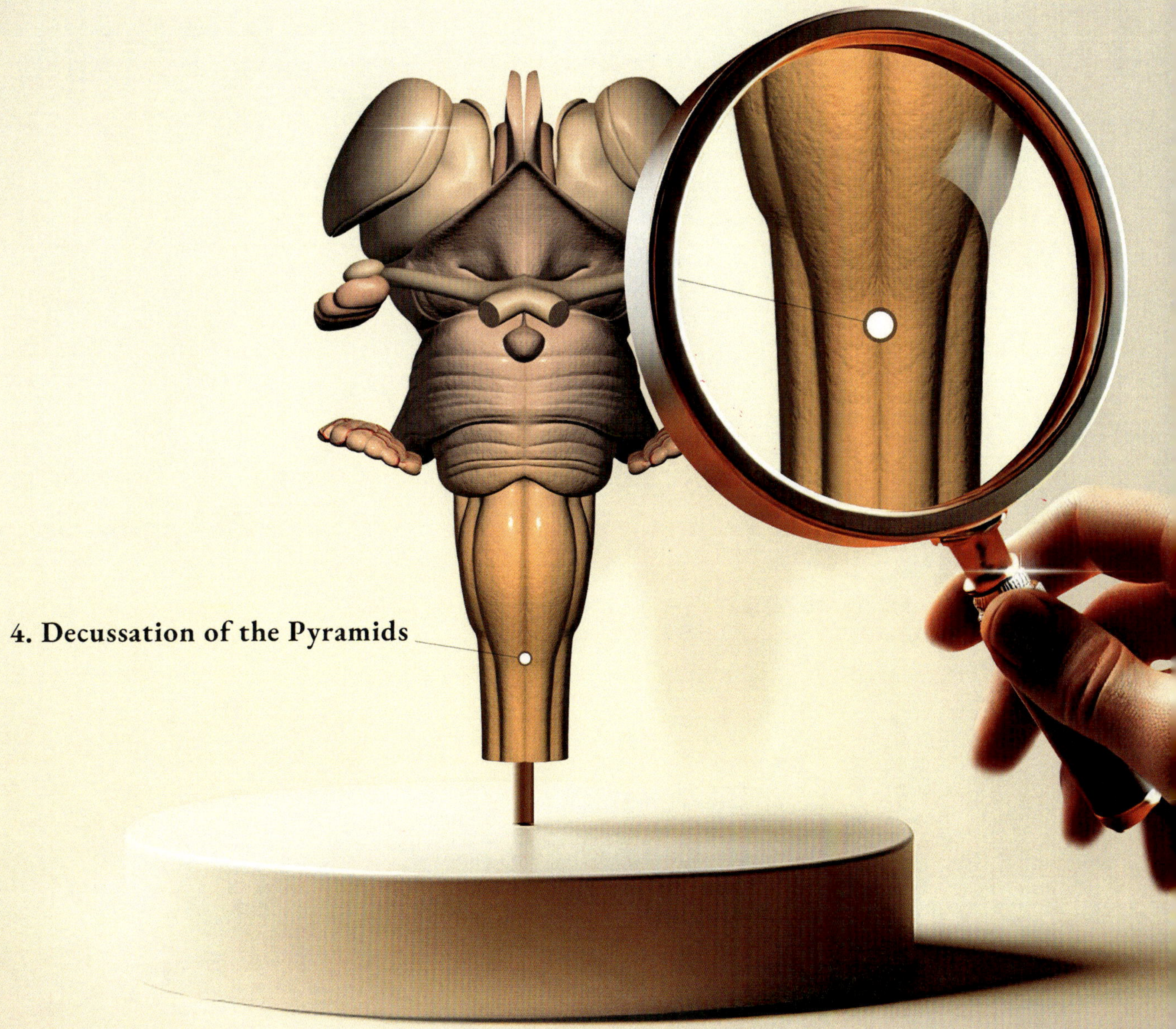

5. Anterolateral Sulcus

The anterolateral sulcus is a shallow groove located lateral to the pyramids on the anterior side of the medulla oblongata. It serves as the exit point for several cranial nerves, including the hypoglossal nerve (XII). This sulcus helps identify the boundaries of important motor pathways and neural structures within the medulla. Damage around the anterolateral sulcus can affect cranial nerve function, leading to motor control and sensory deficits. Proper identification of the anterolateral sulcus is crucial for understanding medulla anatomy.

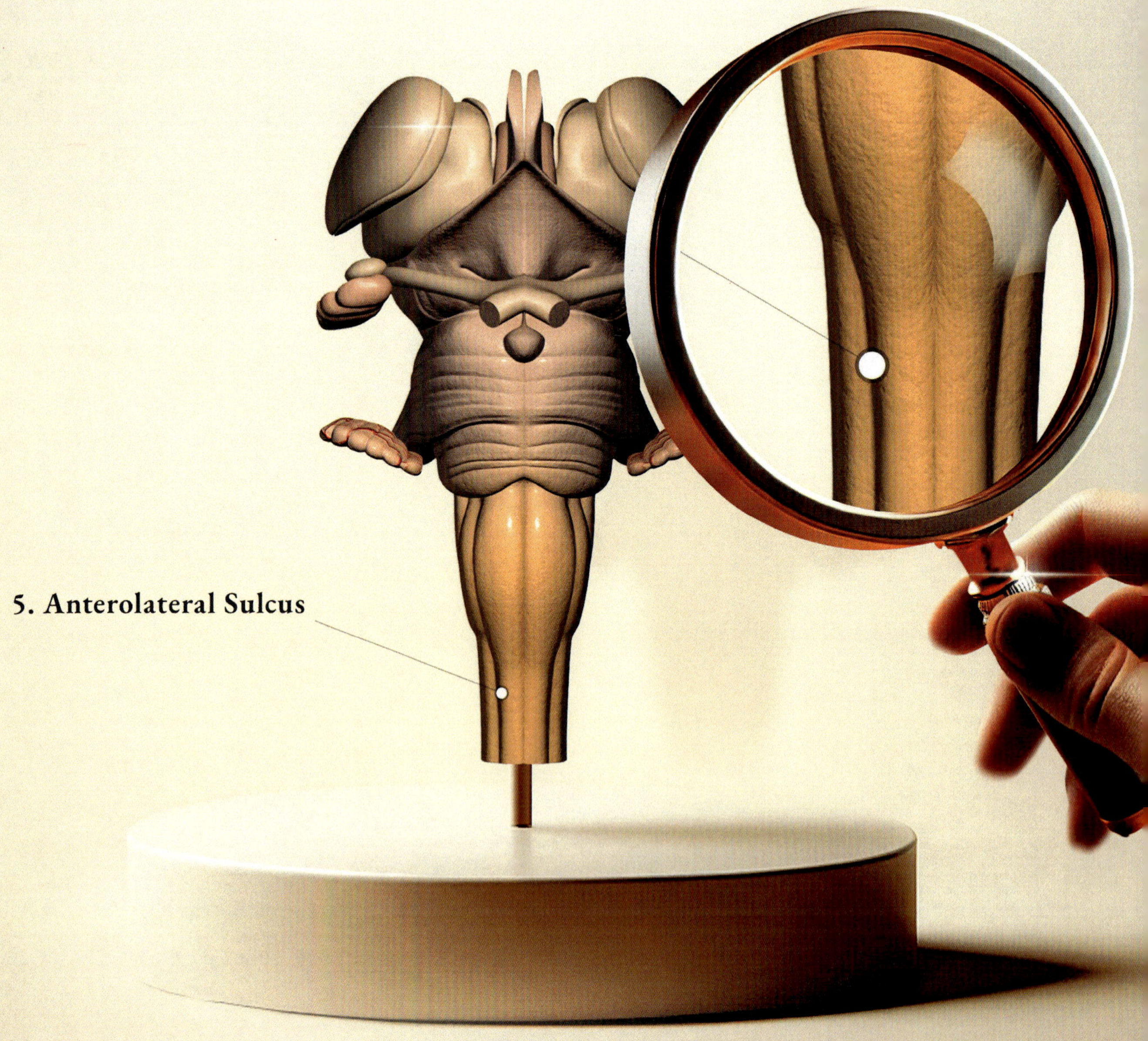

Medulla oblongata - Posterior View

The posterior view of the medulla oblongata reveals crucial anatomical structures for sensory functions. Key features include the gracile and cuneate fasciculi, part of the dorsal column-medial lemniscus pathway, responsible for transmitting fine touch, vibration, and proprioceptive information to the brain. The posterior surface also contains the floor of the fourth ventricle, essential for the cerebrospinal fluid system. This area integrates sensory information and coordinates autonomic functions.

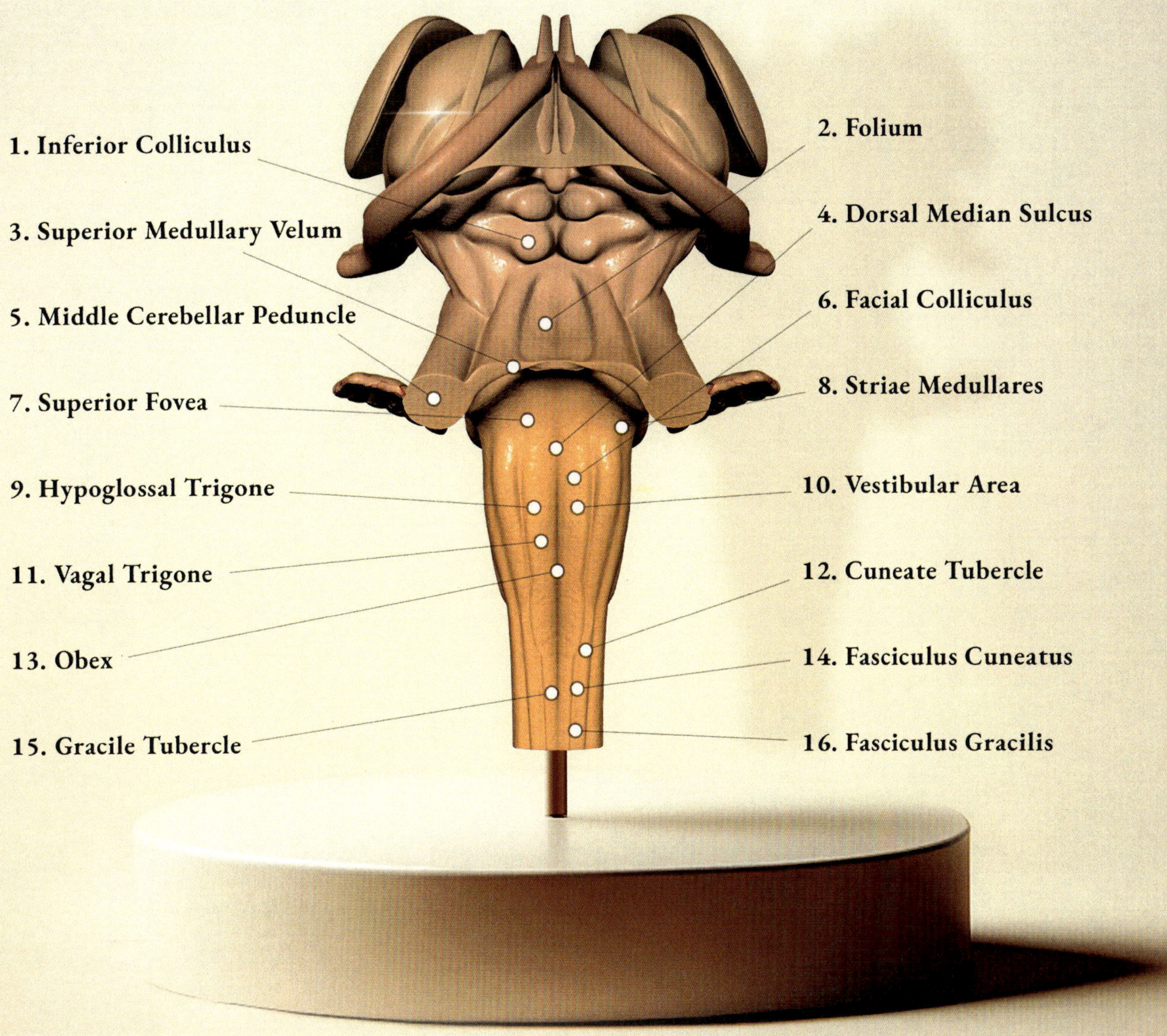

1. Inferior Colliculus

The inferior colliculus is a part of the midbrain that plays a crucial role in auditory processing. It acts as a primary relay station for auditory signals, receiving input from various auditory pathways and integrating these signals to aid in sound localization and auditory reflexes. Damage to the inferior colliculus can result in auditory deficits and difficulty in determining the spatial location of sounds. Proper functioning of the inferior colliculus is essential for accurate hearing and auditory reflexes.

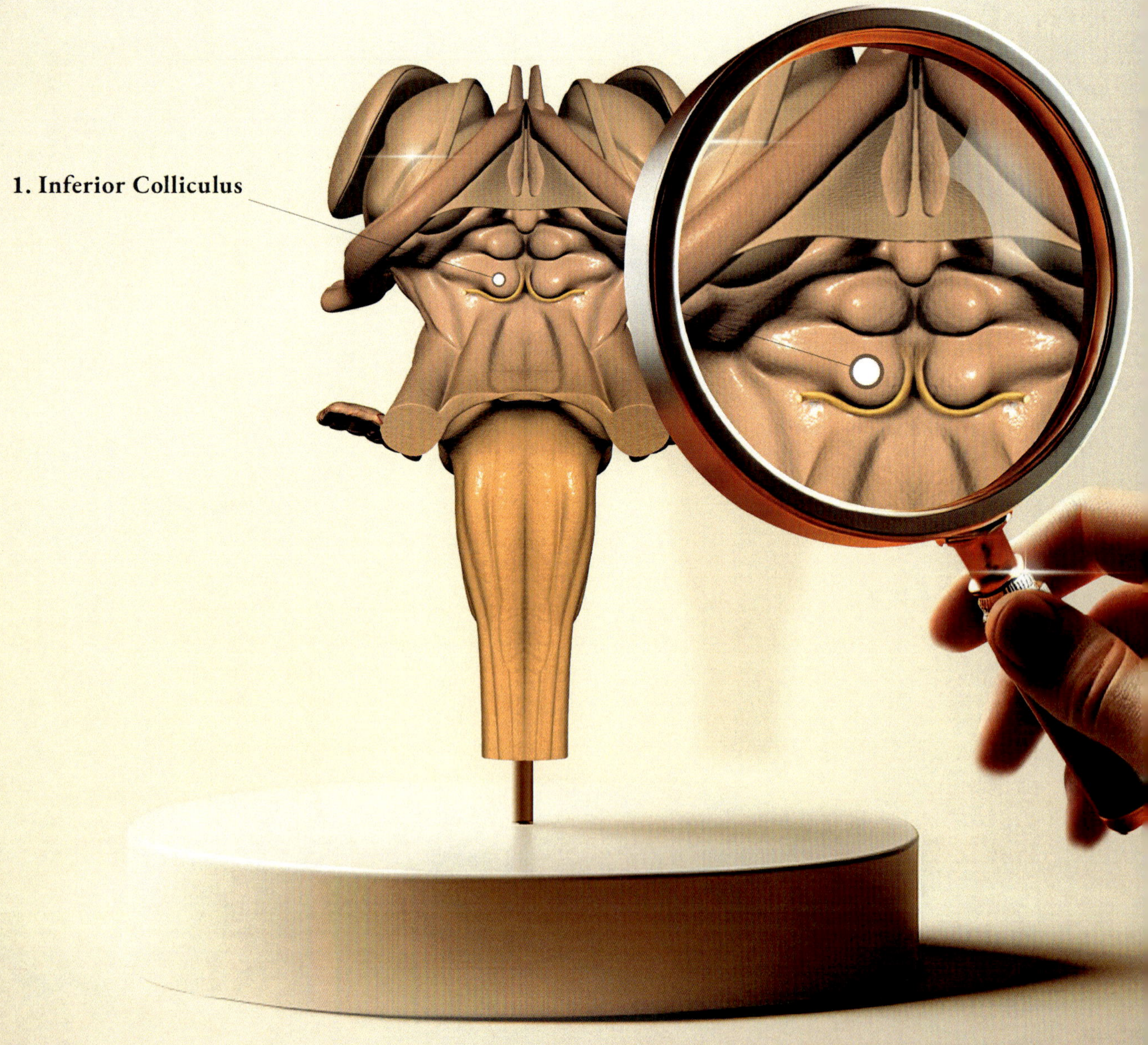

2. Folium

The folium is a part of the cerebellum involved in coordinating motor movements. It plays a crucial role in fine motor control, balance, and coordination by processing input from various parts of the brain and spinal cord. The folium enables precise movements, such as writing or grasping objects, and helps maintain stability during movement. Damage to the folium can lead to significant motor coordination deficits and balance problems, including ataxia and unsteady gait.

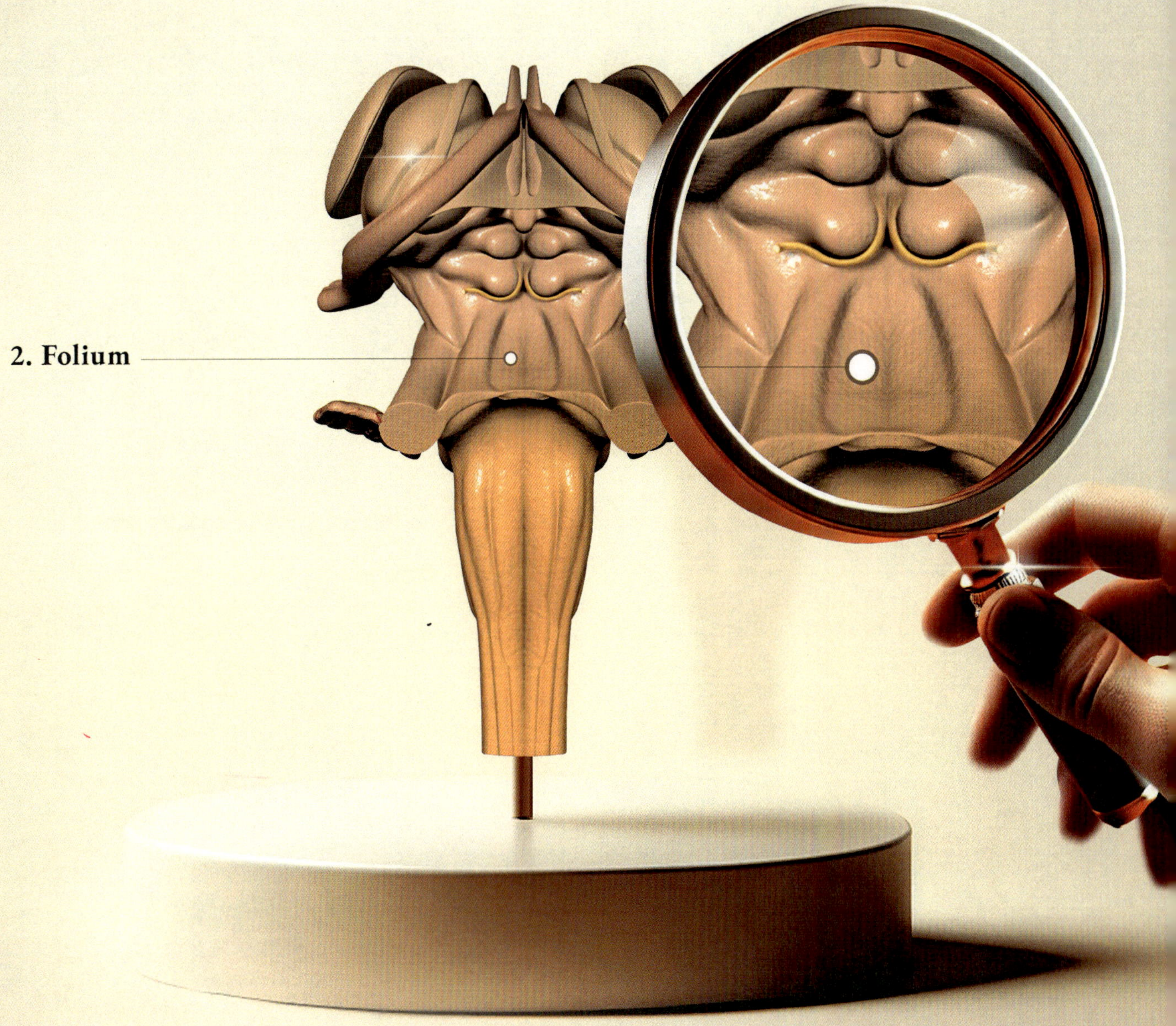

3. Superior Medullary Velum

The superior medullary velum connects the cerebellum to the brainstem, playing a role in transmitting motor and sensory information between these structures. It is important for the coordination of voluntary movements and the integration of sensory input. Damage to the superior medullary velum can affect motor coordination and sensory processing. Proper functioning of this structure is essential for efficient communication between the cerebellum and brainstem.

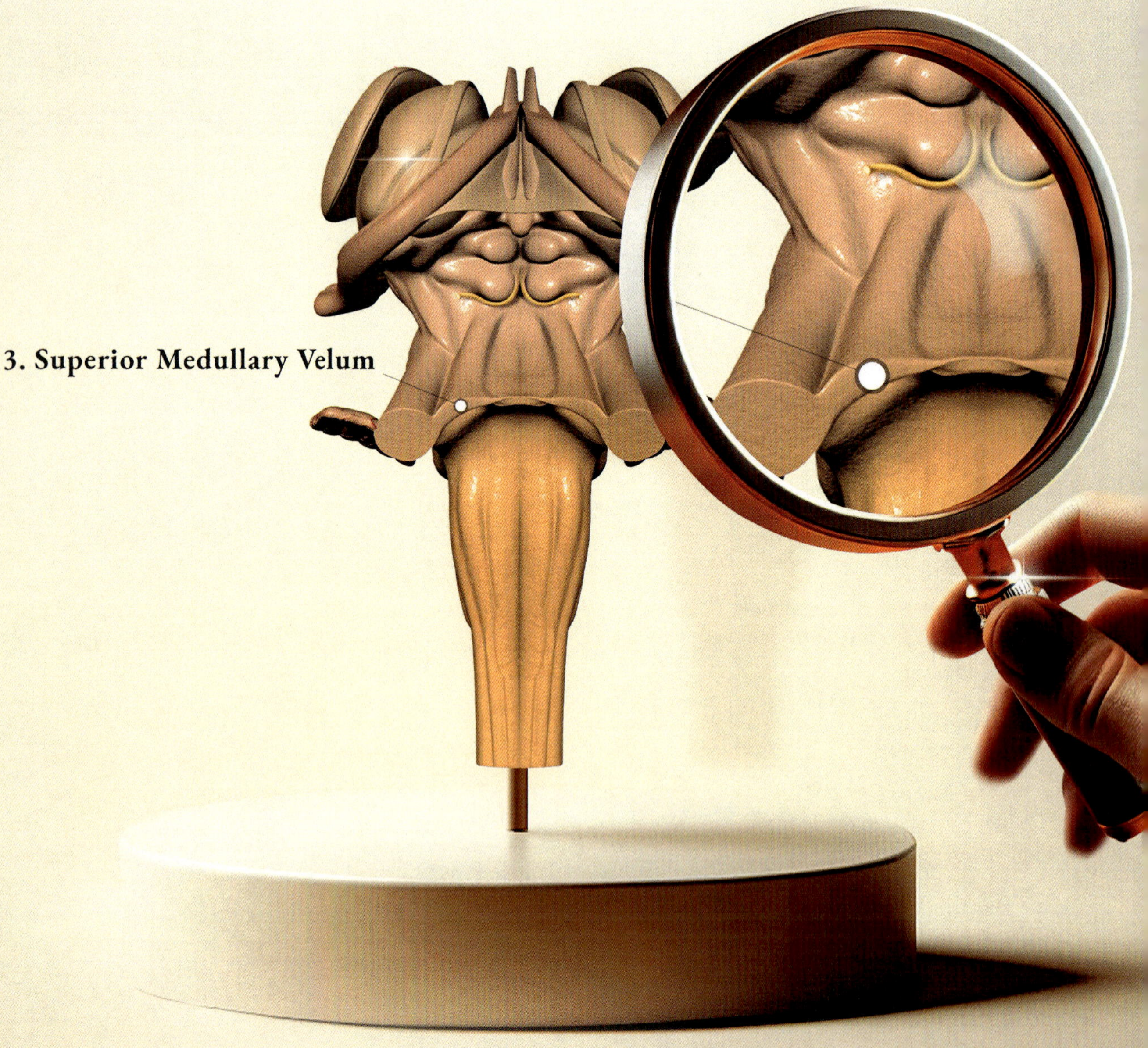

4. Dorsal Median Sulcus

The dorsal median sulcus is a groove on the dorsal (posterior) side of the medulla oblongata, separating its two halves. Though it lacks direct sensory or motor function, it is a crucial anatomical landmark. It aids in identifying and organizing nearby neural structures, such as the fasciculus gracilis and fasciculus cuneatus, which convey sensory information to the brain. The sulcus is essential in neurosurgical procedures and diagnostic imaging for accurate localization of lesions.

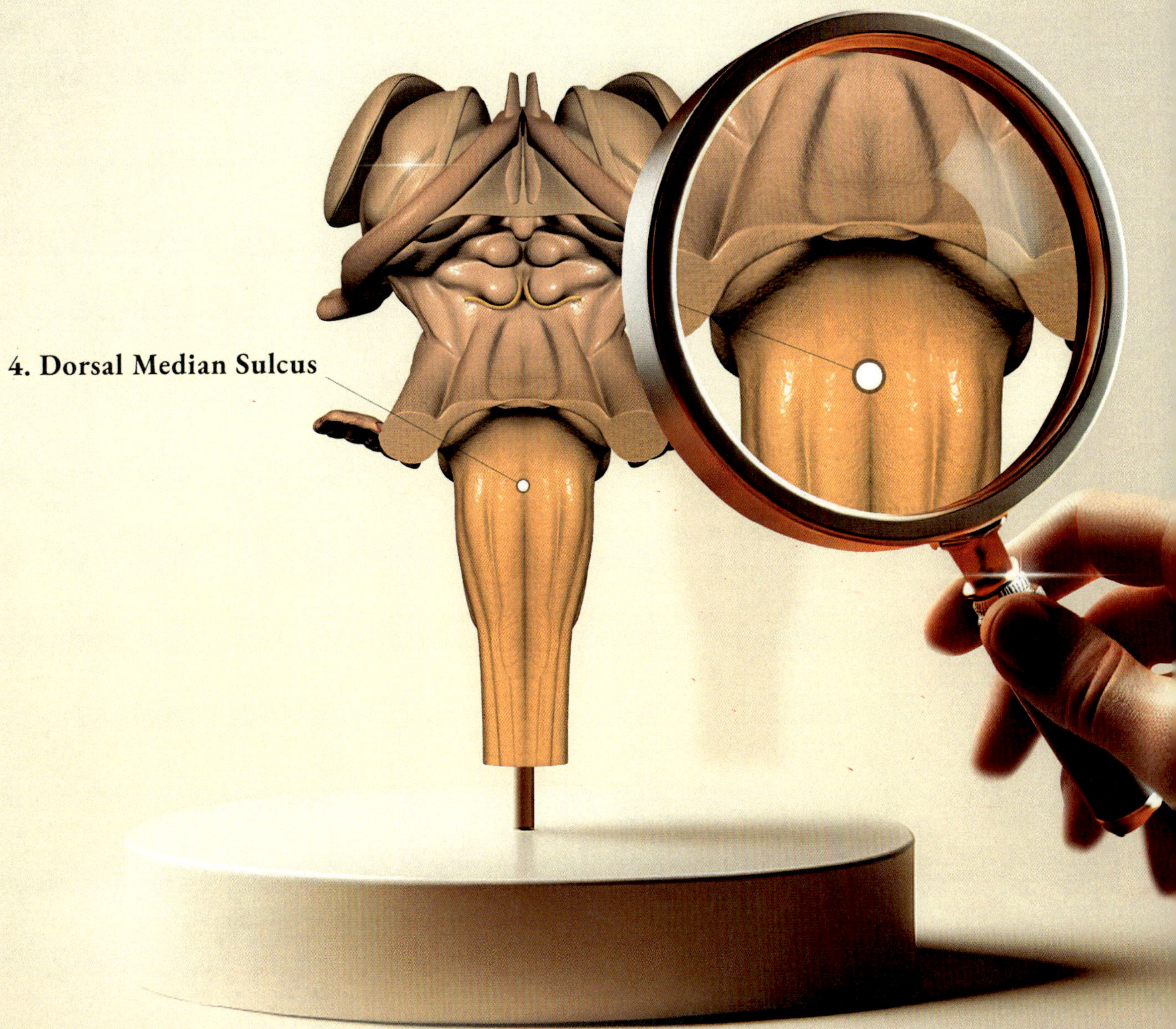

5. Middle Cerebellar Peduncle

The middle cerebellar peduncle connects the cerebellum to the pons and is involved in the transmission of information about voluntary motor control. It carries afferent fibers from the cerebral cortex and pontine nuclei to the cerebellum. Damage to the middle cerebellar peduncle can result in ataxia and coordination issues. Proper functioning of this peduncle is crucial for precise motor control. It plays a vital role in the coordination of complex motor tasks.

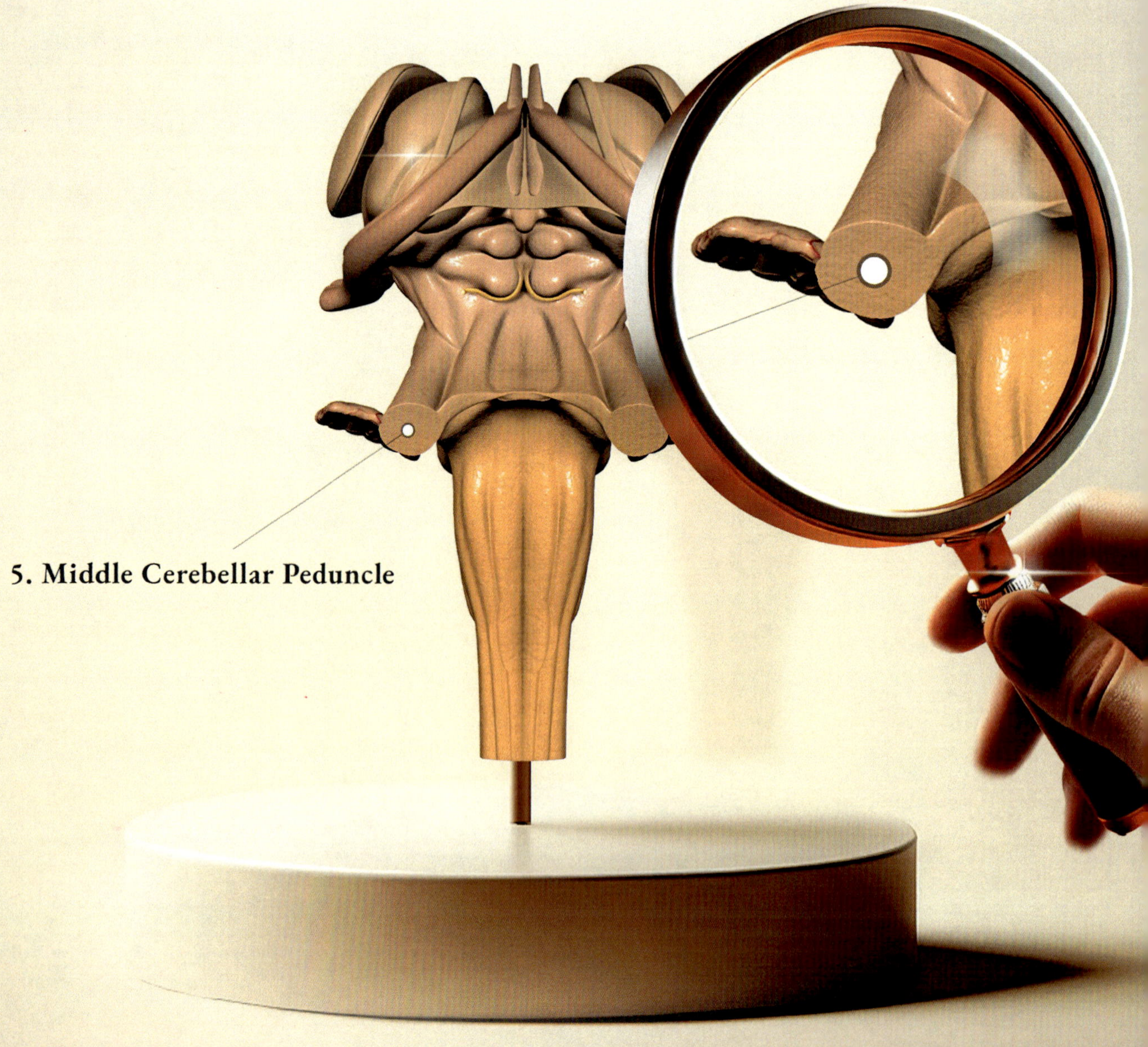

6. Facial Colliculus

The facial colliculus is a protrusion on the dorsal aspect of the pons caused by the underlying fibers of the facial nerve and the abducens nucleus. It is involved in facial expressions and lateral eye movement. Damage to the facial colliculus can result in facial paralysis and problems with eye movement. Proper functioning of the facial colliculus is essential for coordinated facial and eye movements. It is also important for maintaining proper visual tracking and facial symmetry.

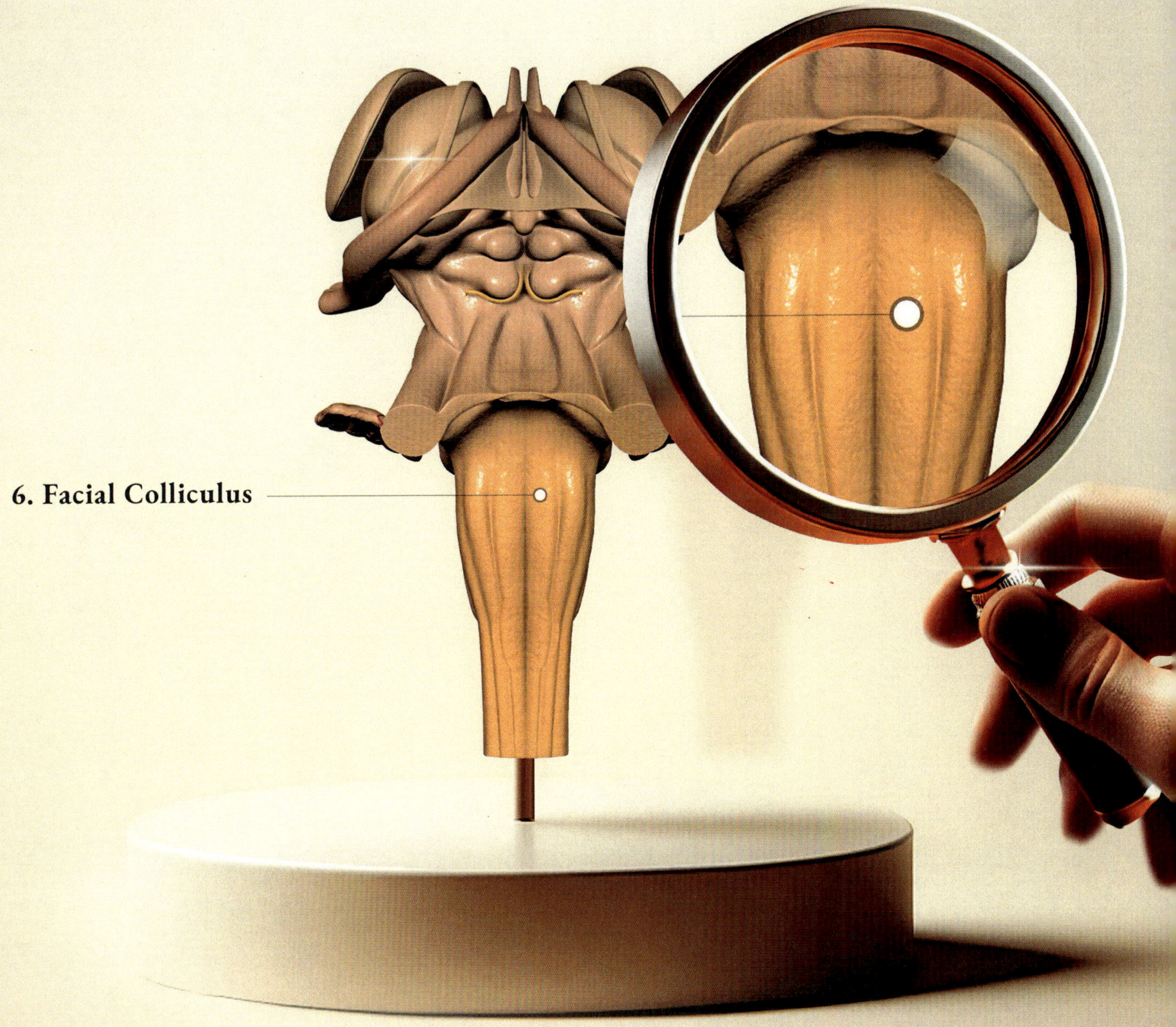

7. Superior Fovea

The superior fovea is a prominent feature in the floor of the fourth ventricle, serving as an important anatomical landmark. Although it lacks direct sensory function, it aids in identifying and distinguishing neural structures within the fourth ventricle. This is crucial for neuroanatomical studies and understanding cerebrospinal fluid (CSF) pathways. In surgical procedures, the superior fovea helps neurosurgeons navigate brain structures with precision, reducing risks to critical areas.

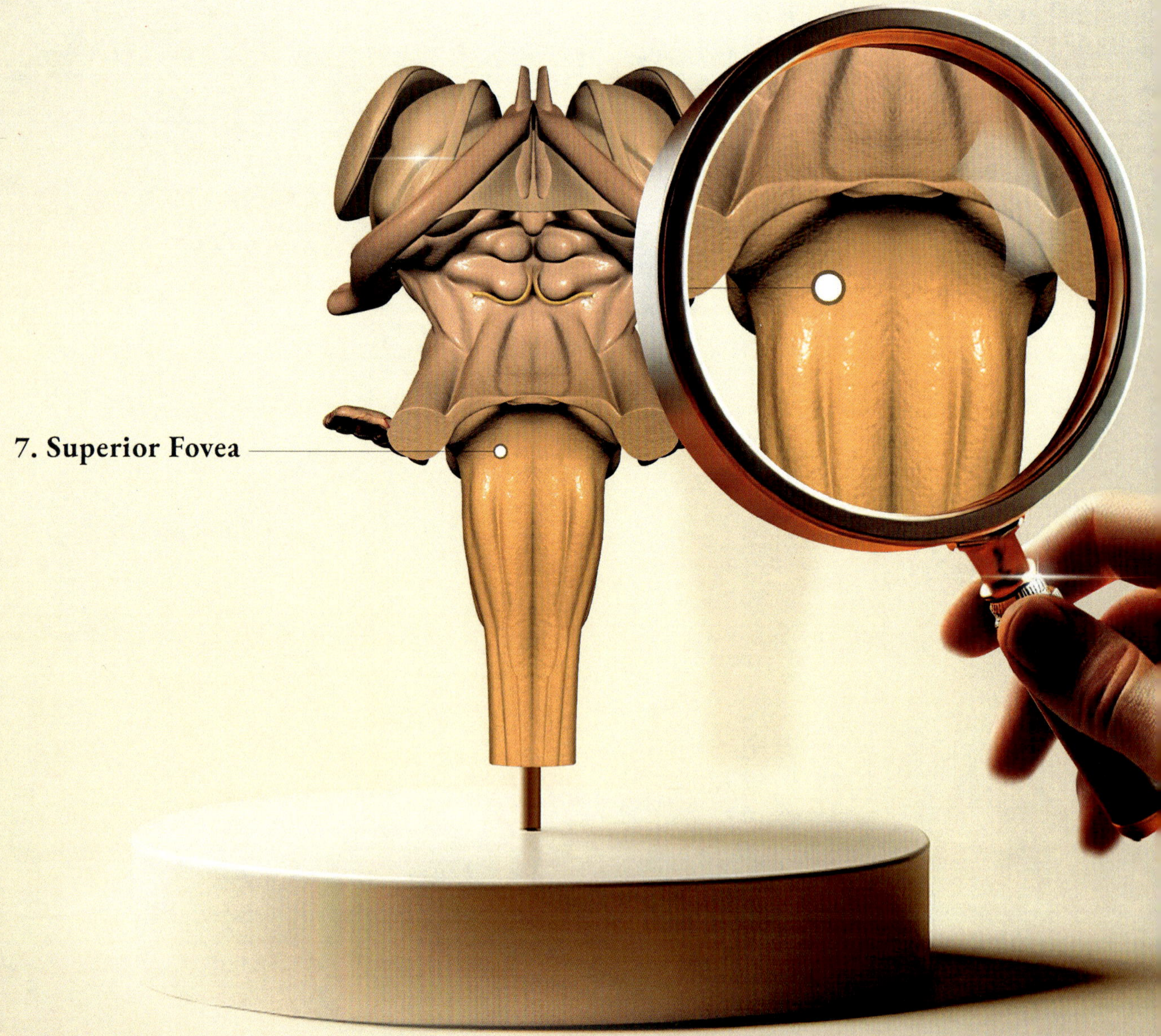

8. Striae Medullares

The striae medullares are bands of nerve fibers that run across the floor of the fourth ventricle and are associated with auditory pathways. They help in the transmission of auditory information from the cochlear nuclei to higher auditory centers. Damage to the striae medullares can affect hearing and auditory processing. Proper functioning of these fibers is essential for effective auditory signal transmission. They also play a role in integrating auditory signals within the brainstem.

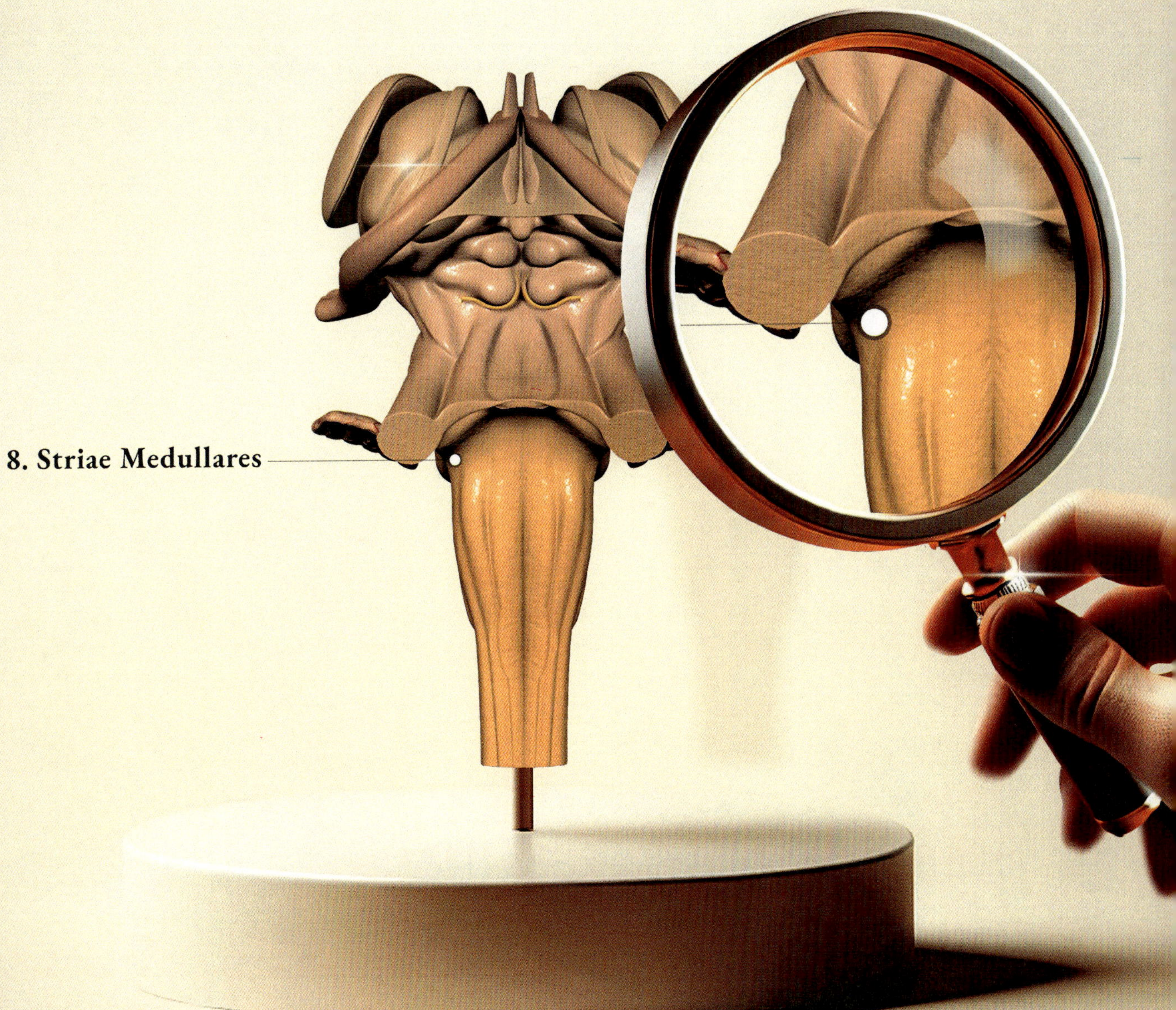

9. Hypoglossal Trigone

The hypoglossal trigone is an area in the floor of the fourth ventricle where the hypoglossal nucleus is located. This nucleus controls the muscles of the tongue, which are essential for speech and swallowing. Damage to the hypoglossal trigone can result in tongue weakness or paralysis, affecting speech and swallowing. Proper functioning of the hypoglossal trigone is crucial for effective tongue movements. It is also involved in coordinating reflexive actions of the tongue.

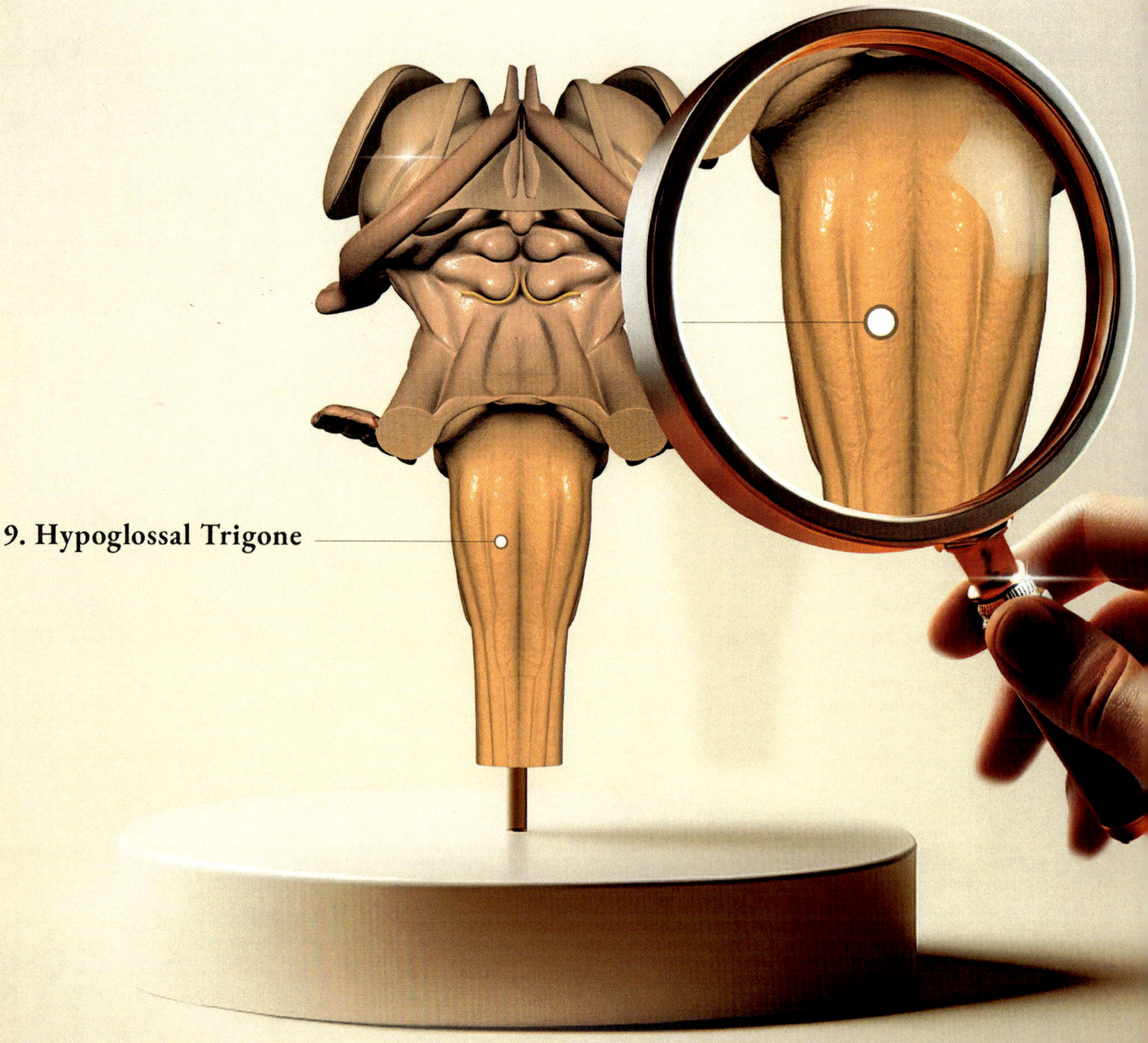

10. Vestibular Area

The vestibular area contains the vestibular nuclei, which are involved in balance and spatial orientation. These nuclei receive input from the inner ear and help coordinate head and eye movements. Damage to the vestibular area can result in dizziness, vertigo, and balance disorders. Proper functioning of the vestibular area is essential for maintaining equilibrium and spatial orientation. It also plays a role in stabilizing vision during head movements.

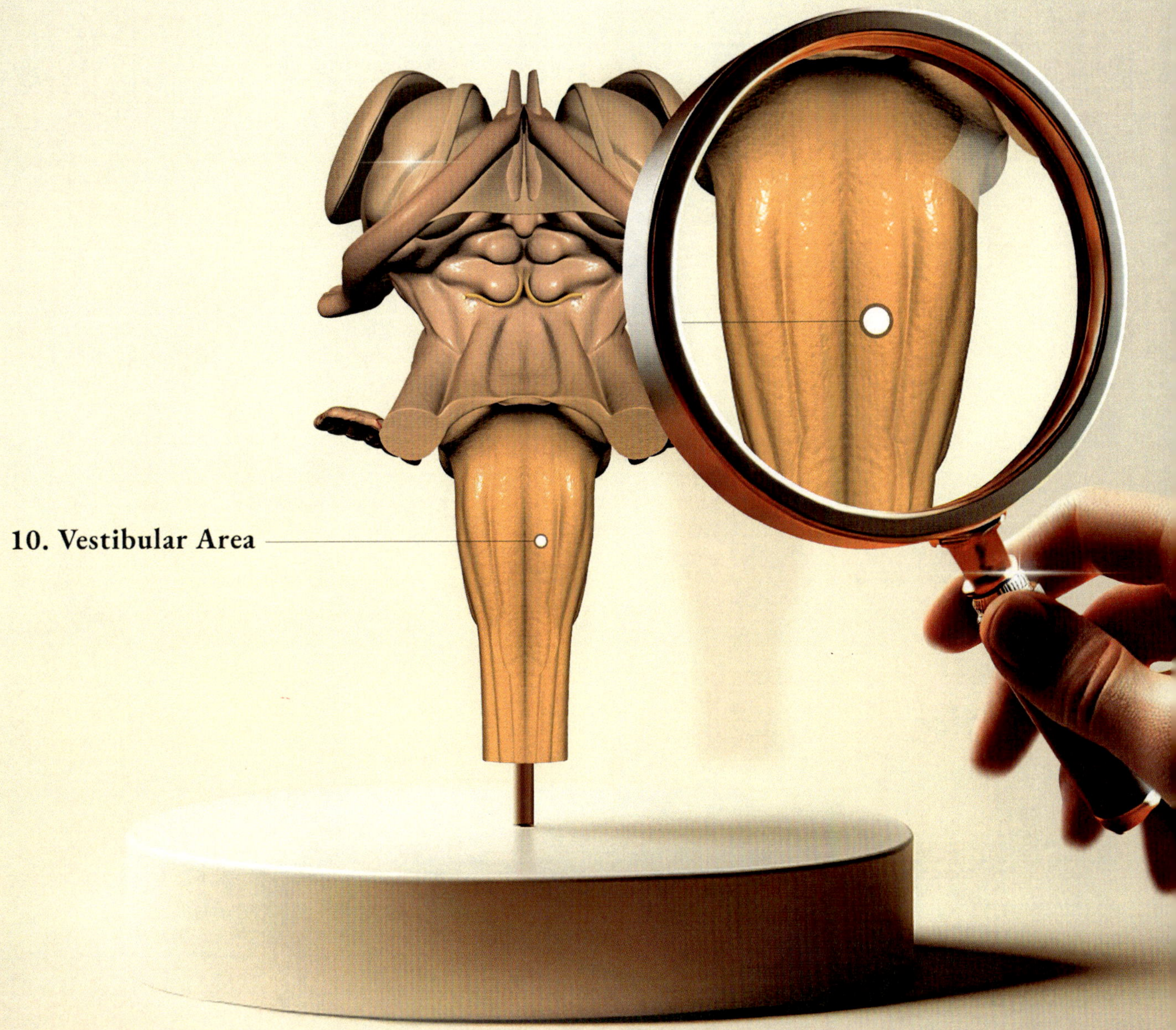

11. Vagal Trigone

The vagal trigone is the region in the floor of the fourth ventricle where the dorsal motor nucleus of the vagus nerve is located. This nucleus plays a role in autonomic control of the heart, lungs, and digestive tract. Damage to the vagal trigone can result in autonomic dysfunction, affecting heart rate, breathing, and digestion. Proper functioning of the vagal trigone is essential for autonomic regulation. It is also critical for maintaining homeostasis within the body.

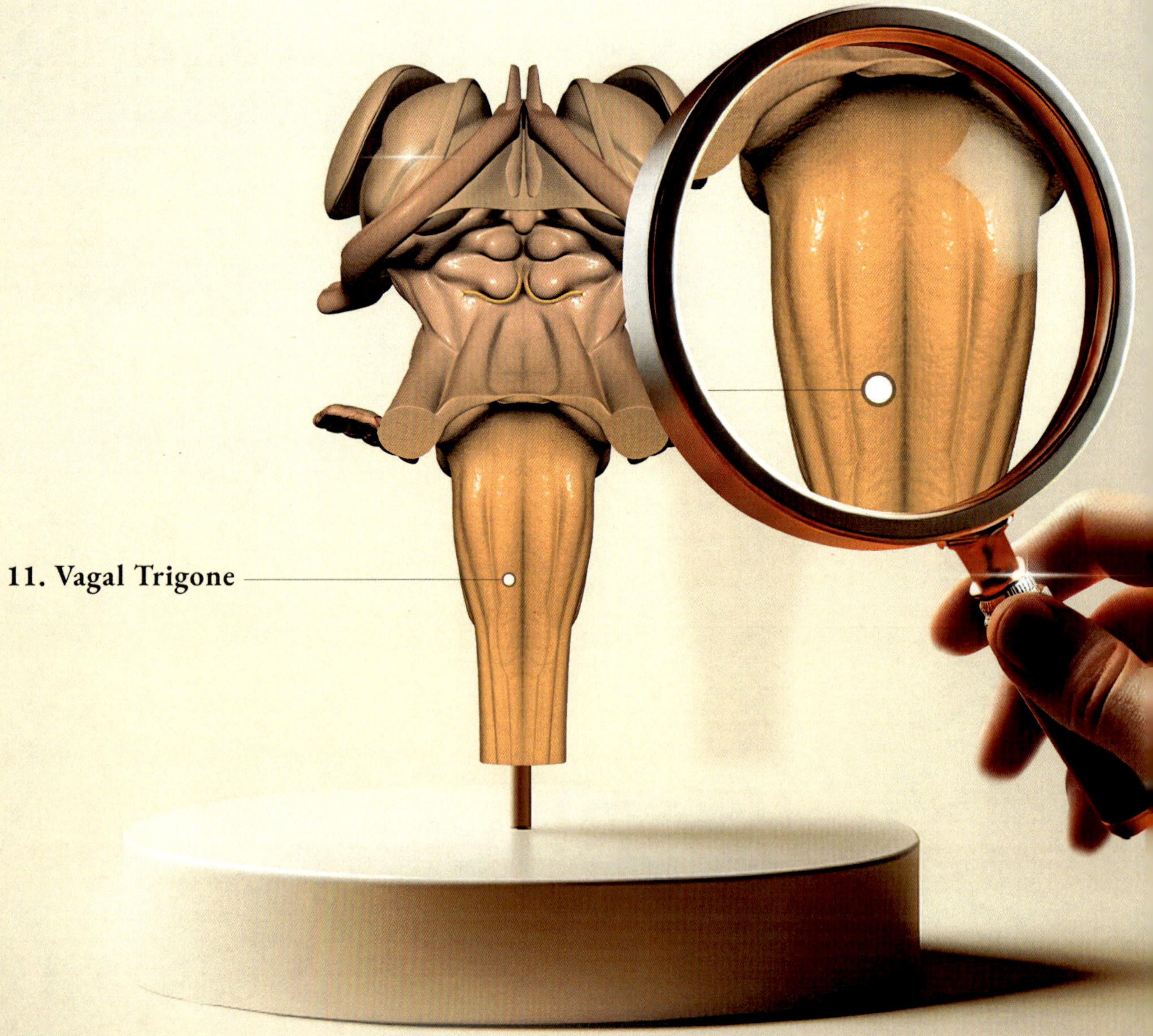

12. Cuneate Tubercle

The cuneate tubercle contains the cuneate nucleus, which processes sensory information from the upper body, including fine touch and proprioception. It is part of the dorsal column-medial lemniscus pathway. Damage to the cuneate tubercle can result in loss of fine touch and proprioception from the upper body. Proper functioning of the cuneate tubercle is essential for accurate sensory perception. It also plays a role in coordinating movement based on sensory feedback.

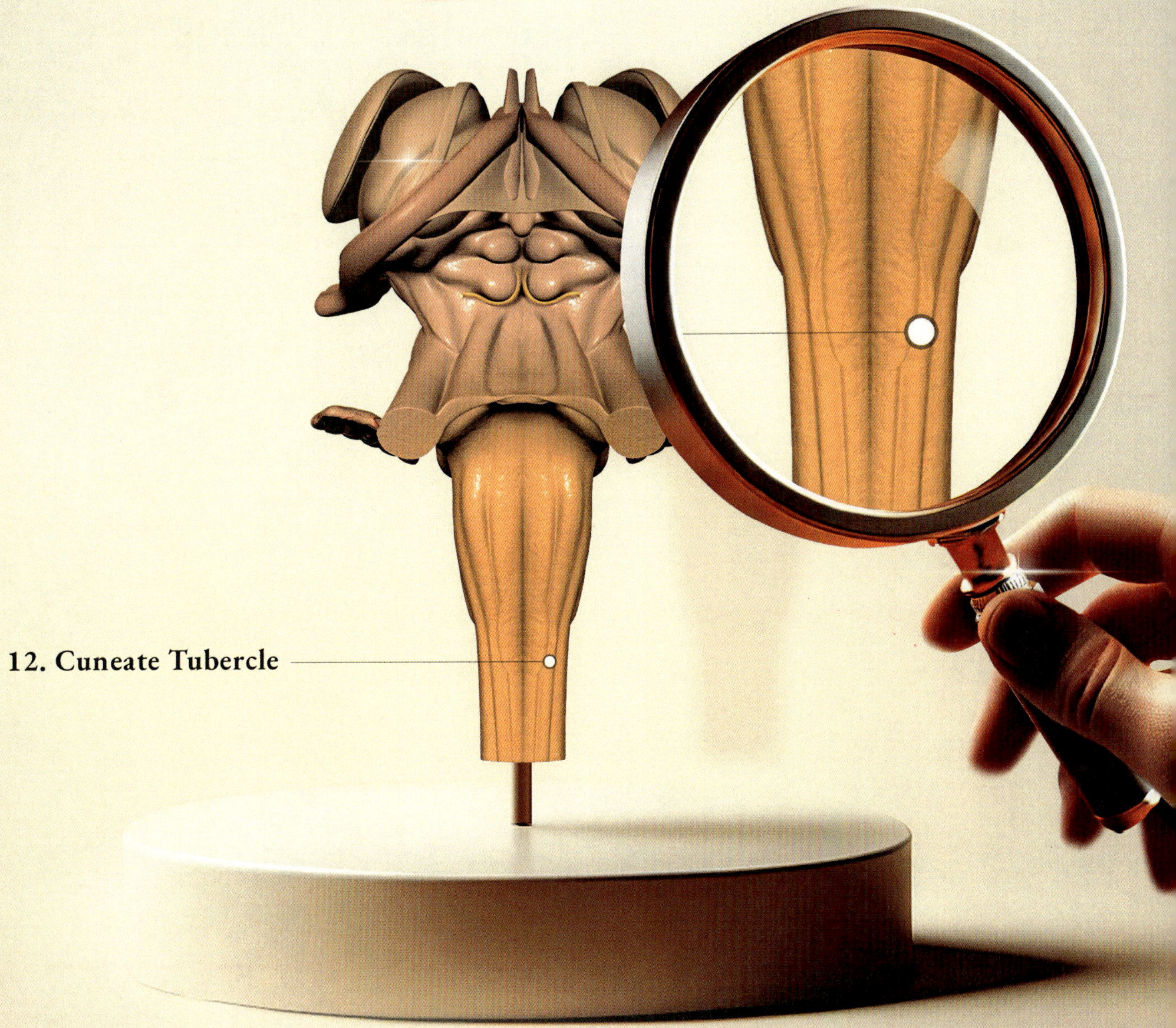

13. Obex

The obex is the point at which the fourth ventricle narrows to become the central canal of the spinal cord. It serves as an important anatomical landmark and is involved in the regulation of cerebrospinal fluid flow between the brain and spinal cord. Damage to the obex can affect cerebrospinal fluid dynamics and result in neurological deficits. Proper functioning of the obex is essential for maintaining normal cerebrospinal fluid circulation. It also helps drain excess cerebrospinal fluid to prevent buildup.

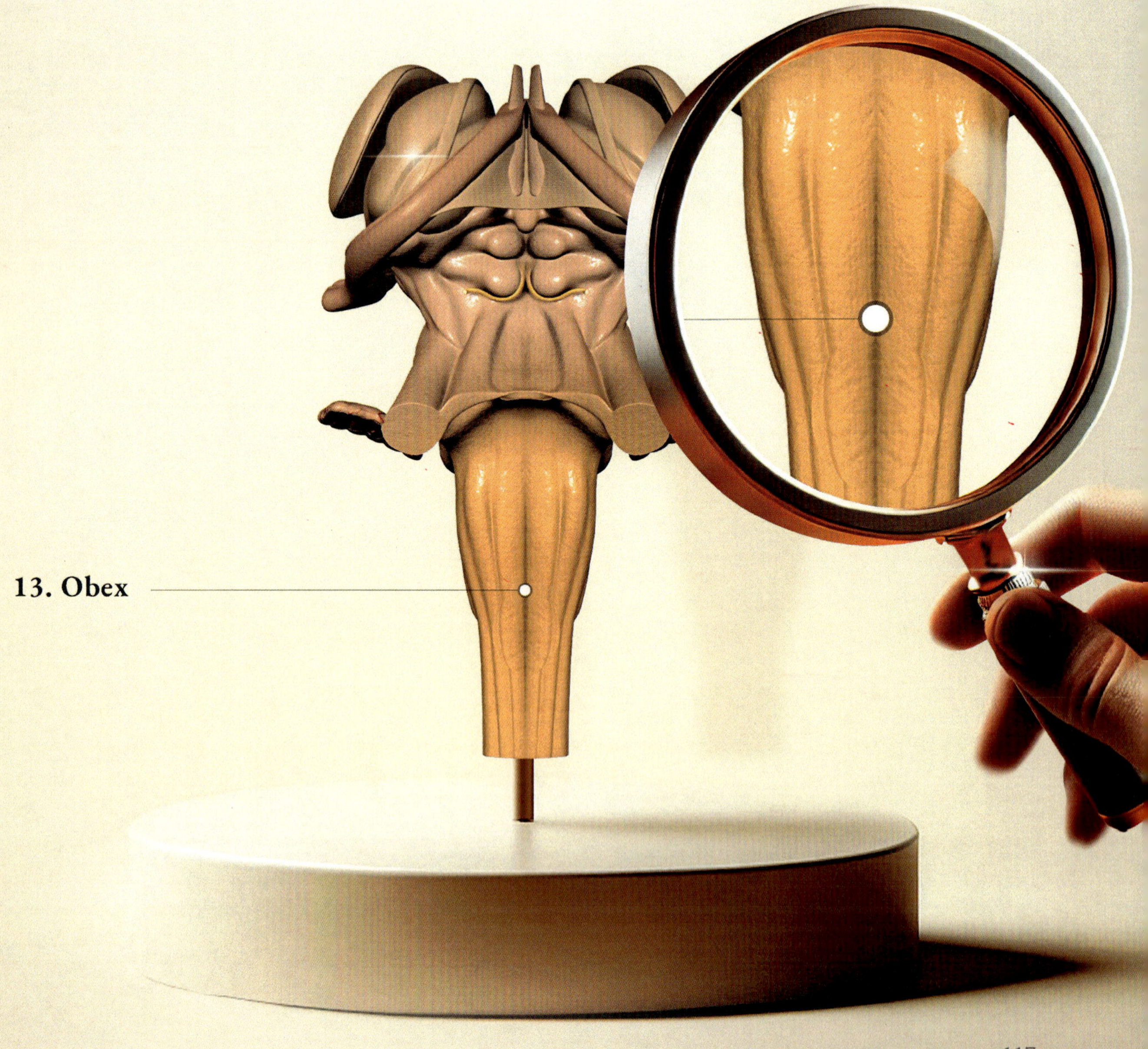

14. Fasciculus Cuneatus

The fasciculus cuneatus is a bundle of nerve fibers that carries sensory information about fine touch, vibration, and proprioception from the upper body to the brain. It is part of the dorsal column-medial lemniscus pathway. Damage to the fasciculus cuneatus can result in loss of these sensory modalities from the upper body. Proper functioning of the fasciculus cuneatus is crucial for accurate sensory perception. It also helps in coordinating movements based on sensory input.

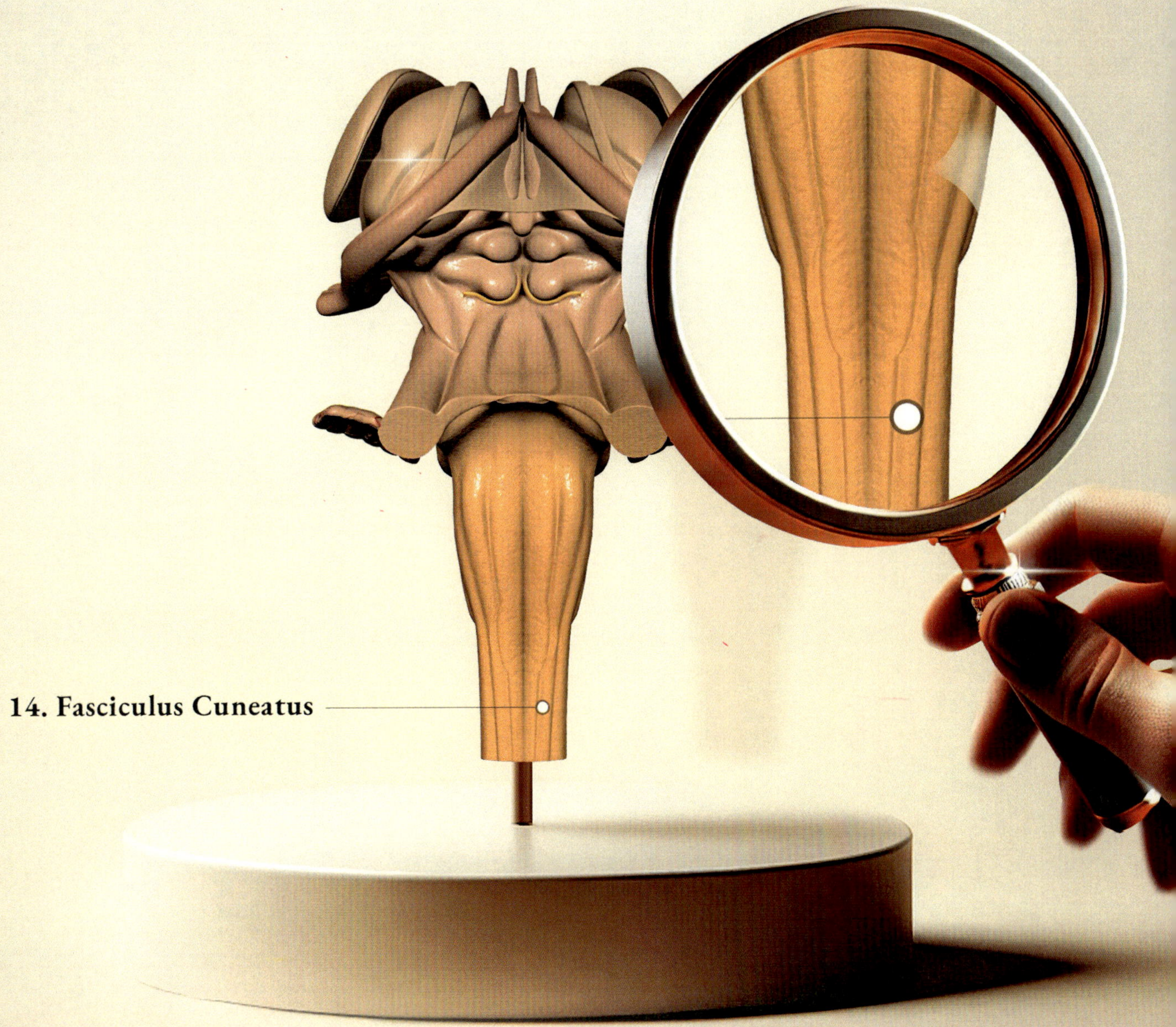

15. Gracile Tubercle

The gracile tubercle contains the gracile nucleus, which processes sensory information from the lower body, including fine touch and proprioception. It is part of the dorsal column-medial lemniscus pathway. Damage to the gracile tubercle can result in loss of fine touch and proprioception from the lower body. Proper functioning of the gracile tubercle is essential for accurate sensory perception. It also aids in maintaining posture and balance through sensory feedback.

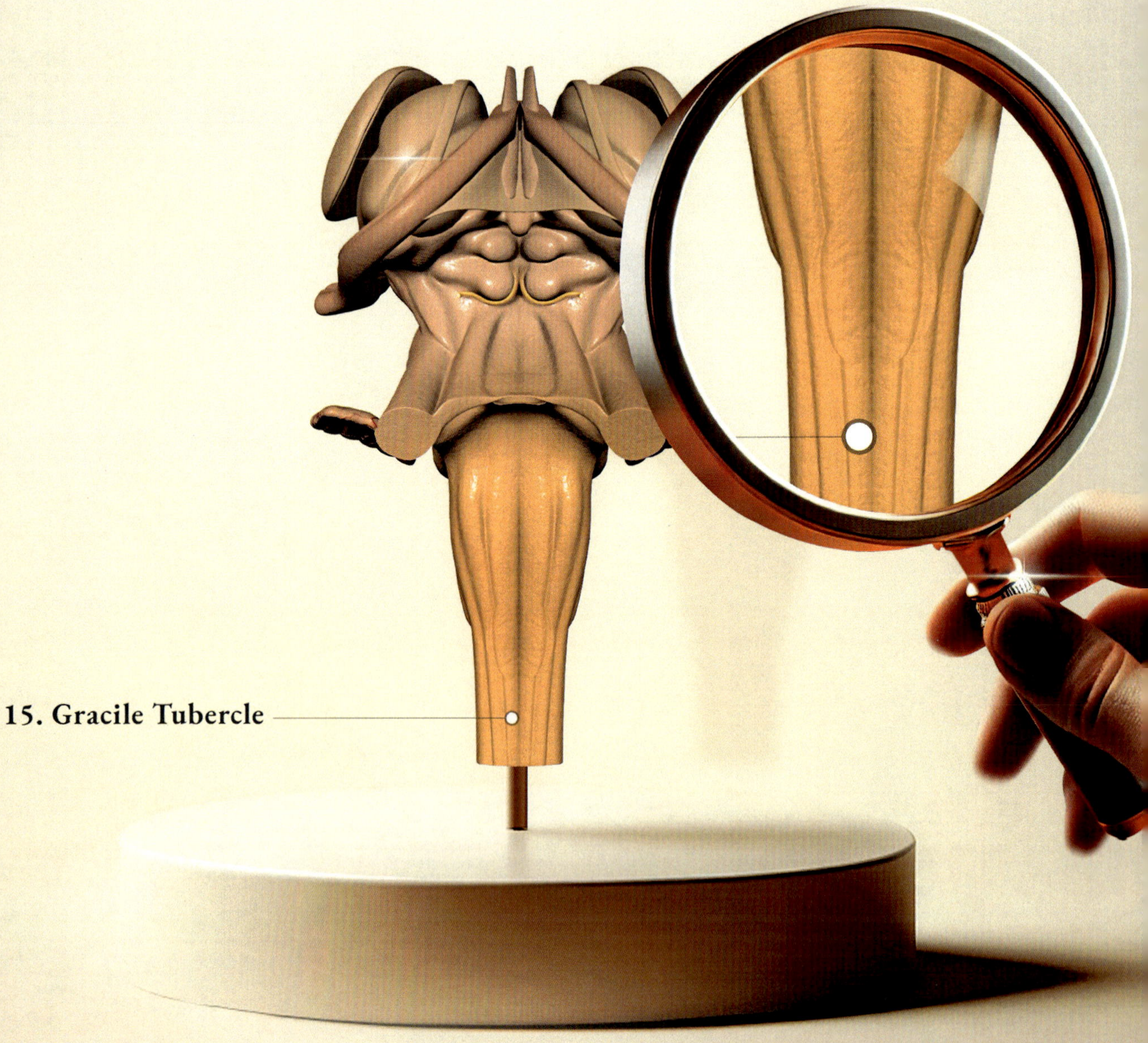

16. Fasciculus Gracilis

The fasciculus gracilis is a bundle of nerve fibers that carries sensory information about fine touch, vibration, and proprioception from the lower body to the brain. It is part of the dorsal column-medial lemniscus pathway. Damage to the fasciculus gracilis can result in loss of these sensory modalities from the lower body. Proper functioning of the fasciculus gracilis is crucial for accurate sensory perception. It also supports coordinated movement and balance.

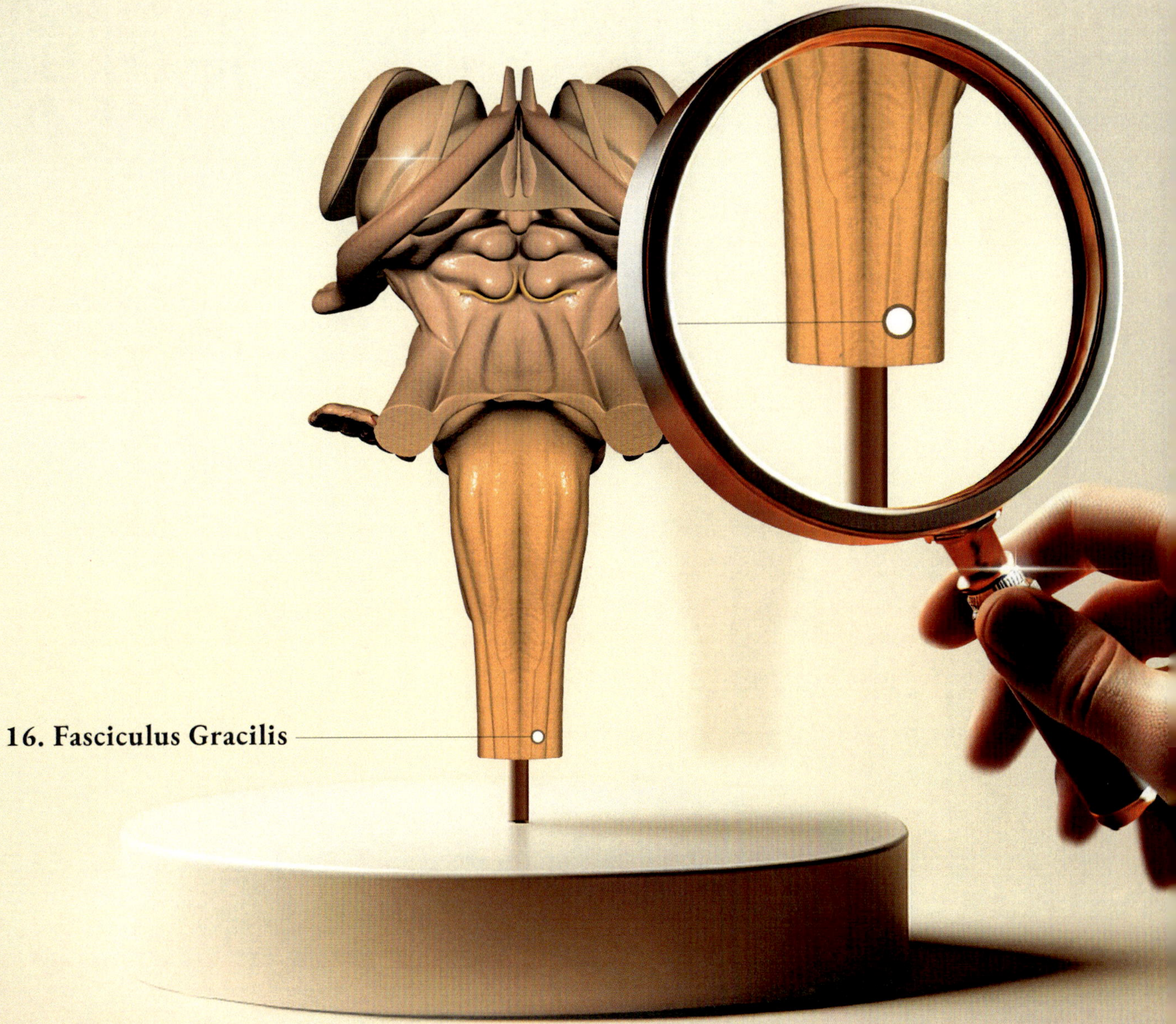

Cranial Nerves

Cranial Nerves in the Region of the Atlas Vertebra

Cranial nerves are a group of 12 pairs of nerves that emerge directly from the brain and have various functions, including sensory, motor, and autonomic functions. Here is an overview of all 12 cranial nerves and their primary functions:

1. Olfactory Nerve (I) - This nerve is responsible for the sense of smell.

The olfactory nerve, known as the I cranial nerve, plays a crucial role in our sense of smell. It consists of a set of sensory cells, olfactory receptors, located in the olfactory epithelium, a specialized tissue within the olfactory region of the upper part of the nasal cavity [Image 1]. These receptor cells have cilia (microscopic hair-like structures) exposed to the air that capture odor molecules we inhale.

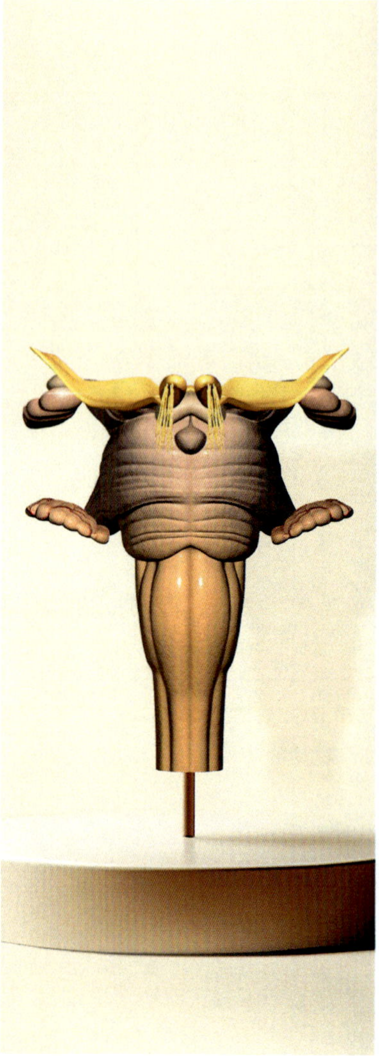

[Image 1] Olfactory Nerve

The axons (nerve fibers) of the olfactory receptors pass through tiny openings in the cribriform plate of the ethmoid bone, forming the olfactory tract. These tracts then group together and form the olfactory bulb, located beneath the frontal lobe of the brain. When odor molecules reach the olfactory epithelium, they bind to the receptors, triggering a cascade of biochemical reactions that generate a nerve signal. These signals are sent through the olfactory bulbs to the olfactory tracts and further to the brain.

The information about smells is first processed in the olfactory cortex, which is part of the limbic system. This region of the brain is responsible for the perception and identification of smells but is also important for emotional reactions and memory related to smells.

1. Olfactory nerve

The olfactory nerve (I) is the first cranial nerve, crucial for the sense of smell. It consists of sensory fibers originating in the olfactory epithelium of the nasal cavity. These fibers pass through the cribriform plate of the ethmoid bone to the olfactory bulb. The olfactory nerve transmits odor information to the brain, enabling smell perception. Damage to this nerve can lead to anosmia (loss of smell), affecting taste and quality of life. Proper functioning of the olfactory nerve is essential for detecting hazards and enjoying flavors and scents.

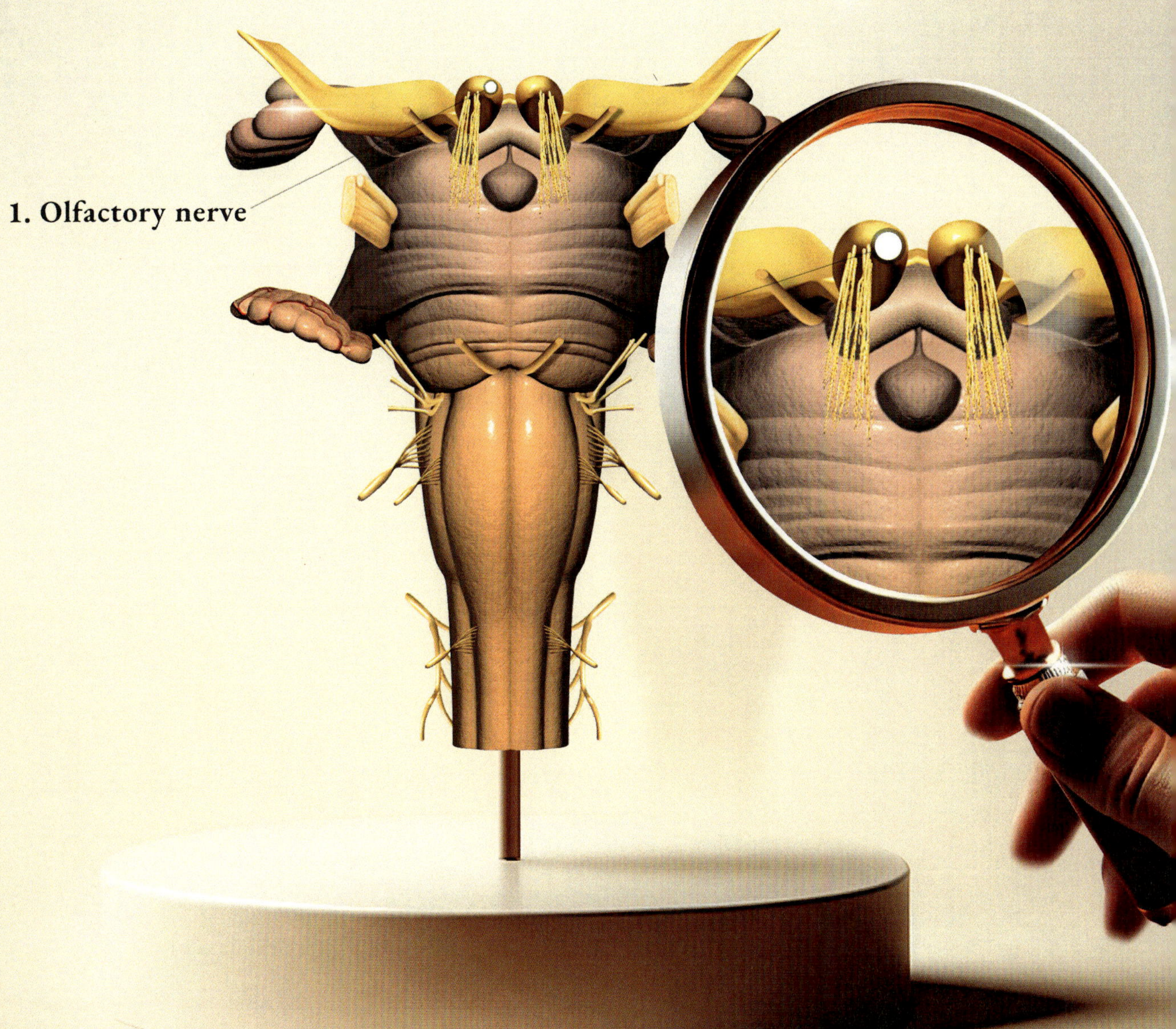

Damage or diseases affecting the olfactory nerve can lead to problems with the sense of smell (anosmia), reduced sense of smell (hyposmia), or distorted sense of smell (parosmia). These changes can result from various conditions, including head trauma, upper respiratory infections, neurodegenerative diseases such as Alzheimer's and Parkinson's disease, or as a side effect of certain medications.

Disorders of the sense of smell can significantly impact the quality of life, as smell plays an important role in detecting dangers, enjoying food and drinks, and interpersonal interactions involving a sense of closeness and attraction.

2. Optic Nerve (II) - Transmits visual information from the retina to the brain.

The optic nerve, known as the II cranial nerve, is a key component of the visual system, transmitting visual information from the retina to the brain [Image 1]. This nerve is not a typical peripheral nerve but an extension of the central nervous system. Its structure consists of the axons of ganglion cells located in the retina. These axons group together to form the optic nerve, which exits the eye at its back, passes through the orbit, and passes through the optic canal into the skull.

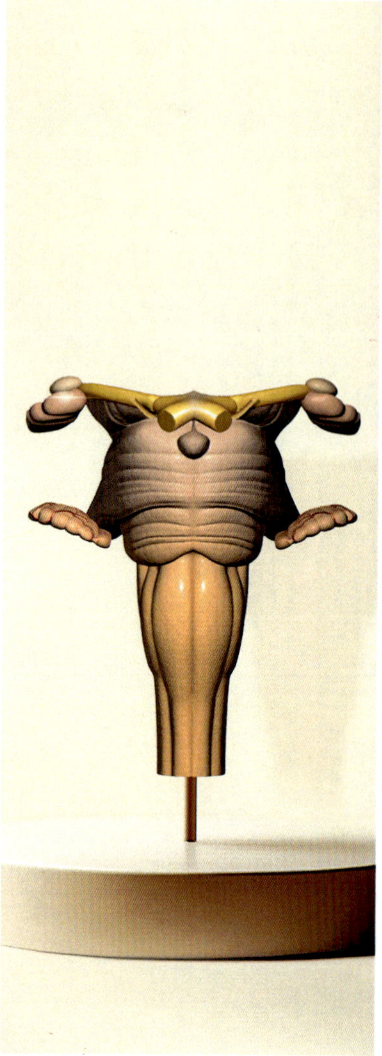
[Image 1] Optic Nerve

The optic nerves from both sides converge at the optic chiasm, located above the pituitary gland. In the optic chiasm, the axons carrying information from the temporal (outer) halves of both eyes continue directly, while the axons from the nasal (inner) halves cross to the opposite side. After the chiasm, the pathway continues as optic tracts to the thalamus, specifically to the lateral geniculate nucleus, from where the information is sent to the visual cortex in the occipital lobe.

2. Optic Nerve

The optic nerve (II) is the second cranial nerve, essential for vision. It consists of sensory fibers originating in the retina of the eye. These fibers form the optic nerve, which passes through the optic canal to the optic chiasm, where some fibers cross to the opposite side. This crossing allows visual information from both eyes to be processed in the brain. The optic nerve transmits visual information to the brain, enabling sight. Damage to the optic nerve can result in vision loss or blindness. Proper functioning of the optic nerve is crucial for visual perception.

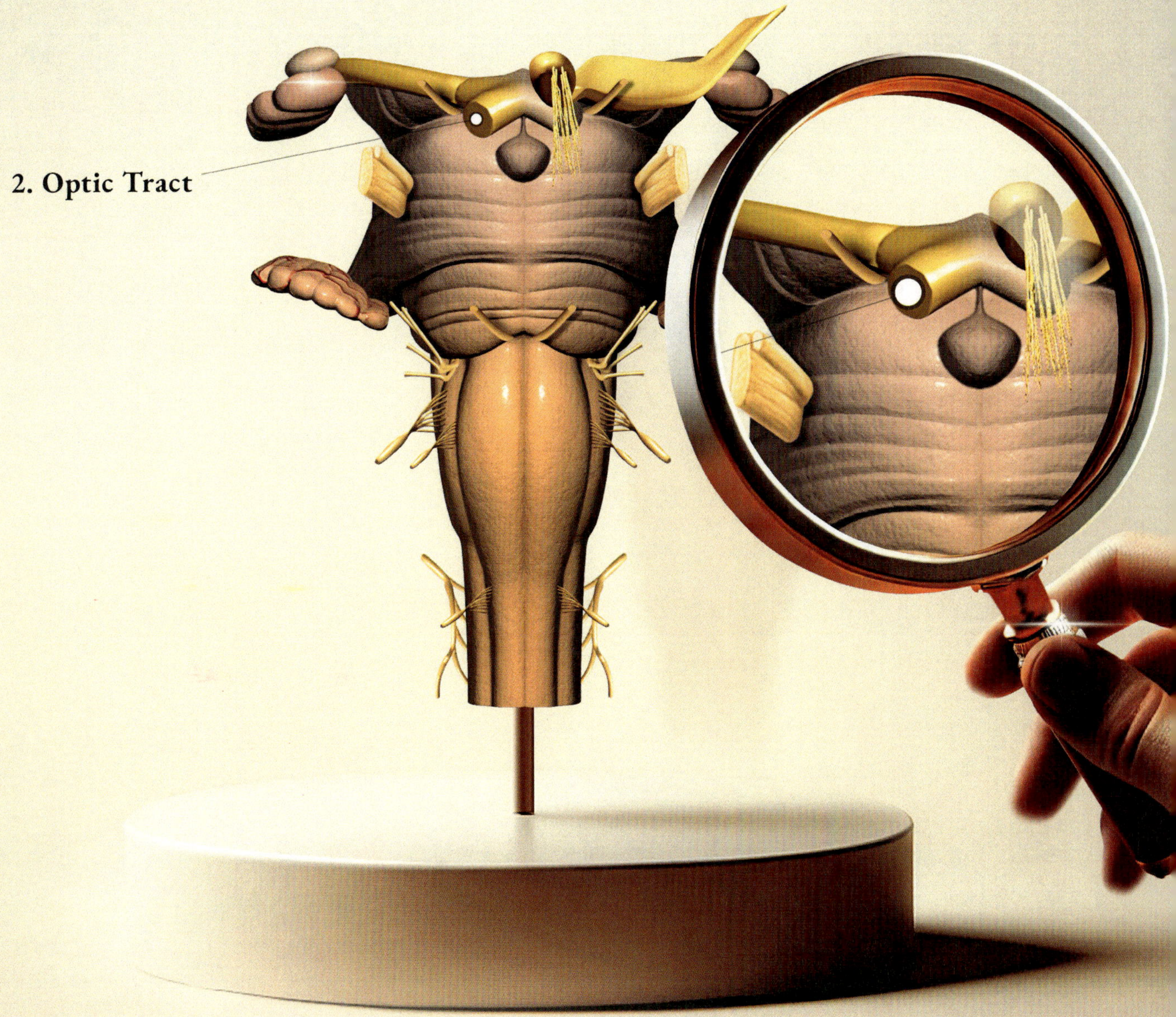

The primary function of the optic nerve is to transmit visual information from the retina to the brain. Each nerve transmits information from one eye, but due to the partial crossing in the optic chiasm, each optic tract carries information from both halves of the visual field (i.e., the right tract carries information from the left half of the visual field and vice versa). This complex process enables precise processing of visual information, which is crucial for our ability to perceive the world around us.

Disorders of the optic nerve can lead to various forms of vision loss, including complete or partial blindness in one eye, such as in cases of optic neuropathy. Multiple sclerosis, glaucoma, and trauma are among the common causes of damage to this nerve. Optic neuropathy can lead to changes in color perception, reduced visual acuity, and visual field abnormalities. Diagnostic tests for assessing optic nerve function include fundus examination, visual field tests, and imaging techniques such as magnetic resonance imaging (MRI) and computed tomography (CT) of the head.

Disorders of the optic nerve require careful medical evaluation to determine the cause and the best treatment, which may include treating the underlying disease or, in some cases, surgical intervention.

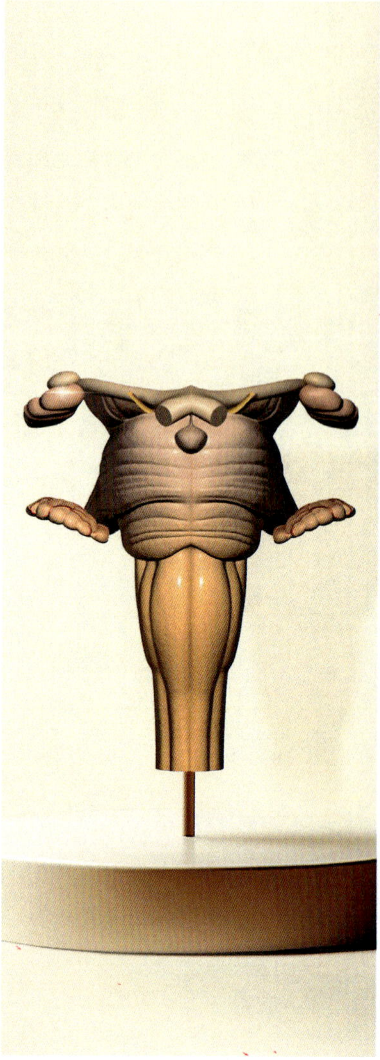

[Image 1] Oculomotor Nerve

3. Oculomotor Nerve (III) - Controls most of the muscles that move the eye, raise the eyelid, constrict the pupil, and control focusing [Image 1].

The oculomotor nerve, known as the III cranial nerve, plays a crucial role in controlling most of the muscles of the eye, enabling various movements and functions of the eye. This nerve originates in the midbrain, specifically in the oculomotor nucleus. From there, the nerve passes through the midbrain, exits the brain in front of the pons, passes through the skull cavity, and then enters the orbit of the eye through the superior orbital fissure.

The oculomotor nerve innervates several key muscles. Among them is the levator palpebrae superioris, the muscle that raises the upper eyelid, allowing the eye to open. It also innervates four of the six muscles that control eye movements: superior rectus, medial rectus, inferior rectus, and inferior oblique. These muscles allow the eye to move in various directions, providing a wide range of movements and enabling precise tracking of objects.

Additionally, the oculomotor nerve innervates the sphincter pupillae, the muscle that constricts the pupil, allowing miosis or narrowing of the pupil. The nerve also contains autonomic (parasympathetic) fibers responsible for accommodation of the eye, which involves adjusting the eye for viewing at different distances. These functions are essential for normal vision, enabling the eyes to adapt to different lighting conditions and focus on objects at various distances.

Disorder or damage to the oculomotor nerve can lead to various symptoms. Diplopia, or double vision, occurs due to the loss of coordination between the eyes. Ptosis, or drooping of the eyelid, occurs due to weakness of the muscle that raises the eyelid. Strabismus, a condition where the eyes are not aligned when looking at an object, can also result from weakness of the eye muscles. Mydriasis, or dilated pupil, can occur due to damage to the parasympathetic fibers, which can impair the eye's ability to properly respond to light conditions.

3. Oculomotor Nerve

The oculomotor nerve (III) is the third cranial nerve, crucial for eye movement and pupil constriction. It innervates the superior, medial, and inferior rectus muscles, as well as the inferior oblique muscle, controlling most eye movements. It also innervates the levator palpebrae superioris muscle, which raises the upper eyelid, and carries parasympathetic fibers to the iris sphincter for pupil constriction. Damage to this nerve can result in double vision, drooping eyelid (ptosis), and pupil dilation. Proper functioning of the oculomotor nerve is essential for coordinated eye movement and vision.

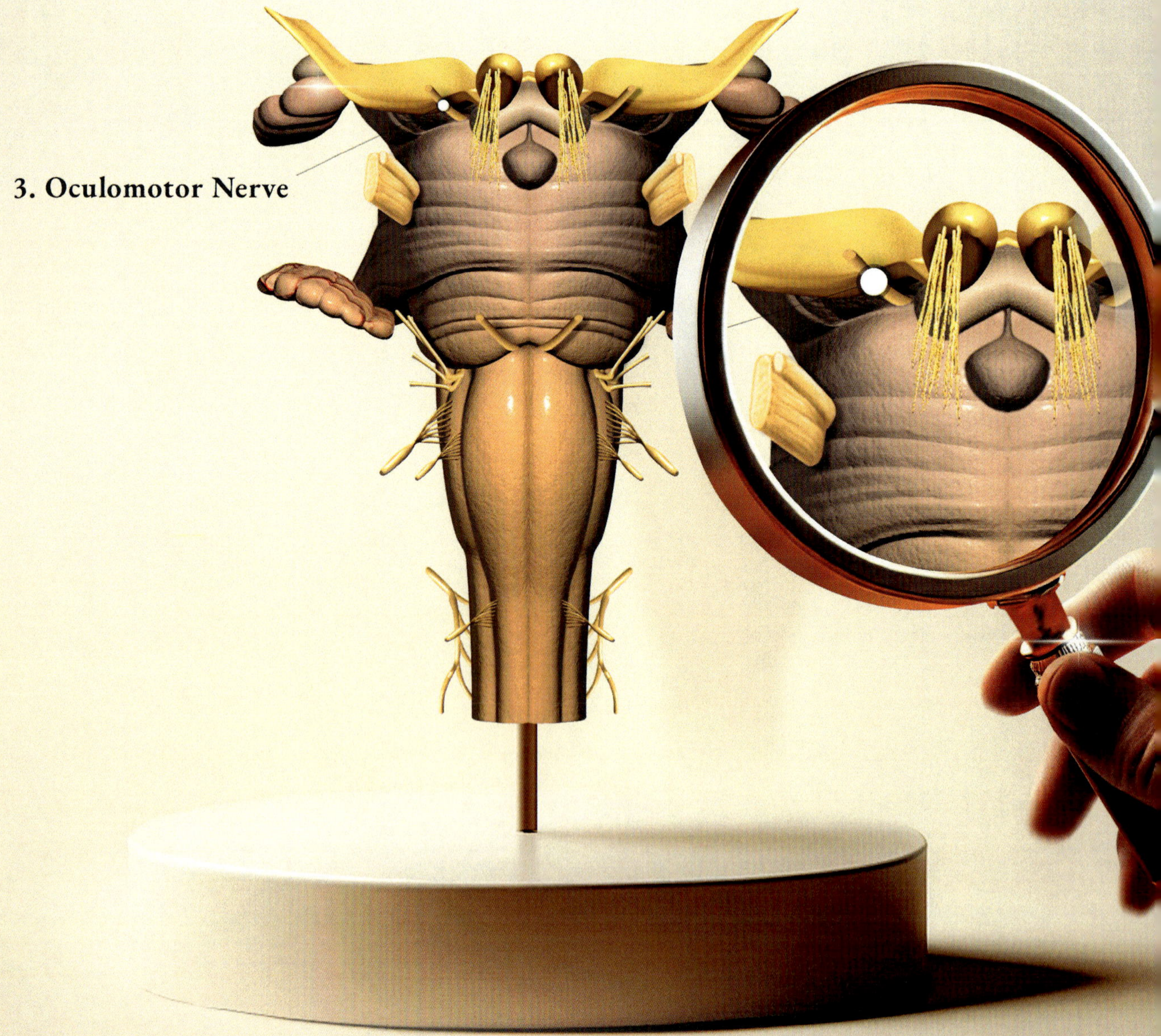

Disorders of the oculomotor nerve can be caused by various conditions, including head trauma, infections, tumors, strokes, or aneurysms. Diagnosis of these disorders involves a neurological examination, imaging studies such as MRI or CT of the head and eyes, and detailed examination of eye functions.

4. Trochlear Nerve (IV) - Innervates the superior oblique muscle of the eye, allowing rotation of the eye downward and toward the nose.

The trochlear nerve, known as the IV cranial nerve, has a specific function in the ocular system [Image 1]. This nerve is the thinnest and longest cranial nerve and the only one that exits from the dorsal, or back, side of the brainstem, specifically from the midbrain. Its uniqueness also lies in the fact that it is the only cranial nerve that crosses, meaning that the fibers of each nerve control the muscle on the opposite side.

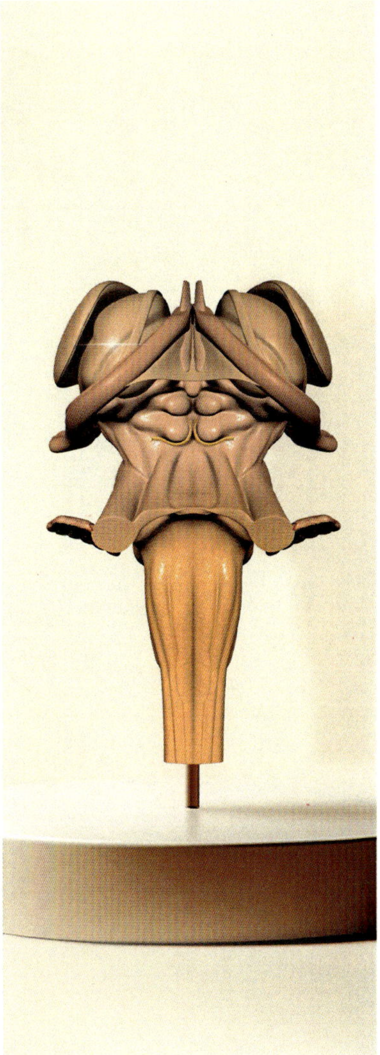

[Image 1] Trochlear Nerve

After exiting the midbrain, the trochlear nerve passes around the brainstem, crosses below the cerebrum, and enters the orbit of the eye through the superior orbital fissure. This path leads it to the only muscle it innervates, the superior oblique muscle. This muscle plays a crucial role in moving the eye downward and toward the nose, which is particularly important for activities such as reading or viewing objects located lower than the eye level.

The main function of the trochlear nerve is to allow precise eye movements, specifically rotation of the eye downward and inward. These movements are essential for binocular vision and coordination of eye movements, enabling clear and focused viewing.

4. Trochlear Nerve

The trochlear nerve (IV) is unique as the only cranial nerve emerging from the dorsal side of the brainstem. It innervates the superior oblique muscle of the eye, enabling downward and lateral movement. This nerve plays a crucial role in precise eye alignment. Damage to the trochlear nerve can result in double vision and difficulty with tasks requiring downward gaze, such as reading or descending stairs. Proper functioning of the trochlear nerve is essential for coordinated and accurate eye movements.

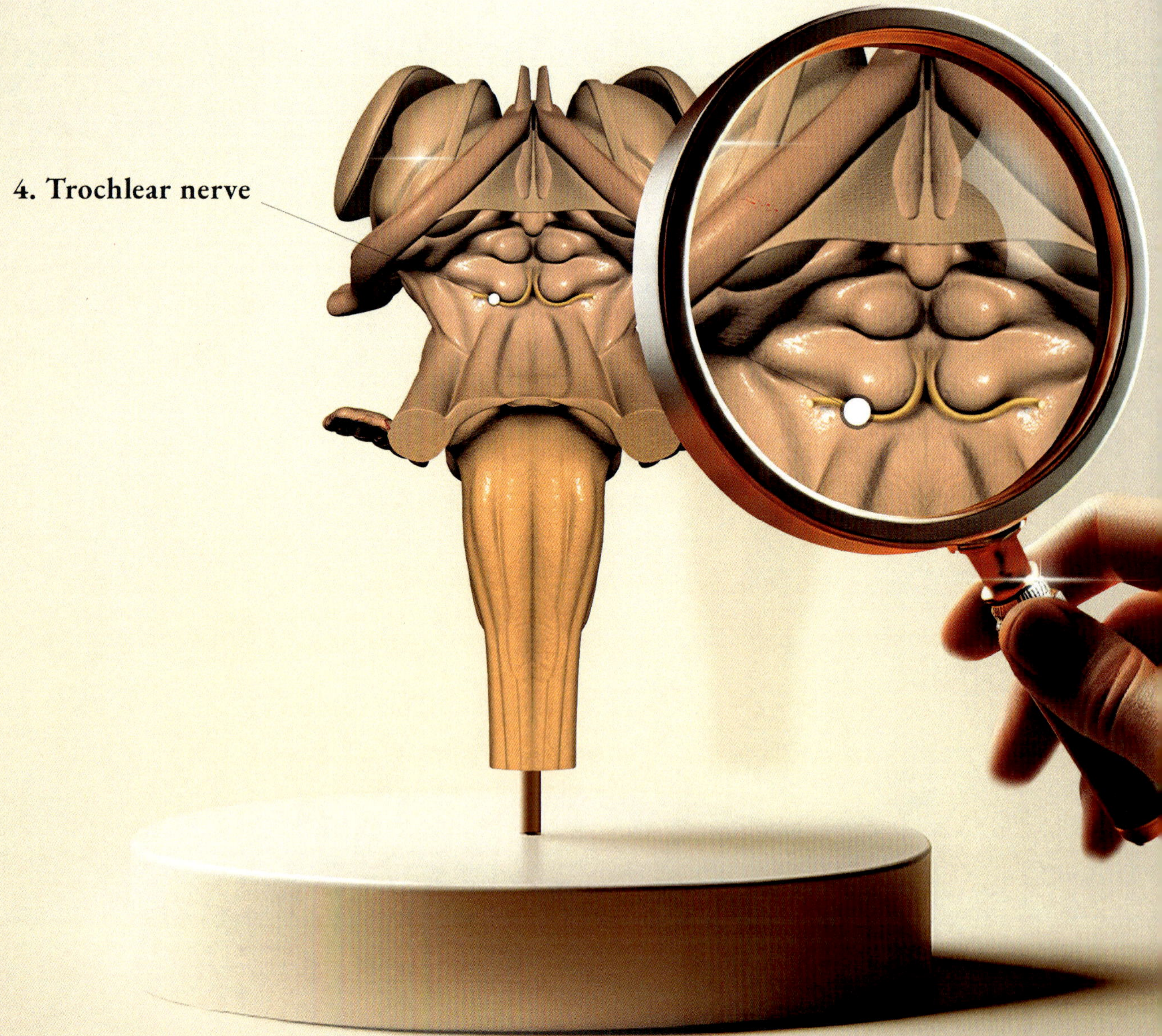

Damage or dysfunction of the trochlear nerve can lead to a condition known as trochlear palsy. This condition is characterized by vertical diplopia, or double vision, because the eyes cannot properly align. People with this disorder often have difficulty looking downward, which can be particularly problematic when descending stairs or reading. To compensate for the visual disturbance, a head tilt toward the healthy side often occurs.

Diagnosis of this disorder includes a neurological examination, eye mobility tests, and imaging techniques such as MRI or CT scans to identify the cause of the damage. Treatment depends on the underlying cause and may include physical therapy, prismatic glasses to correct double vision, or, in some cases, surgical intervention to correct the position of the eye muscle.

5. Trigeminal Nerve (V) - This nerve has three branches that transmit sensory information from the face to the brain and control the muscles responsible for chewing.

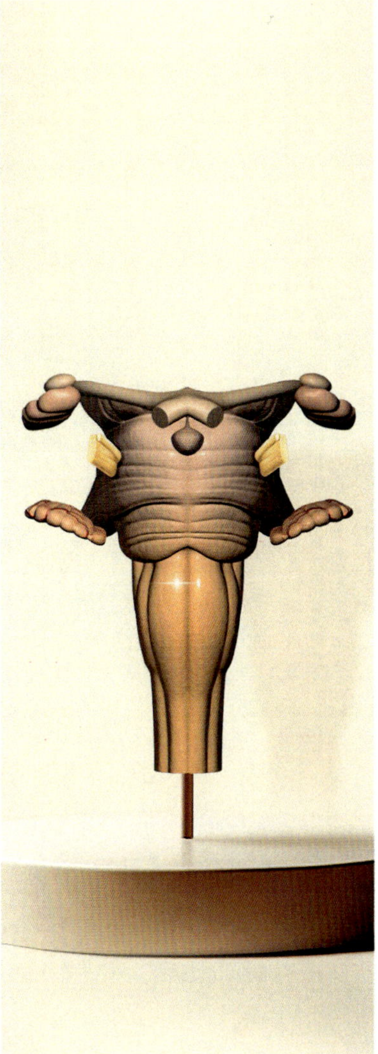

[Image 1] Trigeminal Nerve

The trigeminal nerve, known as the V cranial nerve, is one of the largest and most complex cranial nerves, playing a crucial role in both sensory and motor functions of the face [Image 1]. This nerve originates from the pons, a part of the brainstem, and has a large trigeminal ganglion, known as the Gasserian ganglion, located in the Meckel's cave within the skull. From this ganglion, the nerve divides into three main branches: the ophthalmic branch (V1), the maxillary branch (V2), and the mandibular branch (V3).

The ophthalmic branch (V1) is sensory and innervates the forehead, upper eyelid, and nose. The maxillary branch (V2) is also sensory and innervates the middle part of the face, including the upper lip, upper teeth, and cheek. The mandibular branch (V3) has both sensory and motor functions. Sensory-wise, it innervates the lower part of the face, including the lower lip, lower teeth, and part of the cheek, while motor-wise, it innervates the muscles of mastication, such as the temporalis, masseter, and other muscles involved in chewing and speaking.

The sensory functions of the trigeminal nerve include transmitting sensations such as touch, pain, and temperature from the face to the brain. The motor component, which is dominant in the mandibular branch, allows control of the muscles responsible for chewing, speaking, and other jaw movements.

Disorders of the trigeminal nerve can profoundly affect the quality of life. Trigeminal neuralgia is an extremely painful condition characterized by electric shock-like pain in the areas innervated by one or more branches of the trigeminal nerve. The pain can be triggered by minimal stimuli such as talking, chewing, or even touching. Herpes zoster, also known as shingles, can affect the trigeminal ganglion, causing painful facial rashes. Facial injuries can also damage the trigeminal nerve, leading to loss of sensation or motor function in parts of the face.

Diagnostic procedures for assessing the trigeminal nerve include neurological examinations, MRI to identify structural anomalies or compressions, and electromyography (EMG) to test motor functions. Treatment may involve medications, such as anticonvulsants or analgesics, physical therapy, or surgical interventions in severe cases. For trigeminal neuralgia, neurosurgical procedures such as microvascular decompression or radiofrequency ablation may be considered to reduce

5. Trigeminal Nerve

The trigeminal nerve (V) is the fifth cranial nerve, crucial for facial sensation and chewing. It has three branches: ophthalmic (V1), maxillary (V2), and mandibular (V3). The ophthalmic and maxillary branches provide sensory information from the forehead, eyes, upper lip, and cheeks. The mandibular branch provides sensory input from the lower jaw and controls muscles involved in chewing. Damage to the trigeminal nerve can result in loss of sensation, facial pain, or difficulty chewing. Proper functioning of the trigeminal nerve is essential for facial sensation and mastication.

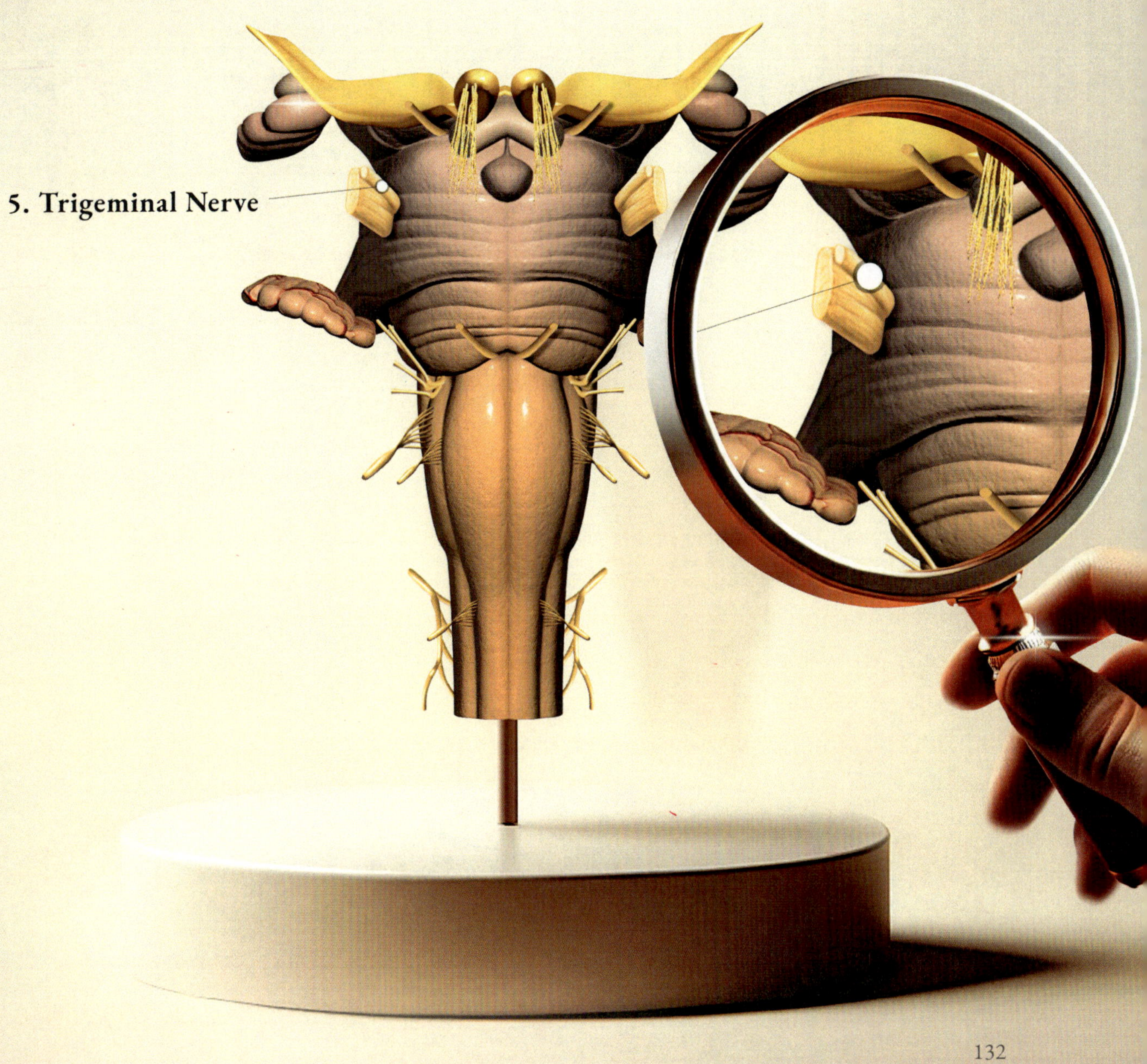

nerve pressure or destroy painful nerve branches.

6. Abducens Nerve (VI) - Controls the lateral rectus muscle, which moves the eye outward.

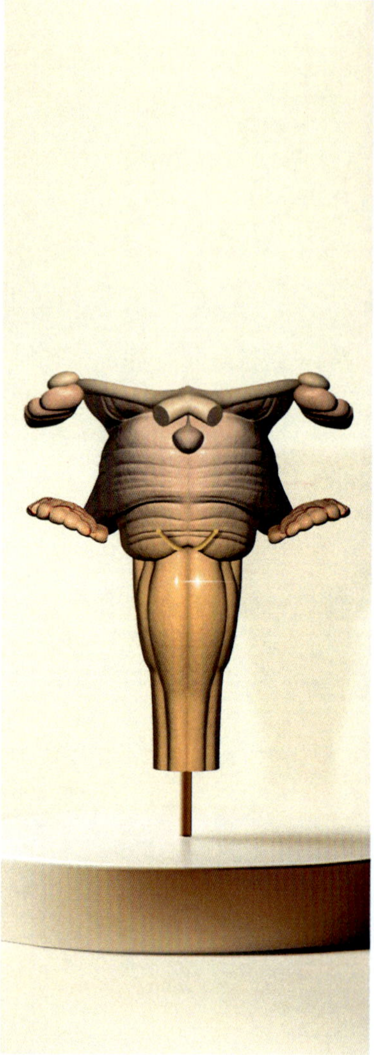

[Image 1] Abducens Nerve

The abducens nerve, known as the VI cranial nerve, plays a specific role in eye movement, enabling the lateral movement of the eye, or abduction [Image 1]. This nerve originates in the abducens nucleus, located in the lower part of the pons in the brainstem. From there, the nerve travels through the brainstem, exits at the base of the brain, and follows a long path within the skull, passing through the petroclival angle and cavernous sinus before entering the eye socket through the superior orbital fissure.

The abducens nerve innervates one key muscle, the lateral rectus muscle. This muscle is responsible for pulling the eye outward, which is crucial for coordinating and widening the field of vision. The primary function of the abducens nerve is to facilitate horizontal eye movements, especially abduction, meaning moving the eye away from the midline of the nose. This function is extremely important for binocular vision and allows the eyes to track objects horizontally.

Damage or dysfunction of the abducens nerve can lead to a condition known as abducens nerve palsy. This condition manifests as an inability to move the eye outward, resulting in double vision (diplopia) and strabismus (misalignment of the eyes). Patients with this condition often have difficulty focusing and tracking objects, significantly impacting their daily lives.

Damage to this nerve can result from various factors, including head trauma, increased intracranial pressure, stroke,

6. Abducens Nerve

The abducens nerve (VI) is the sixth cranial nerve, essential for eye movement. It innervates the lateral rectus muscle, which abducts the eye, moving it outward. This nerve plays a critical role in coordinating horizontal eye movements and maintaining proper alignment. Damage to the abducens nerve can result in an inability to move the eye outward, causing double vision (diplopia) and inward turning of the eye (esotropia). Proper functioning of the abducens nerve is crucial for maintaining normal eye alignment, coordination, and clear vision.

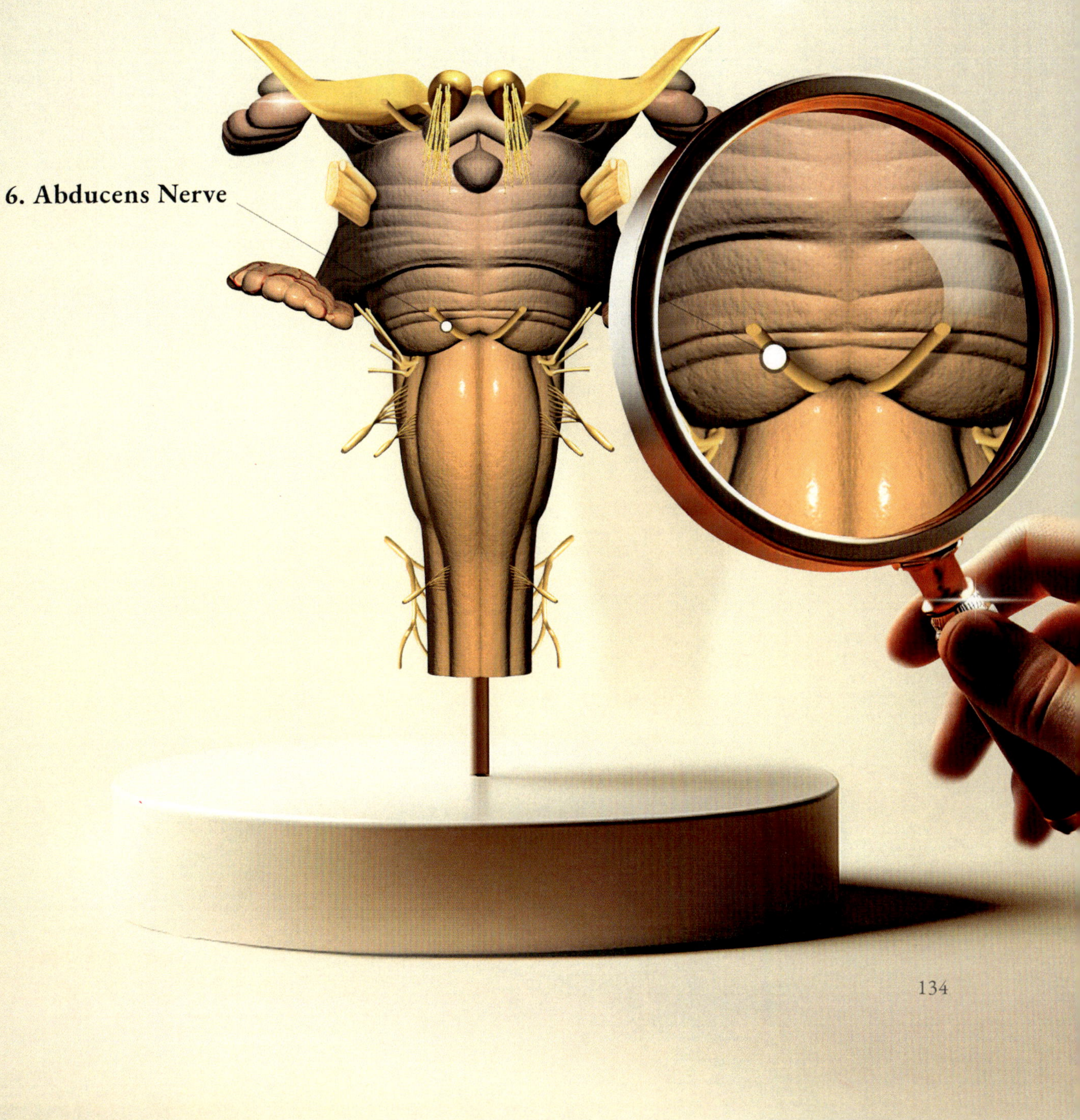

tumors, infections, and neurological diseases such as multiple sclerosis. Diagnosis involves a detailed neurological and ophthalmological examination, tests of eye movement, and imaging studies like MRI or CT scans of the head to identify the causes of damage.

Treatment depends on the underlying cause and may include medication, physical therapy, prismatic glasses to correct double vision, or, in some cases, surgical interventions to correct the position of the eye muscles or decompress the nerve.

7. Facial Nerve (VII) - Innervates the muscles of the face, allowing for facial expressions; also transmits sensory information for taste from the front two-thirds of the tongue and controls some glands (e.g., tear and salivary glands).

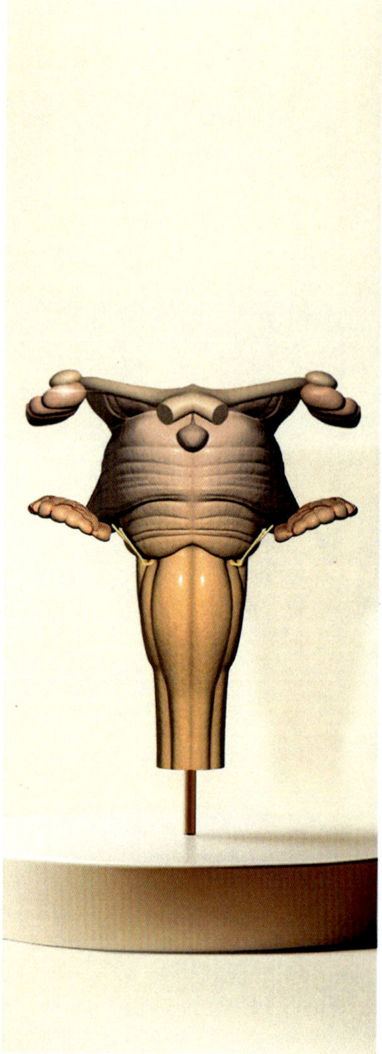

[Image 1] Facial Nerve

The facial nerve, known as the VII cranial nerve, plays a key role in various functions, including facial expressions, taste perception, and autonomic functions [Image 1]. This nerve originates in the facial nucleus within the pons, a part of the brainstem. From there, the nerve travels through the internal auditory meatus, passes through the facial canal in the temporal bone, and exits the skull through the stylomastoid foramen. After exiting, the facial nerve branches into five main branches that innervate different facial muscles: temporal, zygomatic, buccal, mandibular, and cervical.

The motor function of the facial nerve controls the muscles of facial expression, allowing for expressions such as smiling, frowning, blinking, and many others. Additionally, the nerve innervates some muscles in the ear and neck. Although primarily motor, the facial nerve also transmits sensory information for taste from the front two-thirds of the tongue, pro-

7. Facial Nerve

The facial nerve (VII) is the seventh cranial nerve, vital for facial expressions, taste, and glandular functions. It innervates the muscles responsible for facial expressions and transmits taste sensations from the anterior two-thirds of the tongue. Additionally, it controls the lacrimal glands for tear production and the salivary glands. Damage to the facial nerve can result in facial paralysis (Bell's palsy), loss of taste, and reduced tear and saliva production. Proper functioning of the facial nerve is essential for expressive facial movements, taste, and maintaining moisture in the eyes and mouth.

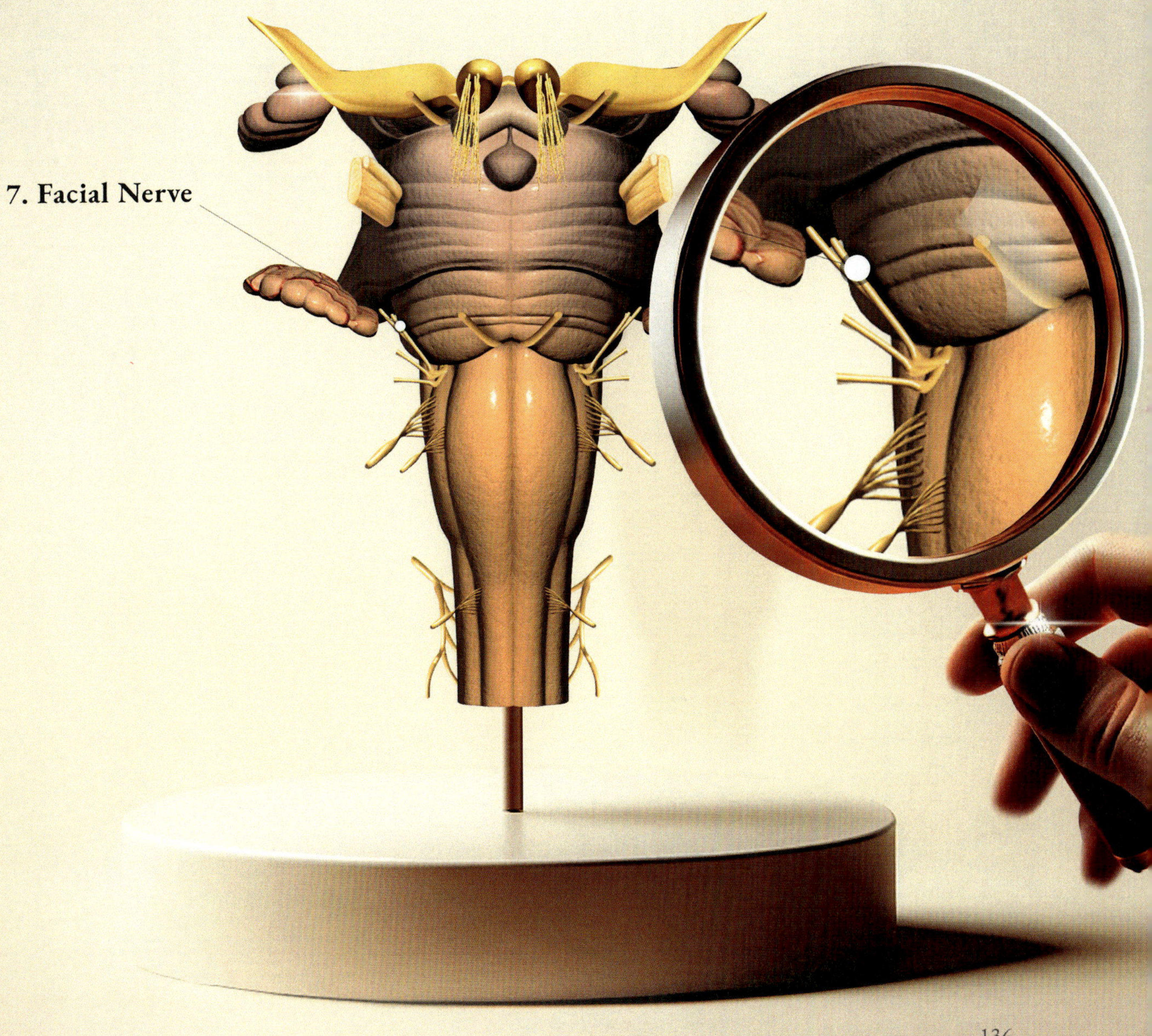

viding a sensory function. Moreover, this nerve has autonomic functions, controlling several glands, including the lacrimal, sublingual, and submandibular glands, responsible for tear and saliva production.

Dysfunction of the facial nerve can cause various symptoms and conditions. One of the most common issues is facial paralysis or Bell's palsy, causing sudden unilateral facial paralysis. This condition can affect the facial muscles, causing one-sided facial drooping, making it difficult to express emotions and perform daily functions such as eating and speaking. Without adequate nerve control, the eyelid may not close properly, leading to dry eye and potential damage. Changes in taste perception are also possible, with a loss or distortion of taste on the front two-thirds of the tongue. Additionally, hyperacusis, or increased sensitivity to sounds on the affected side, can occur due to the innervation of muscles in the middle ear.

Diagnosis of facial nerve problems is based on clinical symptoms, electromyography (EMG), and taste tests. Treatment depends on the cause and extent of the damage. In most cases of Bell's palsy, recovery is possible without treatment, although corticosteroids can help reduce the duration of symptoms. Physical therapy and facial exercises are also recommended to improve muscle mobility. In severe cases, or when the cause is an infection, antiviral or antibacterial medications may be used.

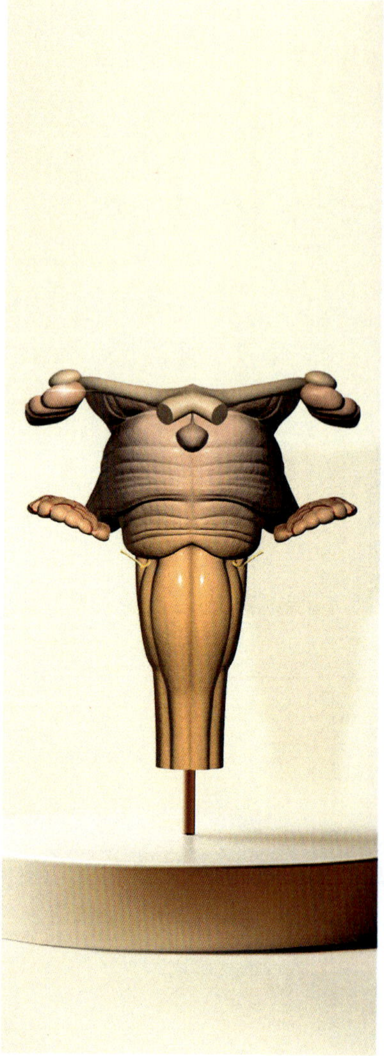

[Image 1] Vestibulocochlear Nerve

8. Vestibulocochlear Nerve (VIII) - Consists of two parts: the vestibular nerve, which helps with balance, and the cochlear nerve, which helps with hearing [Image 1].

The vestibulocochlear nerve, known as the VIII cranial

nerve, is essential for two key functions: hearing and maintaining balance. This nerve emerges from the brainstem at the junction of the pons and medulla oblongata, together with the facial nerve, and enters the inner ear through the internal acoustic meatus. It consists of two distinct parts: the vestibular nerve and the cochlear nerve.

The vestibular nerve innervates structures in the vestibular apparatus of the inner ear, including the three semicircular canals and otolith organs, which are crucial for detecting head movements and gravitational changes. This part of the nerve transmits information about head position and movements, enabling the brain to maintain balance and coordinate movements. Sensors in the vestibular apparatus respond to rotation, tilting, and linear accelerations, sending signals that help maintain the stability of vision and posture.

The cochlear nerve connects the cochlea of the inner ear to the brain. The cochlea is a fluid-filled structure that converts sound waves into electrical signals, which the nerve transmits to the auditory cortex in the brain. This part of the nerve is responsible for sound perception. In the cochlea, sound waves are transformed into electrical impulses that travel to the brain, allowing us to hear and distinguish sounds.

Dysfunction or damage to the vestibulocochlear nerve can cause symptoms such as hearing loss, dizziness and balance problems, and tinnitus. Hearing loss can be partial or complete, depending on the extent of cochlear nerve damage. Disorders of the vestibular nerve can lead to vertigo, disorientation, and difficulties in maintaining balance. Tinnitus, or ringing in the ears, can also be present.

Diagnostic methods include audiometric tests to assess

8. Vestibulocochlear Nerve

The vestibulocochlear nerve (VIII) is the eighth cranial nerve, essential for hearing and balance. It has two main components: the cochlear nerve, which transmits sound information from the inner ear to the brain, and the vestibular nerve, which carries information about balance and spatial orientation. Damage to the vestibulocochlear nerve can result in hearing loss, tinnitus (ringing in the ears), vertigo, and balance disorders. Proper functioning of the vestibulocochlear nerve is crucial for clear hearing and maintaining equilibrium.

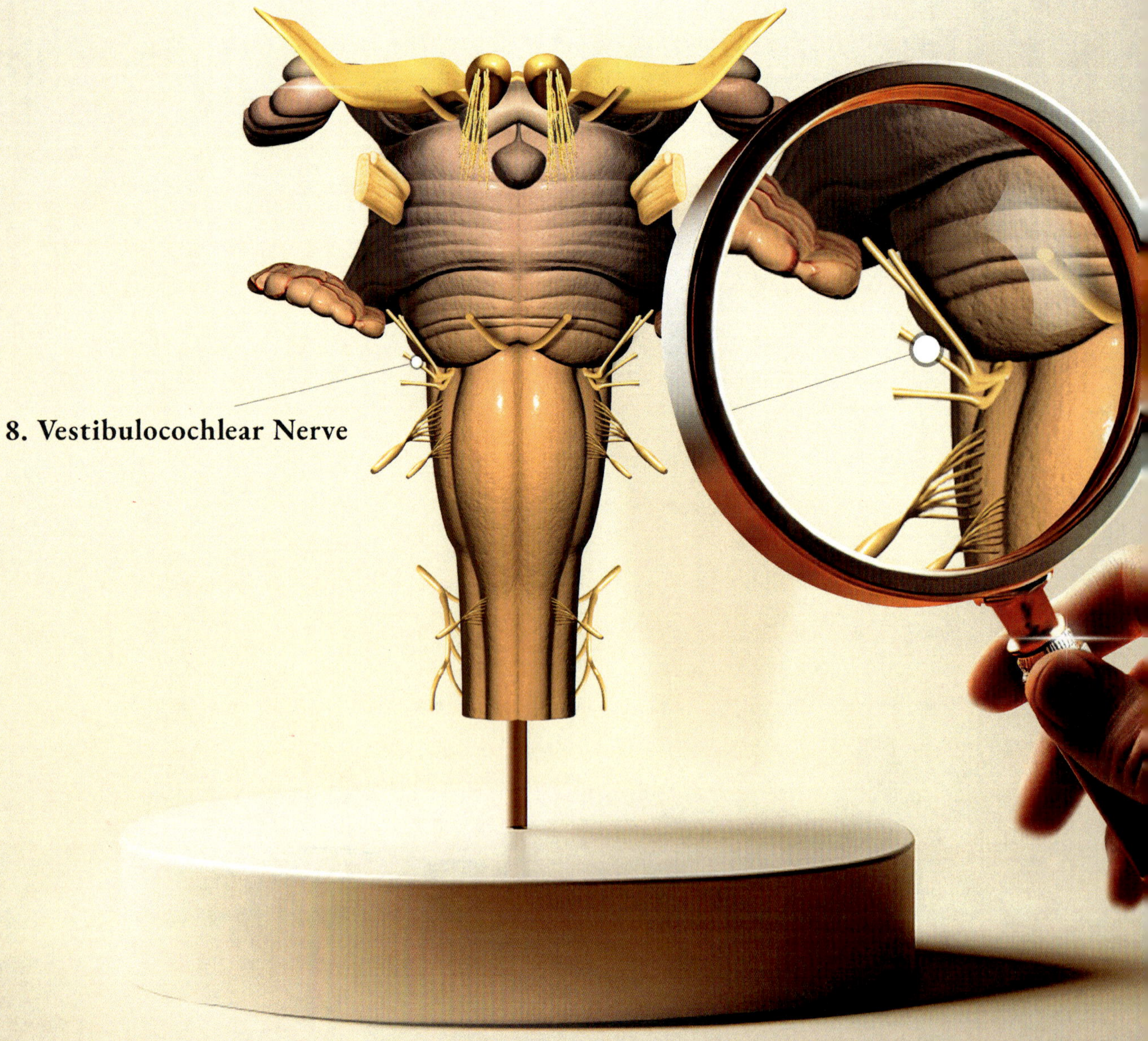

hearing function, vestibular tests such as caloric tests to check the function of the semicircular canals, and imaging studies like MRI or CT scans of the head to identify potential causes of dysfunction. Treatment depends on the diagnosis and may include therapy to restore balance, hearing aids or cochlear implants for hearing loss, and medications to manage symptoms of vertigo and tinnitus.

9. The glossopharyngeal nerve (IX) - Transmits taste from the back third of the tongue and controls swallowing and saliva secretion muscles [Image 1].

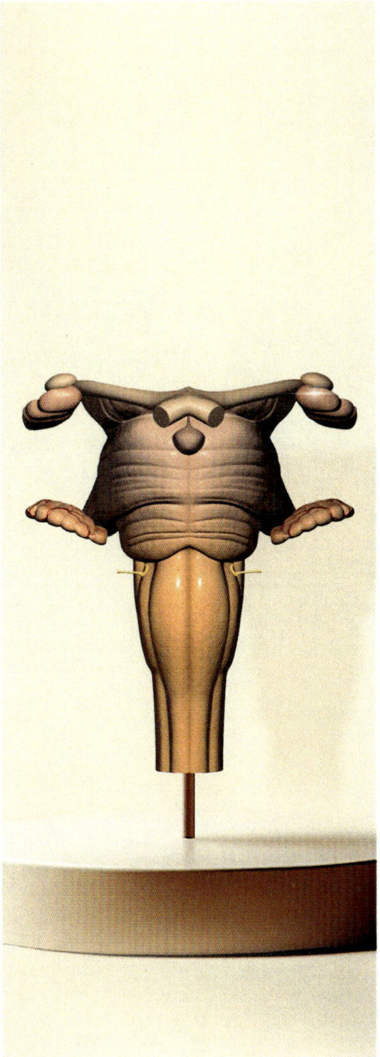

[Image 1] Glossopharyngeal Nerve

The glossopharyngeal nerve, known as the IX cranial nerve, has vital sensory, motor, and autonomic functions essential for swallowing, taste perception, and saliva management. This nerve emerges from the medulla oblongata, a part of the brainstem, and passes through the jugular foramen before entering the pharyngeal region. Its branches extend and innervate various structures within the head and neck.

Sensory functions of the glossopharyngeal nerve include transmitting sensory information from the back third of the tongue, including taste perception. It also conveys sensory information from the upper part of the throat, which is important for the swallowing reflex and the sensation of food or drink in the throat. The motor functions of this nerve involve innervating the stylopharyngeal muscle, which helps elevate the pharynx during speech and swallowing. The autonomic functions of the glossopharyngeal nerve include regulating saliva secretion through the parotid gland, the largest salivary gland, via its tympanic branch, known as Jacobson's nerve. Additionally, this nerve participates in reflexes such as coughing and vomiting and regulates blood pressure and breathing through sensory receptors in the carotid sinus, which detect

9. Glossopharyngeal Nerve

The glossopharyngeal nerve (IX) is the ninth cranial nerve, involved in taste, swallowing, and salivation. It carries sensory information from the posterior third of the tongue, including taste. It also innervates the pharyngeal muscles, aiding in swallowing, and the parotid gland for saliva production. Damage to this nerve can result in loss of taste, difficulty swallowing (dysphagia), and reduced saliva secretion. Proper functioning of the glossopharyngeal nerve is essential for taste, swallowing, and maintaining oral moisture.

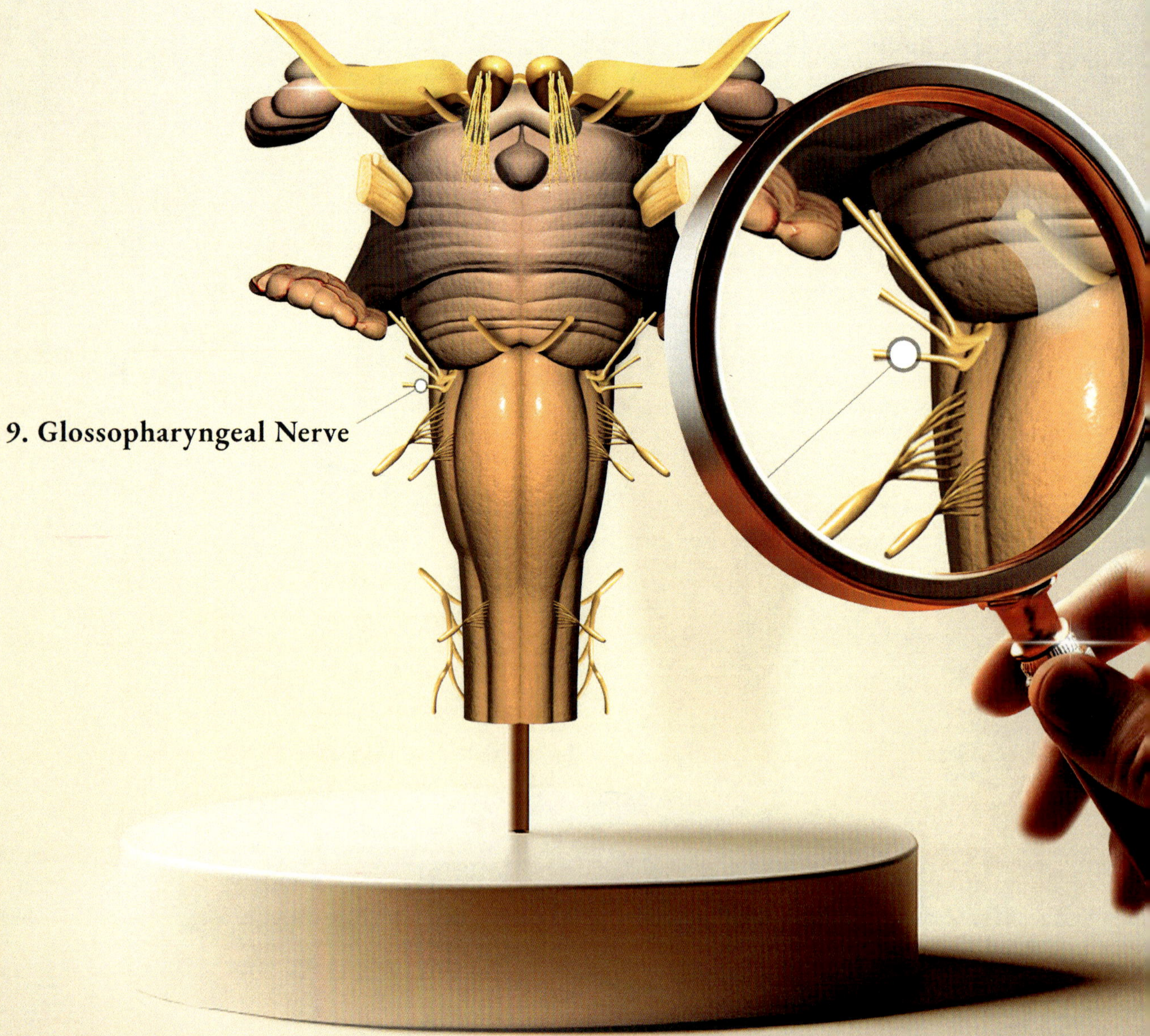

changes in blood pressure, and the carotid body, which responds to changes in oxygen and carbon dioxide levels.

Dysfunction of the glossopharyngeal nerve can cause various symptoms and conditions. Glossopharyngeal neuralgia is an extremely painful condition characterized by episodes of intense pain in the ear, the back third of the tongue, the tonsils, or the throat. Weakness in the muscles innervated by the nerve can make swallowing difficult, while changes in taste perception can lead to a loss or alteration of taste in the back third of the tongue. Reduced saliva production can affect mouth moisture and overall oral health.

Diagnosis of glossopharyngeal nerve problems includes a neurological examination, taste tests, measurement of saliva production, and various imaging techniques such as MRI or CT to identify structural or pathological changes affecting the nerve. Treatment depends on the cause and may include medications to relieve pain, physical therapy to improve swallowing function, or surgical interventions in severe cases.

10. The vagus nerve (X) - This nerve has the broadest range of action, innervating the vocal cords, smooth muscles of internal organs in the thorax and abdomen, and transmitting sensory information from these regions [Image 1].

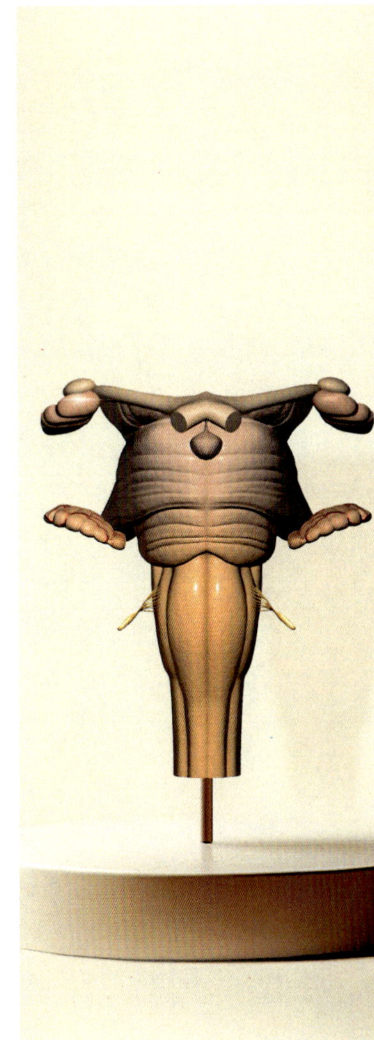

[Image 1] Vagus nerve

The vagus nerve, known as the X cranial nerve, is one of the most important and complex nerves in the human body due to its extensive role in the autonomic nervous system and its ability to reach and influence many organs. This nerve emerges from the medulla oblongata at the base of the brainstem and passes through the jugular foramen. After exiting the skull, the vagus nerve descends down the neck into the thorax and then into the abdomen, branching out to reach and innervate structures in the throat, heart, lungs, and gastrointestinal tract.

The motor functions of the vagus nerve include innervating most of the muscles in the throat, enabling swallowing and speech. It also innervates the vocal cords in the larynx, which is crucial for speaking and singing. The sensory functions of this nerve transmit information from the interior of the throat, larynx, heart, lungs, and gastrointestinal tract, encompassing sensations such as pain, heat, cold, and pressure.

The vagus nerve plays a key role in the autonomic functions of the body. It regulates heart functions by controlling heart rate and blood pressure and also controls breathing by regulating the smooth muscles in the bronchi. In the gastrointestinal tract, the vagus stimulates muscle contractions that enable the movement of food (peristalsis) and the secretion of digestive enzymes. As a major part of the parasympathetic nervous system, the vagus nerve has the ability to "calm" the body after periods of stress, lowering heart rate and promoting recovery and relaxation.

Dysfunction of the vagus nerve can lead to a variety of symptoms and conditions, including gastrointestinal problems such as gastroparesis and difficulty with peristalsis, which can cause constipation or diarrhea. Heart problems, including arrhythmias, may occur due to unregulated parasympathetic control over heart rate. Problems with swallowing and speaking can arise due to the impact on the muscles of the throat and larynx. Vagal syncope, a sudden drop in heart rate and blood pressure, can lead to fainting.

Diagnosis of vagus nerve problems involves a detailed neurological examination and specific tests of the functions of

10. Vagus Nerve

The vagus nerve (X) is the tenth cranial nerve, crucial for autonomic control of the heart, lungs, and digestive tract. It provides sensory and motor innervation to these organs, regulating heart rate, breathing, and digestion. The vagus nerve also influences speech and swallowing. Damage to the vagus nerve can lead to heart rate irregularities, difficulty swallowing, loss of voice, and impaired digestion. Proper functioning of the vagus nerve is essential for maintaining autonomic balance, overall health, and effective communication.

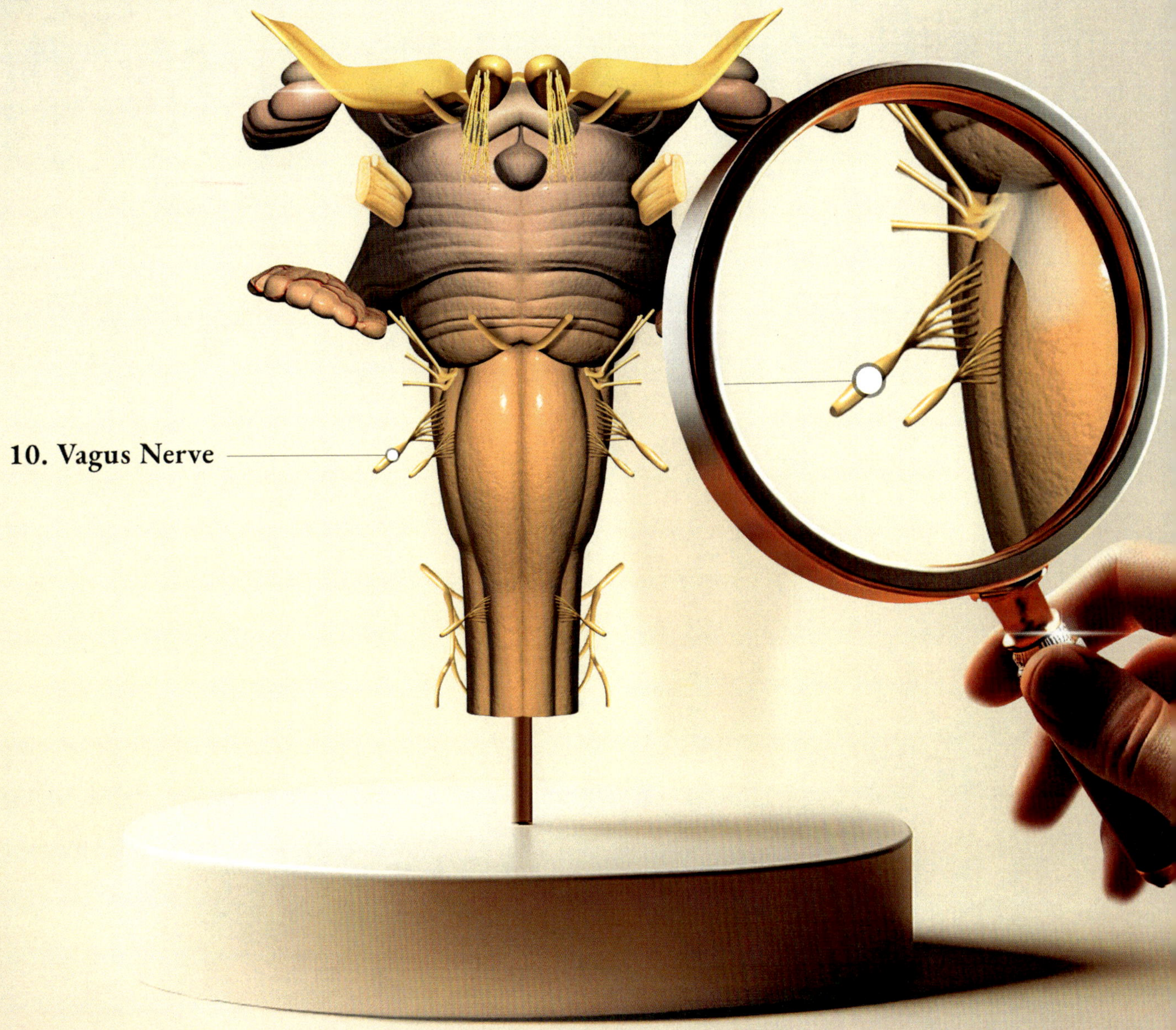

the organs innervated by this nerve. Treatment depends on the specific problem but may include medications that modulate the parasympathetic response or therapeutic interventions on the organs the nerve innervates. In some cases, vagus nerve stimulation (VNS) may be used, particularly in the treatment of certain types of epilepsy and depression.

11. The accessory nerve (XI) - Controls the neck muscles involved in head and shoulder movements.

The accessory nerve, known as the XI cranial nerve, plays a crucial role in the motor control of certain neck and shoulder muscles [Image 1]. This nerve has a unique anatomical structure as it consists of two parts: spinal and cranial. The cranial part begins in the medulla oblongata and quickly merges with the vagus, while the spinal part begins in the cervical spine, at levels C1 to C5. The spinal part ascends through the foramen magnum into the skull, merges with the cranial part, and then exits the skull through the jugular foramen. After exiting, the nerve passes through the posterior part of the neck and innervates specific muscles.

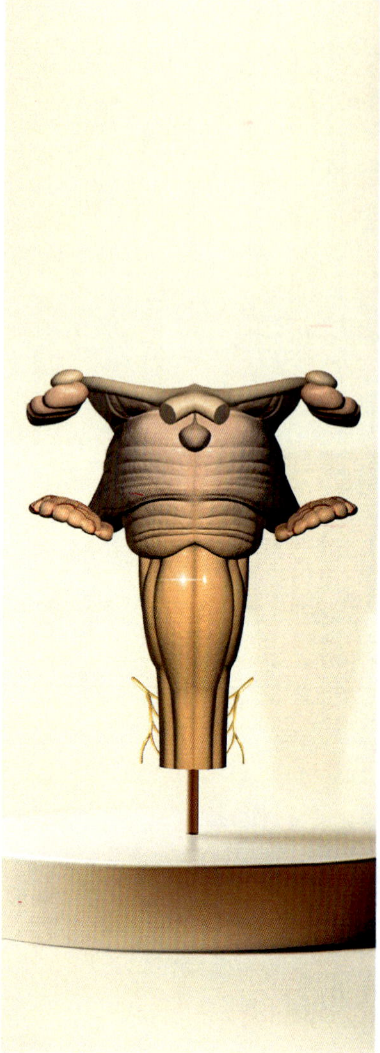
[Image 1] Accessory nerve

The accessory nerve controls two main muscles: the sternocleidomastoid and the trapezius. The sternocleidomastoid is a muscle that runs along the side of the neck from the temporal bone of the skull to the sternum. This muscle enables the rotation and flexion of the head. The trapezius is a broad muscle that covers most of the upper back and shoulders. Innervation of the trapezius muscle allows for the elevation, rotation, and retraction of the scapulae, as well as neck extension.

The primary function of the accessory nerve is to enable head and shoulder movements. The muscles it innervates play

11. Accessory Nerve

The accessory nerve (XI) is the eleventh cranial nerve, essential for controlling certain muscles in the neck and shoulders. It has two parts: a spinal component and a cranial component. The spinal part innervates the sternocleidomastoid and trapezius muscles, enabling head rotation and shoulder elevation. The cranial part assists the vagus nerve in controlling muscles involved in swallowing. Damage to the accessory nerve can result in weakness or paralysis of the neck and shoulder muscles, leading to difficulty in head movement and shoulder drooping.

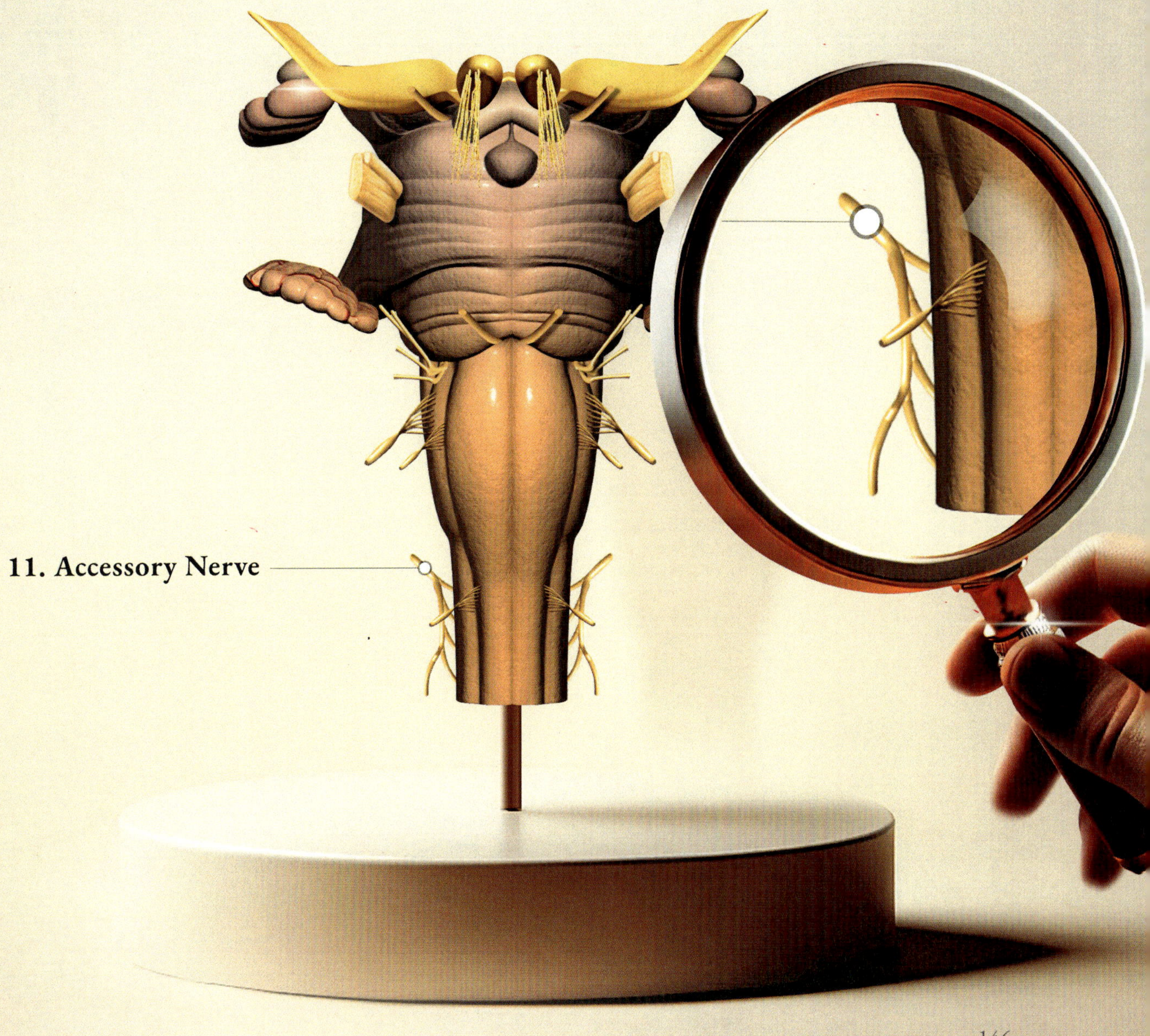

a key role in many everyday activities, such as turning the head, lifting the arms, and breathing through their support of the diaphragm. Damage or dysfunction of the accessory nerve can lead to weakness or paralysis of the sternocleidomastoid, which can result in difficulty turning the head to the opposite side of the injury. Additionally, weakness or atrophy of the trapezius can lead to difficulty lifting the arms above the head and may cause a "drooping shoulder" on the side of the injury.

Diagnosis of accessory nerve problems is often based on physical examination and symptoms and confirmed by electromyography (EMG) or imaging methods such as MRI or CT. Treatment depends on the cause of the damage and may include physical therapy to strengthen and improve muscle function, steroid injections to reduce inflammation, or surgical interventions in cases of severe trauma or nerve compression.

12. Hypoglossal nerve (XII) - Controls the muscles of the tongue, which is important for speech and swallowing.

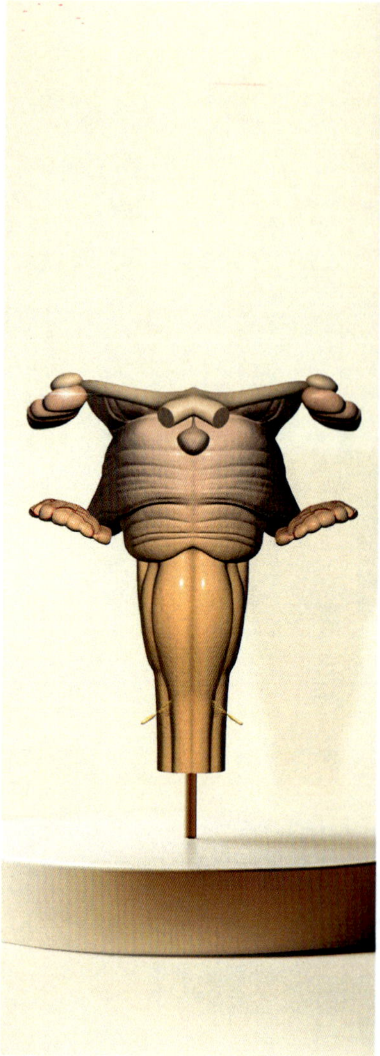
[Image 1] Hypoglossal nerve

The hypoglossal nerve, the XII cranial nerve, plays a key role in controlling the tongue muscles, essential for speech, swallowing, and manipulating food in the mouth [Image 1]. This nerve begins in the hypoglossal nucleus, located in the medulla oblongata, the lower part of the brainstem. The hypoglossal nerve exits the skull through the hypoglossal canal and then descends and spreads along the underside of the tongue. Its path leads it from the medulla oblongata directly to the tongue muscles, without branching to other structures.

The hypoglossal nerve is primarily a motor nerve and innervates all the tongue muscles except for the palatoglossus, which is innervated by the vagus nerve. The muscles it controls include the genioglossus, which helps protrude the tongue; the hyoglossus, which depresses and retracts the tongue; the styloglossus, which elevates and retracts the tongue; and the intrinsic muscles, which fine-tune the shape of the tongue for precise movements needed for speech and chewing.

The function of the hypoglossal nerve enables complex tongue movements essential for clear and effective speech, as well as for chewing and swallowing. Proper functioning of this nerve is crucial for the ability to articulate, produce various speech sounds, and general communication.

Dysfunction or damage to the hypoglossal nerve can lead to various problems, including atrophy of the tongue muscles, causing difficulties in speech and swallowing. Fasciculations of the tongue, which are involuntary muscle contractions visible as twitching under the skin of the tongue, may also be present. If the damage is unilateral, the tongue will deviate towards the side of the damaged nerve upon protrusion.

Diagnosis of hypoglossal nerve problems may include a neurological examination, electromyography (EMG) to assess the electrical activity of the tongue muscles, and imaging techniques like MRI or CT to examine structural causes of the damage. Treatment depends on the cause and may include the use of muscle relaxants, speech and swallowing therapy, and in some cases, surgical intervention for nerve reconstruction or decompression. In situations where the damage is permanent, therapies focused on improving communication abilities and dietary adaptation can be beneficial in managing symptoms.

Each of these cranial nerves has specific roles that are crucial for the normal functioning of the human body, including

12. Hypoglossal Nerve

The hypoglossal nerve (XII) is the twelfth cranial nerve, crucial for tongue movement. It innervates both the intrinsic and extrinsic muscles of the tongue, enabling precise movements for speech, swallowing, and food manipulation. This nerve allows the tongue to change shape and position, essential for articulation and efficient mastication. Damage to the hypoglossal nerve can result in tongue weakness or paralysis, leading to difficulties in speaking, swallowing, and chewing. Proper functioning of the hypoglossal nerve is vital for effective communication and overall oral health.

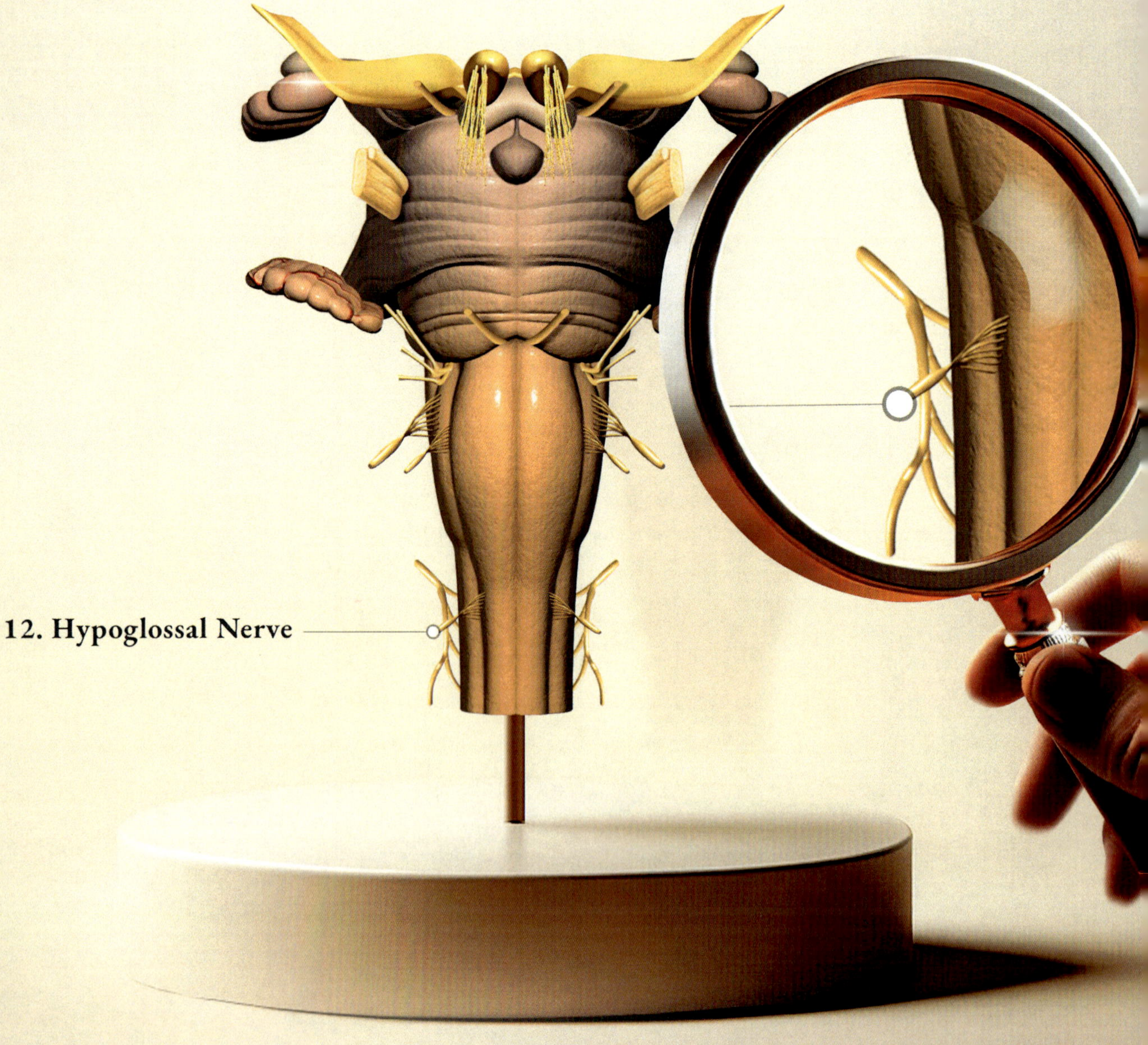

senses, expressions, and control of vital functions.

Cranial nerves, which emerge directly from the brain and brainstem, are different from spinal nerves like C1 that emerge from the spinal cord. However, some cranial nerves can have functional connections with the region where the C1 atlas vertebra is located, particularly through muscular and sensory pathways.

Cranial Nerves with Significant Connections to the Atlas C1 Region

The hypoglossal nerve, known as the XII cranial nerve, primarily innervates the muscles of the tongue, enabling important functions such as speech, swallowing, and manipulating food in the mouth. This nerve has a significant functional connection with C1 through anastomoses formed between the hypoglossal nerve and C1 [Image 1]. This connection allows for the coordination of some neck movements with tongue movements, which is crucial for harmonizing activities between these two regions.

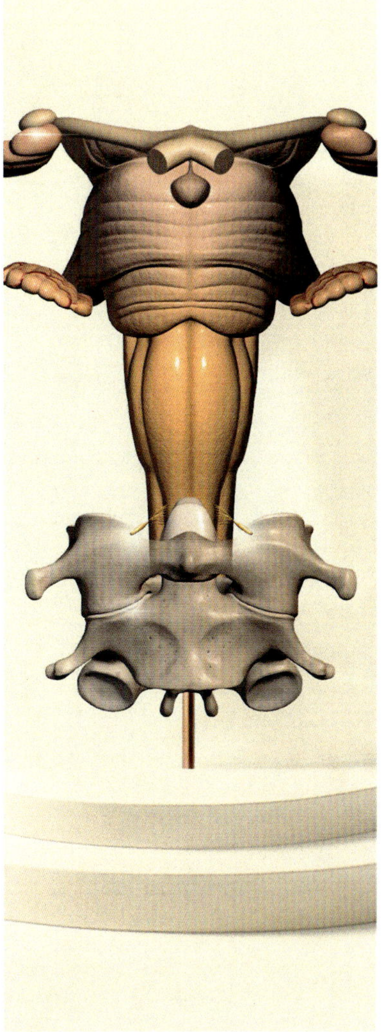

[Image 1] Hypoglossal nerve and C1

The accessory nerve, or XI cranial nerve, has a unique anatomical structure. Its cranial components emerge from the brainstem, while its spinal components emerge from the upper part of the spinal cord, pass through the foramen magnum, and join with the cranial components. This nerve innervates the sternocleidomastoid and upper parts of the trapezius muscles, which are in the vicinity of the atlas [Image 2]. The function of these muscles partially depends on the stability and position of the C1 vertebra, as a stable atlas allows for the proper functioning and coordination of the neck and shoulder muscles.

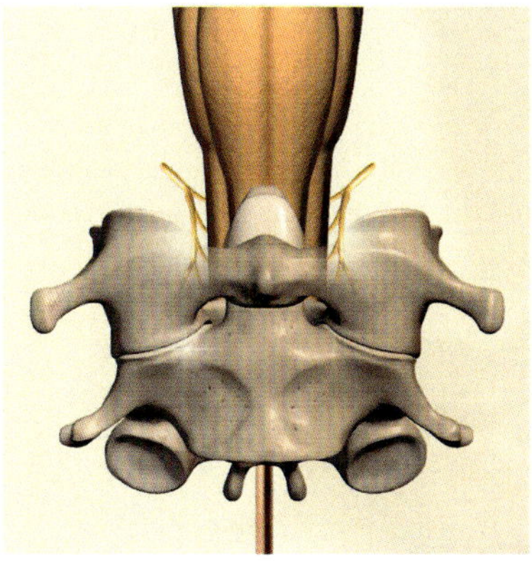

[Image 2] Accessory nerve and C1

The vagus nerve, known as the X cranial nerve, although not directly connected to C1, passes through the neck and has many branches that can be mechanically influenced by the position of the atlas. In the context of cervical manipulations or dislocations, the position of the atlas can affect the functionality of the vagus nerve [Image 1], which can cause various symptoms related to the autonomic functions this nerve controls, including heart rate, breathing, and digestive processes.

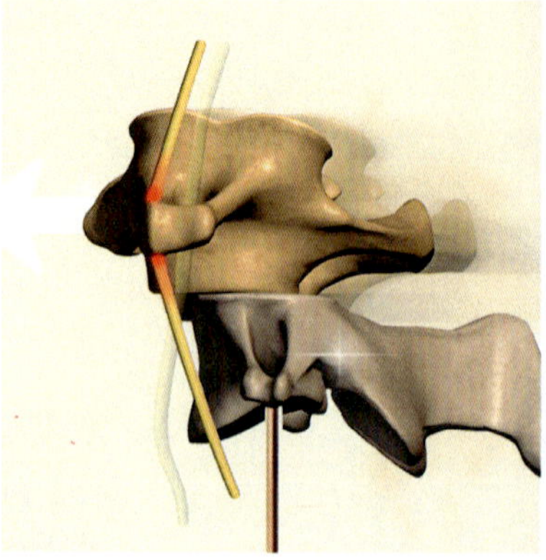

[Image 1] Atlas on vagus nerve

Although cranial nerves are not directly connected to C1 in terms of anatomical emergence, their functions and branches can be indirectly affected by the condition of the atlas vertebra. Disorders in the position of the atlas can cause pain, functional nerve impairments, or even specific neurological symptoms. Understanding these complex relationships is crucial for diagnosing and treating neurological problems that may be associated with the condition of the cervical spine.

Diagnosing through the observation of facial muscle impressions, which are connected to the 12 cranial nerves, provides deep insights into a patient's neurological health. Each cranial nerve has specific functions and innervates certain muscles and structures in the face and head. Observing the movements, tone, and symmetry of facial muscles can reveal important information about the functionality of these nerves.

Cranial nerves play a crucial role in controlling the muscles of the face, eyes, tongue, and neck. For example, the facial nerve (VII cranial nerve) controls facial expressions, while the hypoglossal nerve (XII cranial nerve) innervates the muscles of the tongue. Any dysfunction or asymmetry in the activities of these muscles can indicate problems with the corresponding cranial nerve.

When the atlas vertebra, the first cervical vertebra, is displaced or subluxated, it can put pressure on the nerves passing through the neck, including cranial nerves. This can interfere with the clear and uninterrupted flow of nerve impulses through the cranial nerves, resulting in various neurological symptoms. For example, if the facial nerve is affected by pressure due to atlas subluxation, the patient may exhibit asymmetry in facial expressions or have difficulty controlling facial muscles.

Diagnosing through the observation of facial muscle impressions involves carefully observing the patient's face while performing various movements, such as smiling, frowning, closing the eyes, or moving the tongue. This can accurately reveal the cause of the problem, identifying which nerve has impaired function. For example, an asymmetrical smile may indicate a problem with the facial nerve, while difficulties with tongue movements may indicate a problem with the hypoglossal nerve.

Connecting symptoms to the position of the atlas vertebra can be done through additional diagnostic tests, such as X-rays, magnetic resonance imaging (MRI), or computed tomography (CT) to determine if and to what extent there is atlas subluxation. However, the most precise diagnosis can be obtained through 3D scanning. If the atlas is displaced, therapies such as atlas vertebra adjustments directly address the cause of nerve compression, reducing pressure on the nerves and allowing for better nerve impulse flow.

Understanding the connection between facial muscle symptoms and the position of the atlas vertebra is crucial for a holistic approach to diagnosing and treating neurological disorders. Proper diagnosis and treatment can significantly improve patients' quality of life, allowing them to regain normal functions and reduce symptoms associated with cranial nerve dysfunction.

"Let your light so shine before men, that they may see your good works, and glorify your Father which is in heaven."

(Matthew 5:16)

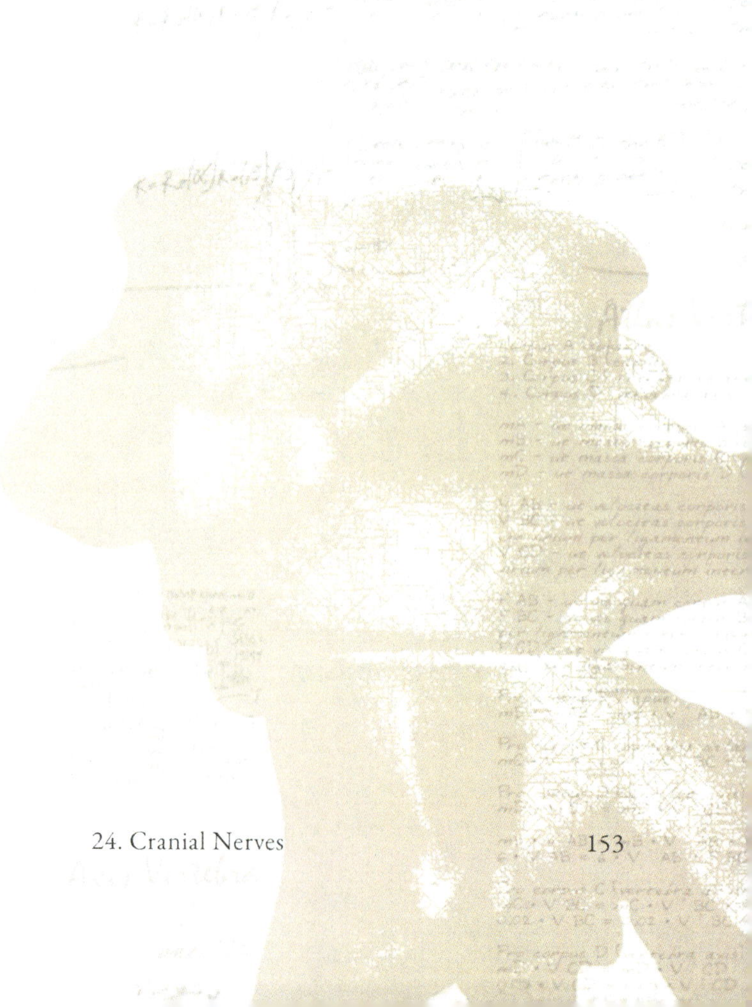

Foramina

Foramina, the openings in the skull, play a crucial role in allowing cranial nerves to pass from the brain to various parts of the head, neck, and body. During embryonic development, these openings form as part of the complex process of skull and head structure formation. In the early stages of embryogenesis, mesenchymal cells form cartilage that gradually mineralizes and shapes the bones of the skull, while the nerve canals and foramina are defined to facilitate the passage of cranial nerves. There are foramina located on both the upper [Image 1] and lower sides of the skull [Image 2].

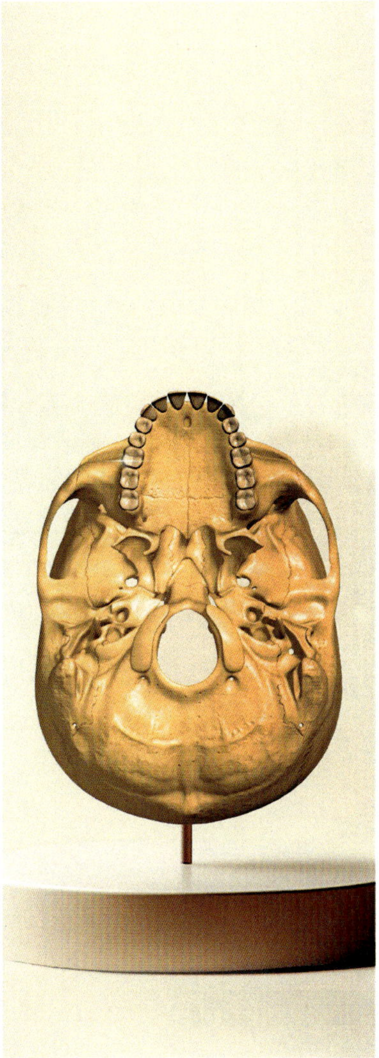

[Image 1] The upper foramina

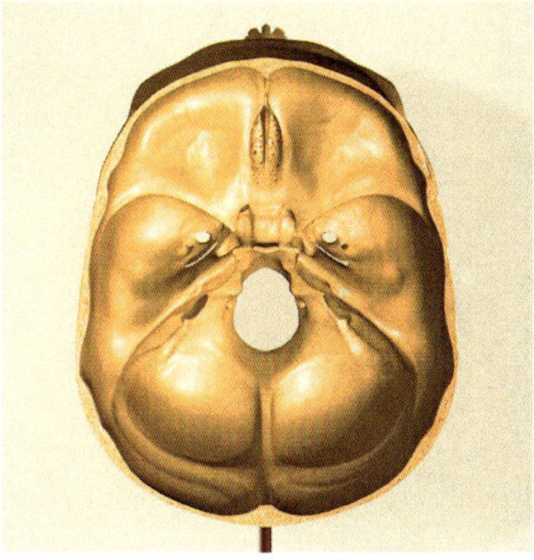

[Image 2] The lower foramina

Cranial nerves passing through specific foramina begin their journey in the brainstem, particularly from the medulla oblongata, and exit the skull to innervate different regions. The key foramina that cranial nerves pass through are:

1. **Foramen magnum:** The spinal accessory nerve (XI) passes through this large opening, innervating muscles of the neck and shoulders. The spinal cord also passes through the foramen magnum.

2. **Jugular foramen:** The glossopharyngeal nerve (IX), vagus nerve (X), and accessory nerve (XI) pass through this foramen. These nerves play essential roles in controlling the muscles of the pharynx, larynx, and tongue, as well as innervating internal organs via the vagus nerve.

3. **Hypoglossal canal:** The hypoglossal nerve (XII) passes through this canal, responsible for the motor innervation of the tongue muscles.

4. **Foramen ovale:** The mandibular branch of the trigeminal nerve (V3) passes through here, innervating the lower jaw and muscles of mastication.

5. Foramen rotundum: The maxillary branch of the trigeminal nerve (V2) passes through this foramen, innervating the upper jaw, teeth, and cheeks.

6. Superior orbital fissure: This fissure allows passage for nerves controlling the muscles of the eye, including the oculomotor nerve (III), trochlear nerve (IV), abducens nerve (VI), and the first branch of the trigeminal nerve (V1), which provides sensory information from the forehead and eyes.

7. Optic canal: The optic nerve (II) passes through this canal, carrying visual information from the eyes to the brain.

It is of utmost importance that our head remains in the correct anatomical position in relation to the atlas vertebra, as a misaligned atlas can lead to serious problems. When the atlas is not properly positioned, it can cause compression of the cranial nerves in the foramina through which they pass from the medulla oblongata to their final destinations. This compression can result in a range of health issues, including pain, reduced nerve function, and dysfunction in the body parts those nerves innervate. Proper atlas alignment is essential for nerve function and health.

In cases where cranial nerves are compressed in the foramina, there can also be physical damage to the Schwann cells that wrap around the nerves. Schwann cells play a crucial role in protecting and regenerating nerves, but when they are subjected to constant pressure and friction due to the misalignment of the atlas, the regeneration process becomes nearly impossible. Damage to these cells further complicates the condition, as without their full function, the nerves can suffer permanent damage, leading to more severe neurological problems and a diminished quality of life for the patient.

1. Foramen Magnum

The foramen magnum, the largest foramen in the skull, is located at the base of the occipital bone. It serves as the passage for the spinal cord, connecting it to the brainstem. Additionally, the vertebral arteries, spinal arteries, and accessory nerves (XI) pass through this opening. The foramen magnum is critical for the central nervous system, providing the main conduit for neural and vascular connections between the brain and spinal cord. Its size and location are crucial for neurological and circulatory functions.

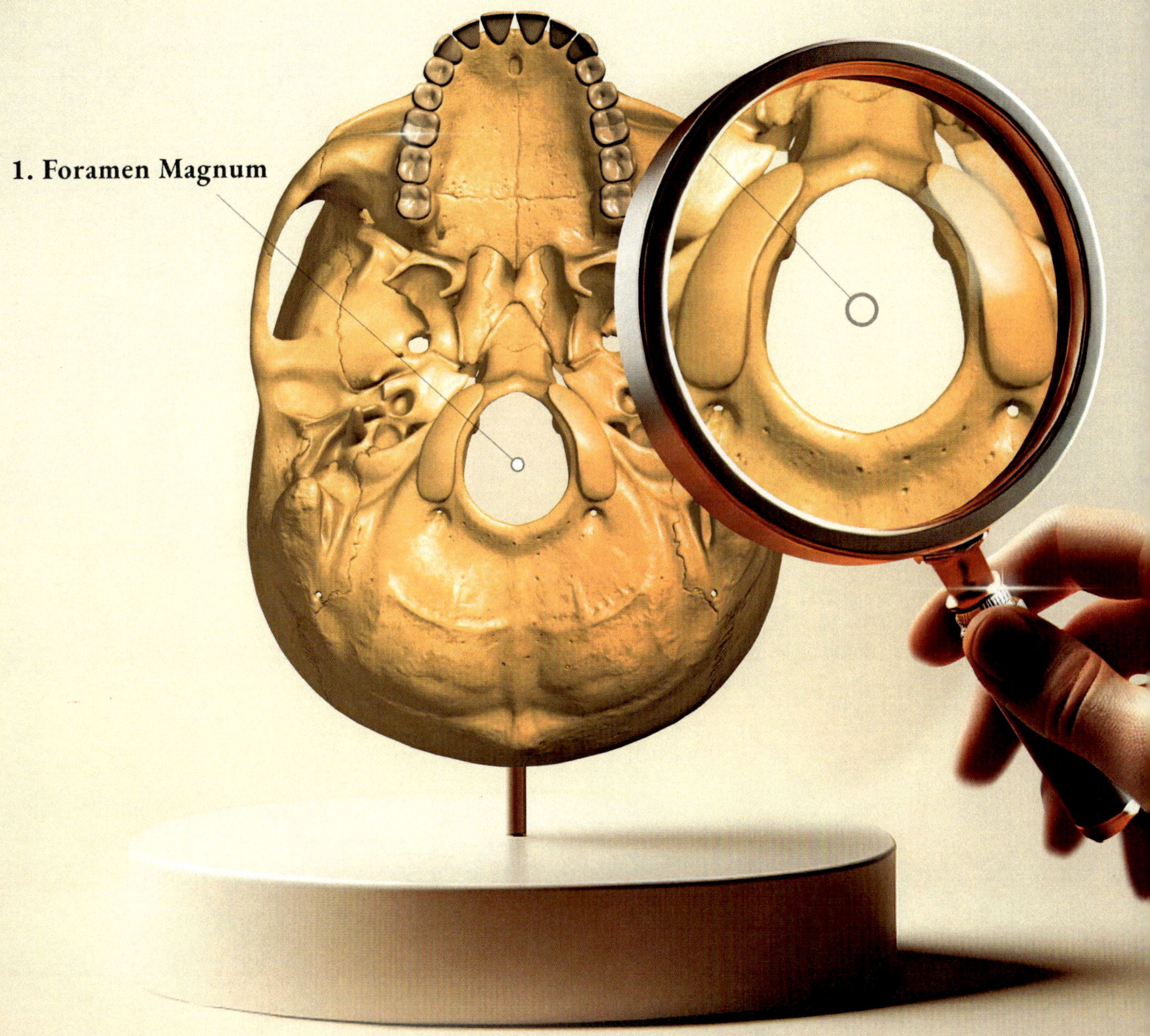

2. Jugular Foramen

The jugular foramen, a large, irregular opening between the temporal and occipital bones, allows passage of the glossopharyngeal nerve (IX), vagus nerve (X), and accessory nerve (XI). The internal jugular vein also exits the skull through this foramen. These nerves are essential for swallowing, speech, and head and shoulder movements. The jugular foramen's complex anatomy and role in neurovascular transmission make it significant in clinical and anatomical studies.

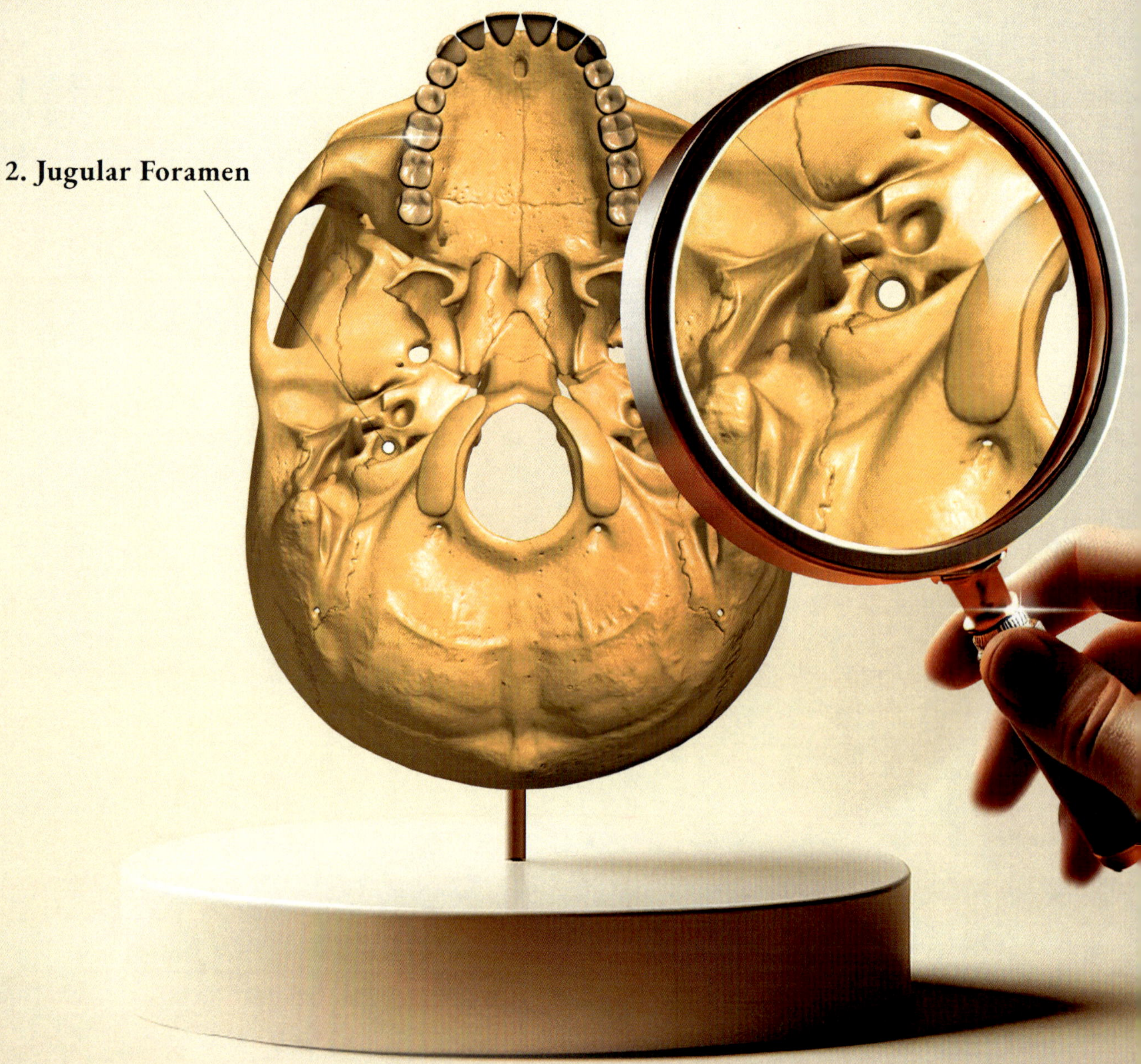

3. Hypoglossal Canal

The hypoglossal canal, an opening in the occipital bone near the foramen magnum, allows passage of the hypoglossal nerve (XII). This nerve provides motor innervation to the tongue muscles, crucial for movements necessary for speech, swallowing, and maintaining tongue position at rest. The canal's precise location and pathway are vital for the hypoglossal nerve's function, making it important in the study of cranial nerve anatomy and understanding tongue motor control.

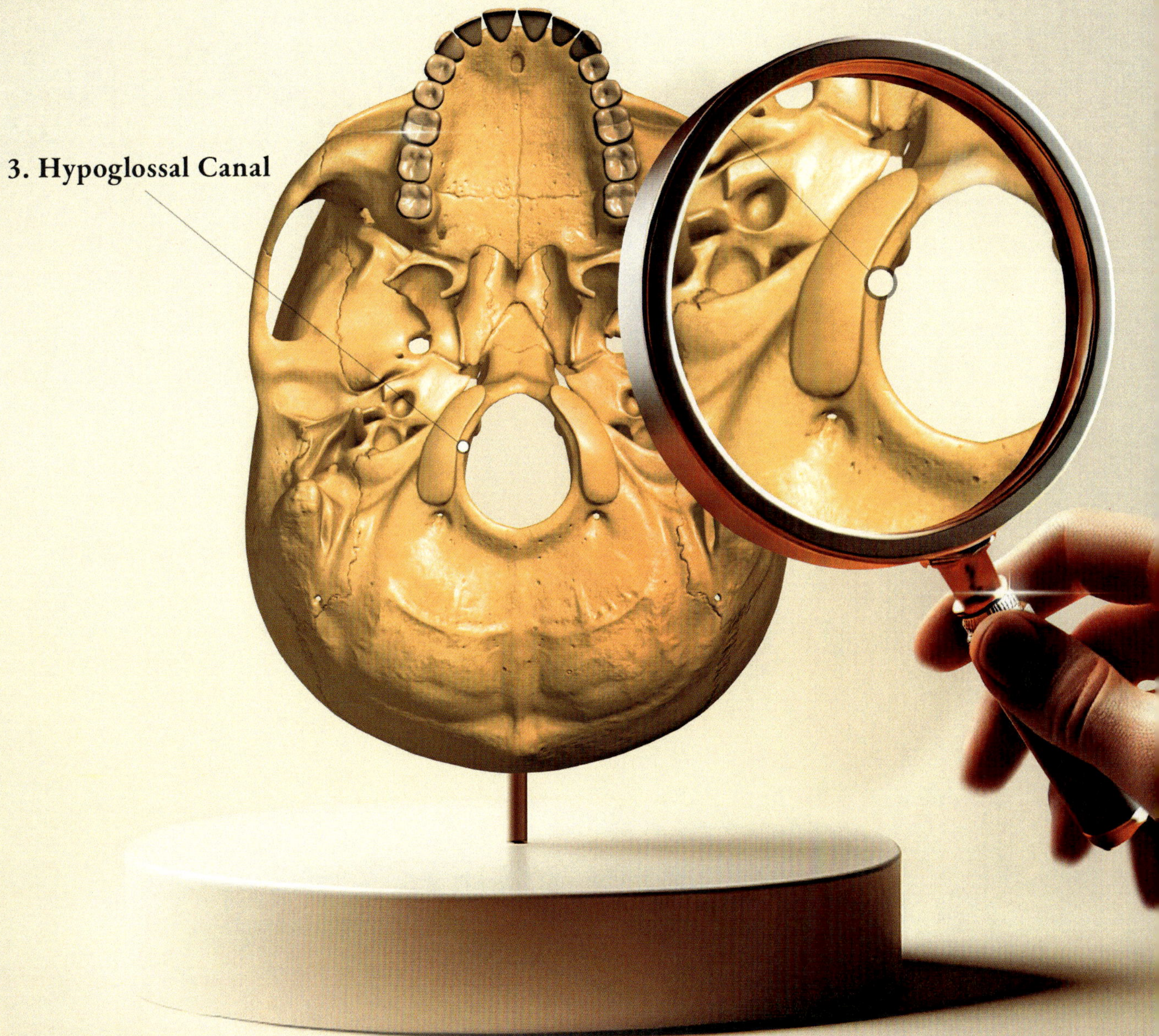

4. Foramen Ovale

The foramen ovale, located in the sphenoid bone at the base of the skull, allows the passage of the mandibular branch of the trigeminal nerve (V3), which is responsible for sensory information from the lower face and motor functions of chewing. It also transmits the accessory meningeal artery and occasionally an emissary vein from the cavernous sinus. This foramen is essential for the innervation of the lower jaw, teeth, and some muscles involved in mastication, supporting both sensory and motor functions.

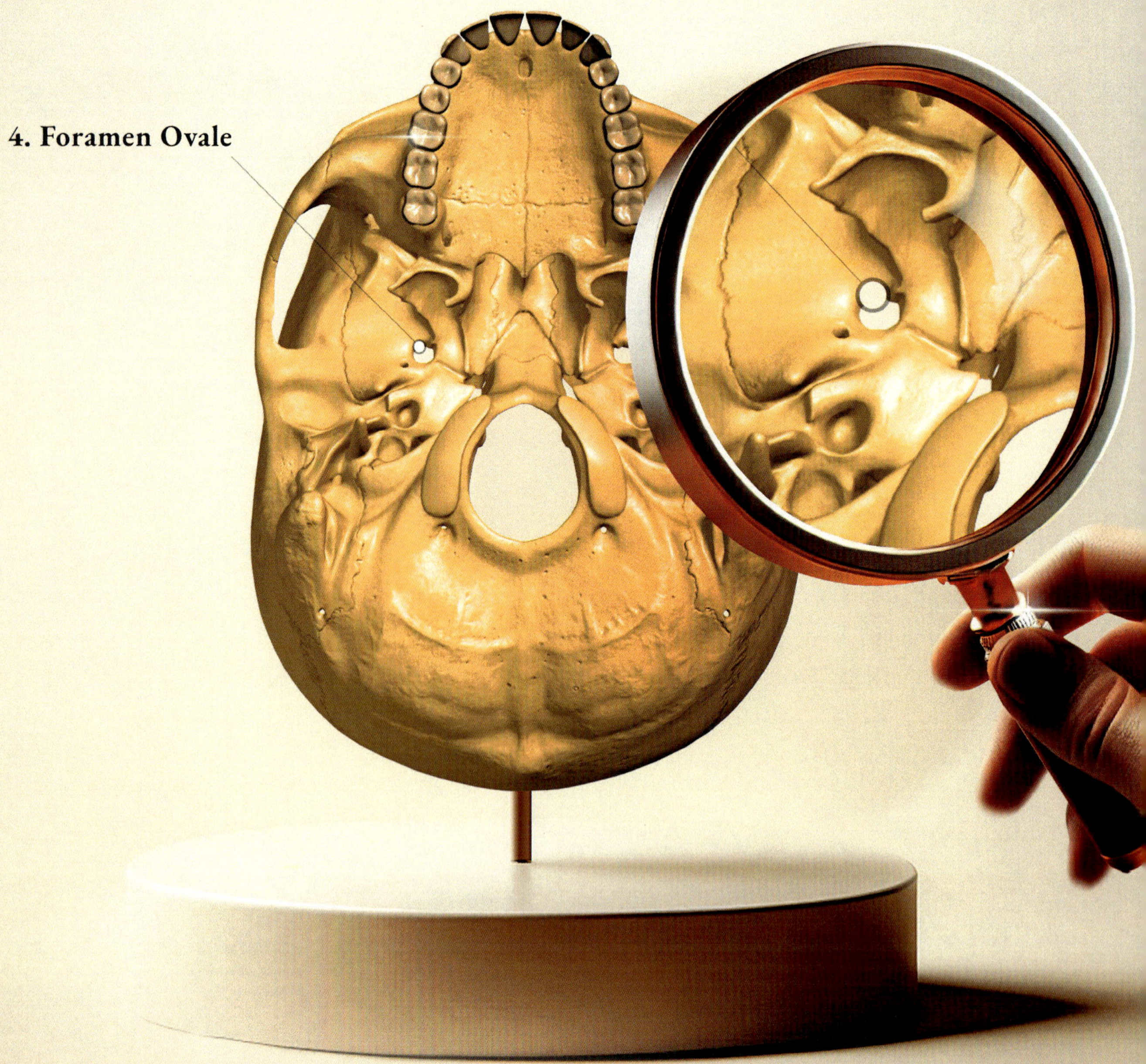

5. Foramen Rotundum

The foramen rotundum, located in the sphenoid bone, allows passage of the maxillary branch of the trigeminal nerve (V2). This nerve transmits sensory information from the midface, including the lower eyelid, upper lip, and cheek. It plays a crucial role in midface innervation, enabling sensations like touch, pain, and temperature. The foramen rotundum is significant in anatomical studies and clinical procedures, serving as a landmark for understanding facial innervation and for treating facial pain.

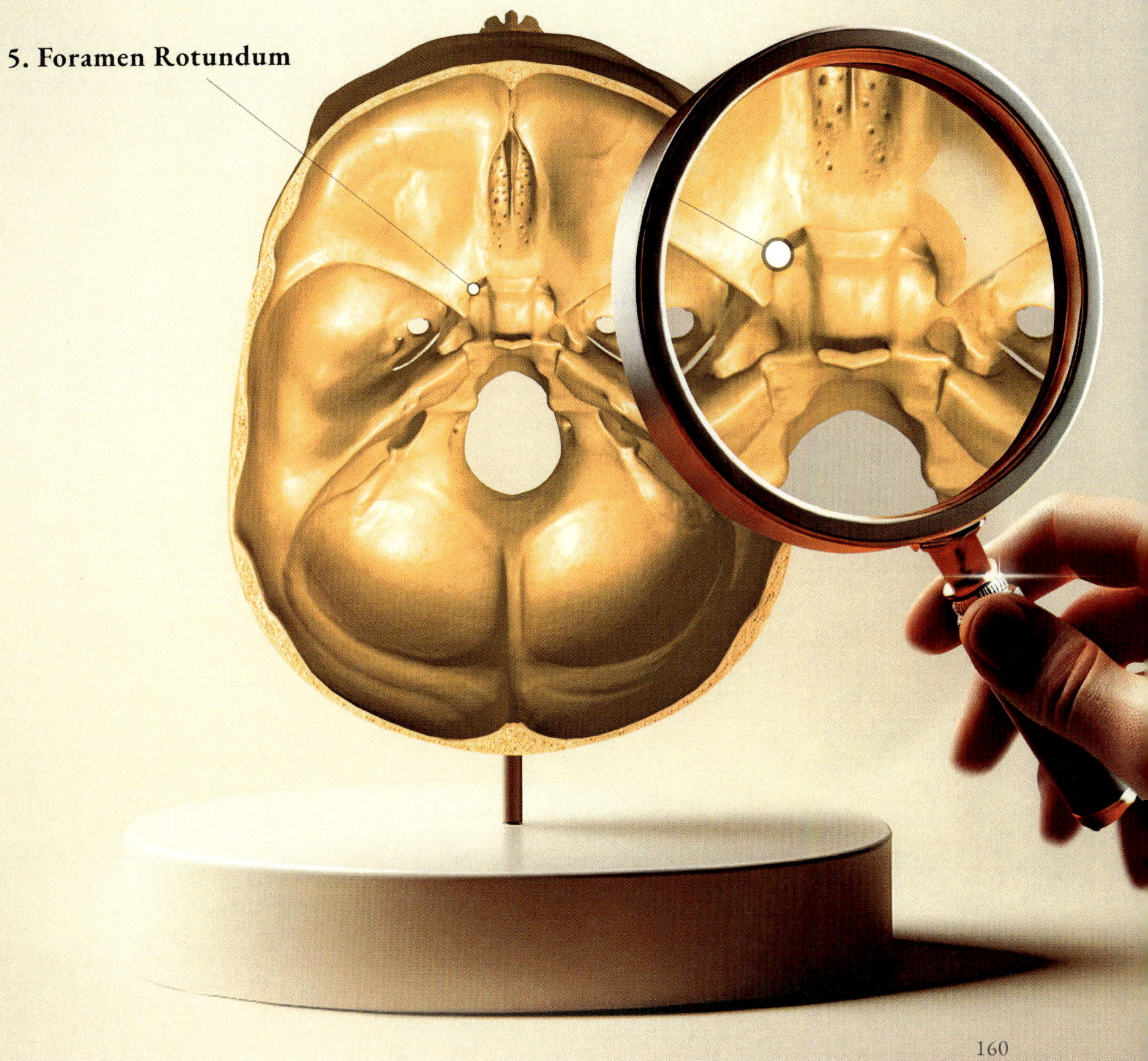

6. Foramen Rotundum

The interior of the skull contains foramina, openings for nerves and blood vessels. Two key foramina are the foramen rotundum, transmitting sensory information from the midface via the maxillary branch of the trigeminal nerve (V2), and the internal acoustic meatus, through which the facial nerve (VII) and vestibulocochlear nerve (VIII) pass, responsible for facial expressions, hearing, and balance. These foramina are essential for the flow of information and nutrients between the brain and the body.

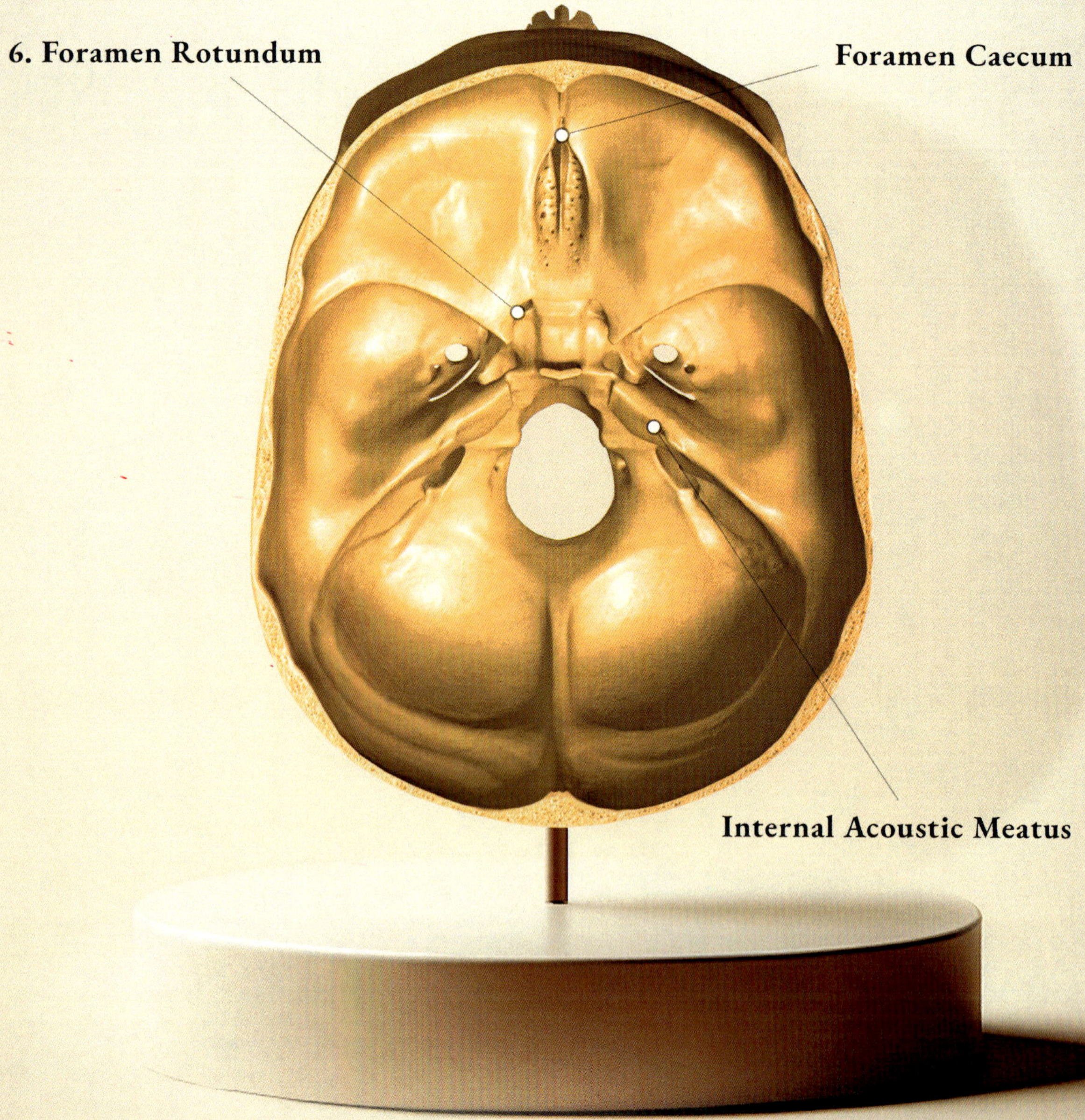

7. Optic canal

The left and right optic canals are crucial openings in the sphenoid bone of the skull, through which the optic nerves (cranial nerve II) pass, allowing them to travel from the eyes to the brain, enabling vision by transmitting visual information. Each optic canal serves as an entry point for the optic nerve, as well as the ophthalmic artery, which supplies blood to the eye. Proper function of these canals is essential for vision, as they provide a clear pathway for nerve signals between the retina and the brain.

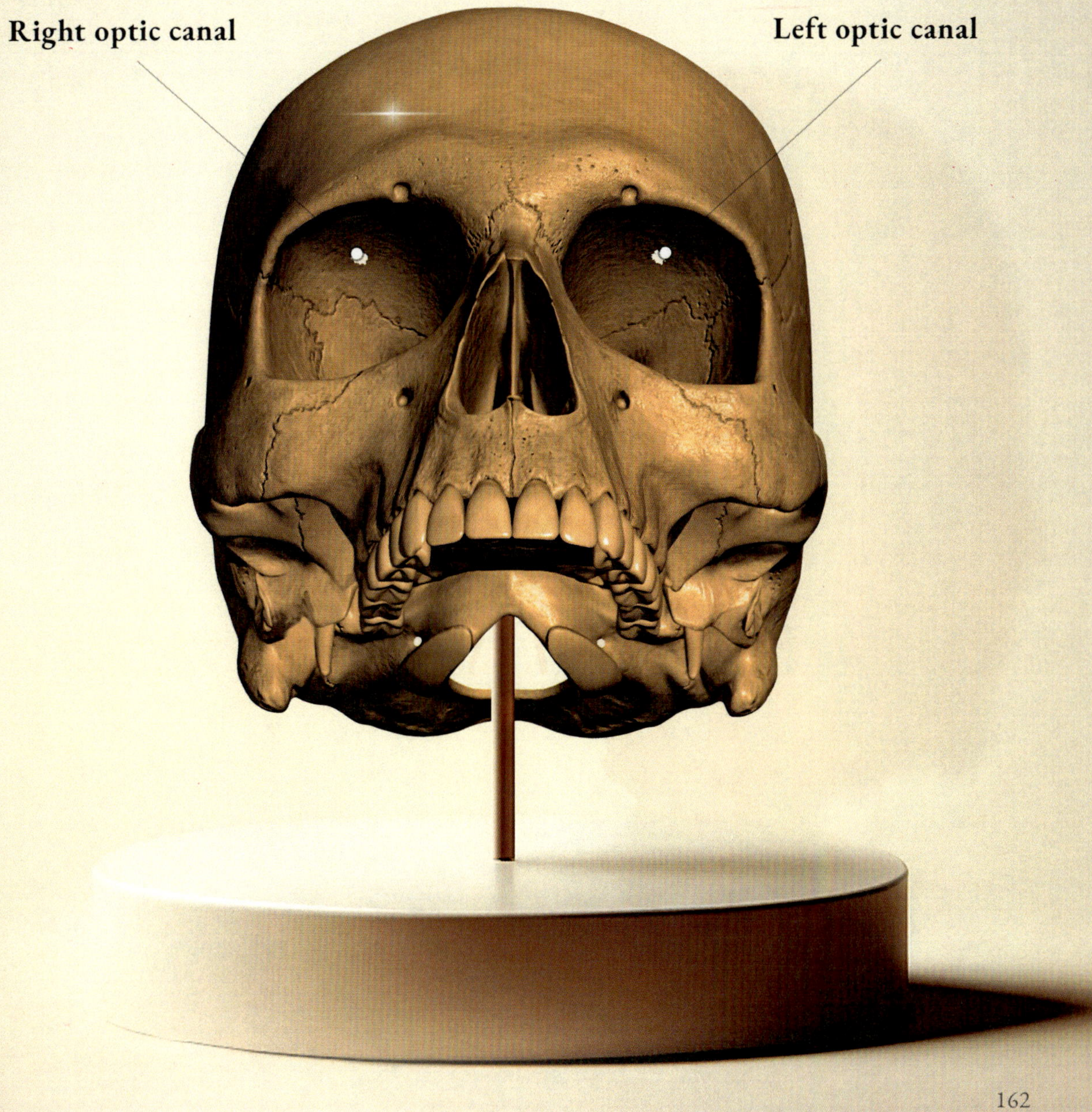

Development and Maturation of the Atlas

Development of the atlas vertebra encompasses a complex process spanning from the embryonic stage to the formation of mature bone, involving bone formation and fusion, as well as anatomical changes throughout the lifespan.

During the embryonic stage, the atlas vertebra begins to take shape as part of early embryogenesis, where mesenchymal cells differentiate and begin to form the cartilaginous groundwork that will later become bone. Throughout embryonic development, neural crest cells play a pivotal role in this process. Originating from the neural crest, these cells migrate into surrounding tissues and provide signals for bone and other structure formation.

As the embryo grows and develops, the cartilaginous foundation of the atlas vertebra gradually mineralizes, transforming into bone. This process of mineralization, known as osteogenesis, is influenced by various factors, including genetic factors and mechanical forces acting on the embryo during development.

During fetal development, different regions of the atlas vertebra begin to fuse, forming mature bones. This fusion process, known as osteofication, results in the formation of distinct anatomical structures such as lateral mass processes, articular surfaces, and the vertebral foramen.

After birth, the atlas vertebra continues to develop and change as the child grows. Gradually, the bones become stronger and denser, while the formation of anatomical features characteristic of the atlas vertebra is completed. During childhood and adolescence, the atlas undergoes further refinement as it adapts to the mechanical demands of movement and posture.

Why the Atlas and Axis Lack an Intervertebral Disc

Unlike the other vertebrae in the spine, there is no intervertebral disc between the atlas and the axis. This absence is not incidental but is instead a specific adaptation to their function. Intervertebral discs serve as shock absorbers between vertebrae, allowing flexibility and mobility while absorbing pressure. However, the atlas and axis do not require this type of cushioning because their primary function is not to bear vertical loads like the lower vertebrae.

Instead, the atlas and axis are designed to provide significant mobility to the head, particularly rotation. As such, their joint is structured to be strong and stable, achieved through direct contact between bony structures supported by strong ligaments. The dens of the axis allows the atlas to rotate around it, creating a specialized joint that would be hindered by the presence of a disc, as discs primarily facilitate bending and flexion rather than rotation.

In the absence of a disc, the stability and mobility of the atlas and axis are maintained by a complex system of ligaments. The atlantoaxial and atlanto-occipital ligaments hold these vertebrae securely in place, allowing them to move in line with the needs of the head without losing stability. These ligaments prevent excessive movement and dislocation, which is especially important given the proximity of the spinal cord and cranial nerves.

The absence of a disc between the atlas and axis can be seen as a creative advantage. Humans and many mammals have this specific anatomy to allow rotational movements of the head, which is crucial for survival. For example, quickly rotating the head enables rapid response to potential threats. A disc between these vertebrae would limit mobility, thereby reducing the efficiency of such movements.

Intervertebral Discs of the Neck

Intervertebral discs of the neck are cartilaginous structures located between the cervical vertebrae (C1-C7). They act as shock absorbers, allowing flexibility and mobility of the spine while absorbing impacts and pressure. These discs also help maintain proper spacing between the vertebrae, protecting the spinal cord and nerve roots. Degeneration or injury to these discs can cause herniation and pain.

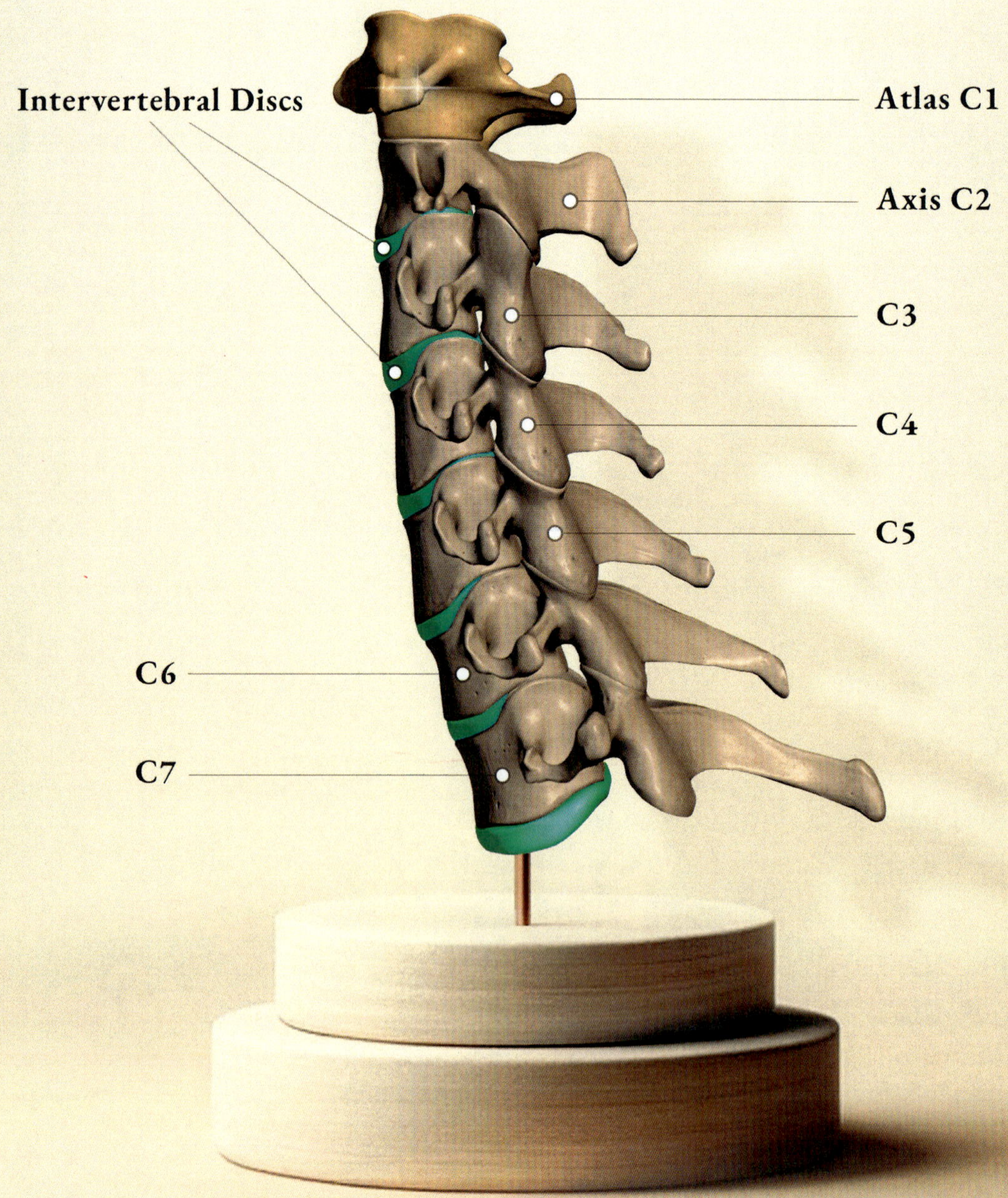

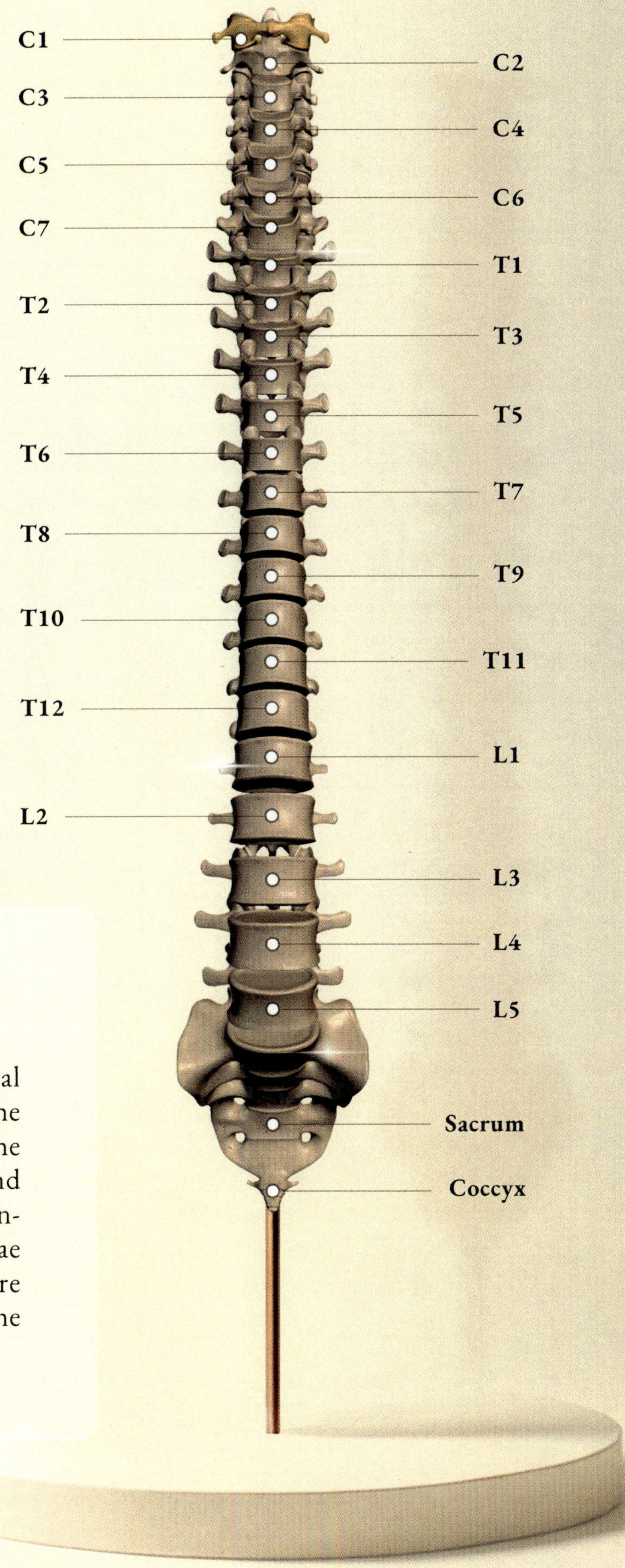

Anterior

The anterior view of the vertebral column shows the front aspect of the spine. This perspective highlights the vertebral bodies, which support and bear the body's weight. The alignment and structure of the vertebrae are crucial for maintaining posture and flexibility. This view shows the correct alignment of the vertebrae.

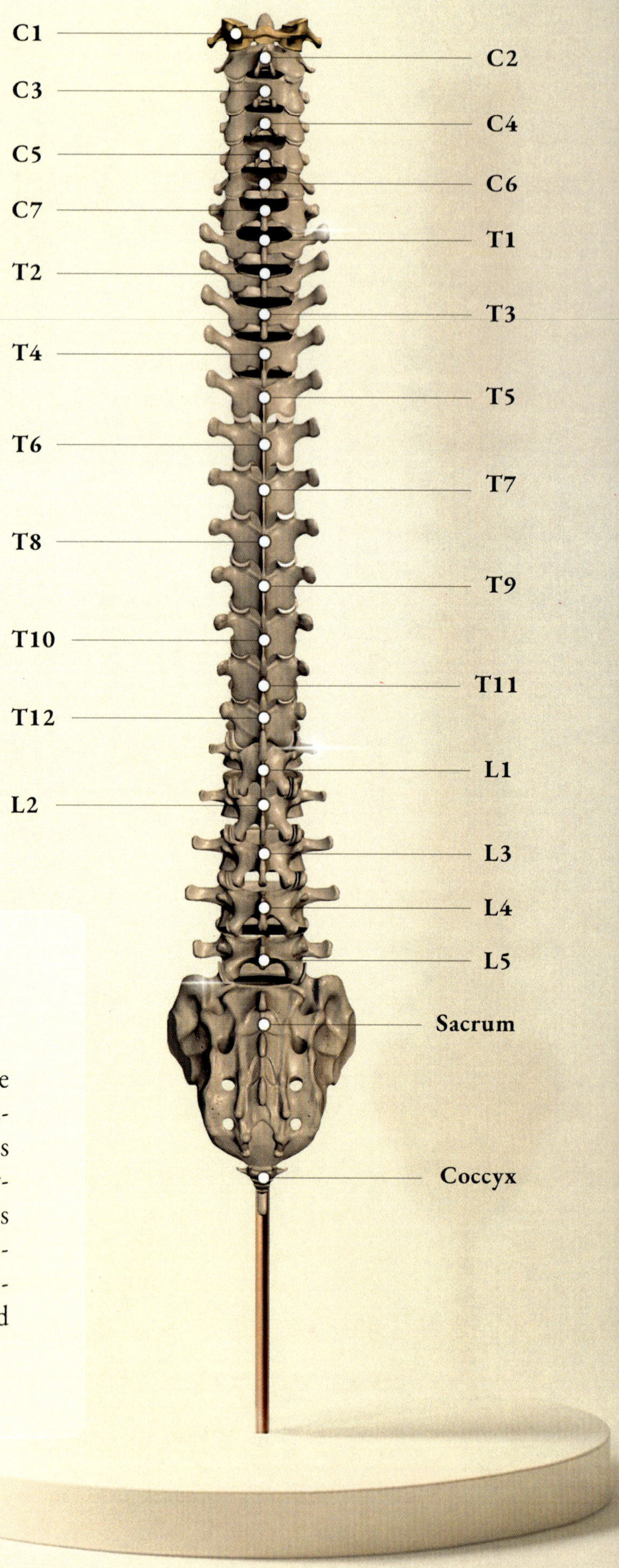

Posterior

This perspective highlights the spinous processes, the bony projections felt along the back. It reveals the alignment of vertebrae and intervertebral foramina, allowing nerves to exit the spinal cord. Proper alignment is crucial for maintaining posture, protecting the spinal cord, and ensuring flexibility and movement.

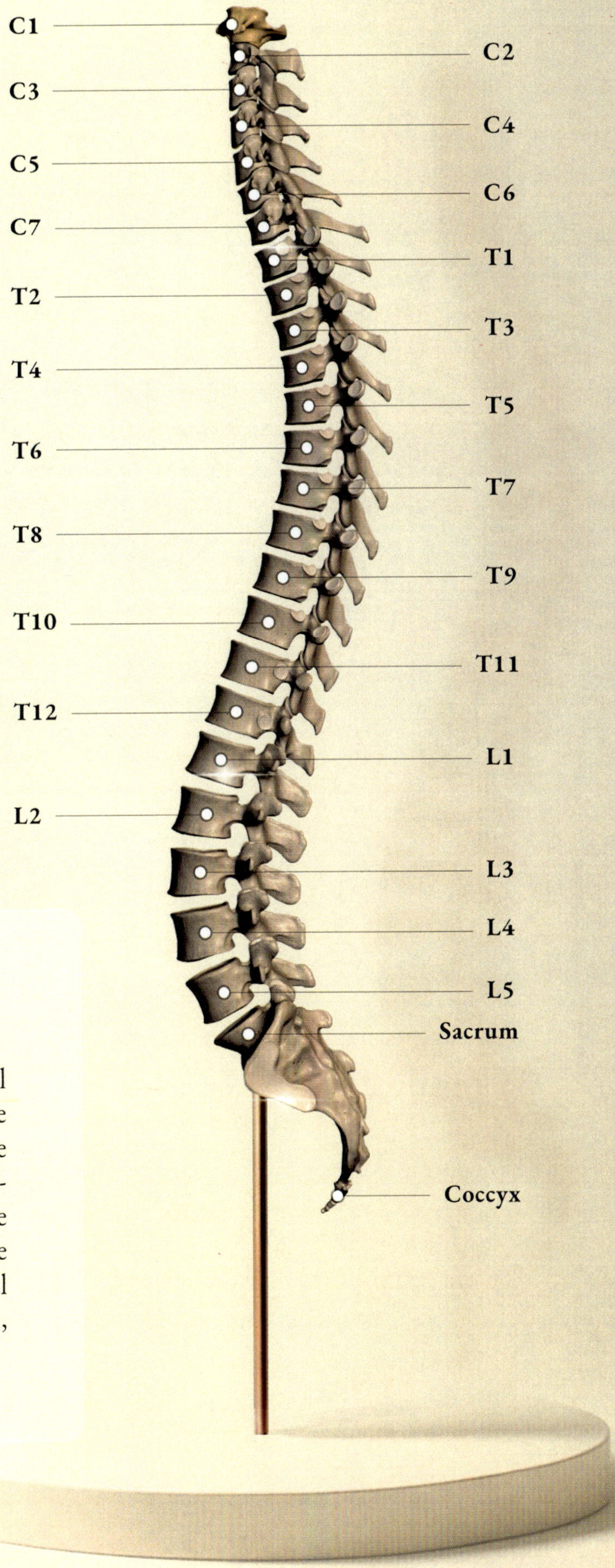

Lateral

In the lateral view of the vertebral column, the correct alignment of the spine is best seen, particularly the proper lordosis and kyphosis. Lordosis is the natural inward curve in the cervical and lumbar regions of the spine, while kyphosis is the natural outward curve in the thoracic region, providing essential support.

Pathologies of the Atlas

Atlas vertebra pathologies encompass a wide range of disorders that can significantly impact the function and structure of this crucial part of the spine. This subsection explores various pathological conditions associated with the atlas vertebra, including congenital abnormalities, traumatic injuries, degenerative changes, and tumor processes.

Congenital abnormalities of the atlas vertebra may manifest as various anatomical variations or developmental defects that can cause dysfunction or irregularities in structure. These disorders may involve underdevelopment of certain parts of the atlas, irregularities in shape or size, as well as other genetically determined anomalies that can affect the function of this vertebra.

Traumatic injuries to the atlas vertebra are often associated with serious consequences, including fractures, dislocations, and ligament injuries. Such injuries can result in destabilization of the atlas, leading to pain, reduced neck mobility, and potential neurological complications.

Degenerative changes, such as osteoarthritis or disc degeneration, can also affect the atlas vertebra over time. Loss of cartilage tissue, the appearance of osteophytes, or ligament degeneration can result in changes in the structure and function of the atlas, leading to pain, stiffness, and reduced neck mobility.

Tumor processes in the vicinity of the atlas vertebra can pose a serious threat to the integrity of this vertebra and surrounding structures. Primary bone tumors or metastases from other tumors can cause compression of nerve structures, destabilization of the atlas, and other serious consequences.

Understanding the various pathological conditions of the atlas vertebra is crucial for timely diagnosis, treatment, and prevention of complications. An interdisciplinary approach involving orthopedic, neurological, and other medical experts is essential for effectively managing these pathologies and preserving spinal and neck function.

"The question is not how severe the illness is, but how strong the person is."

(Paracelsus)

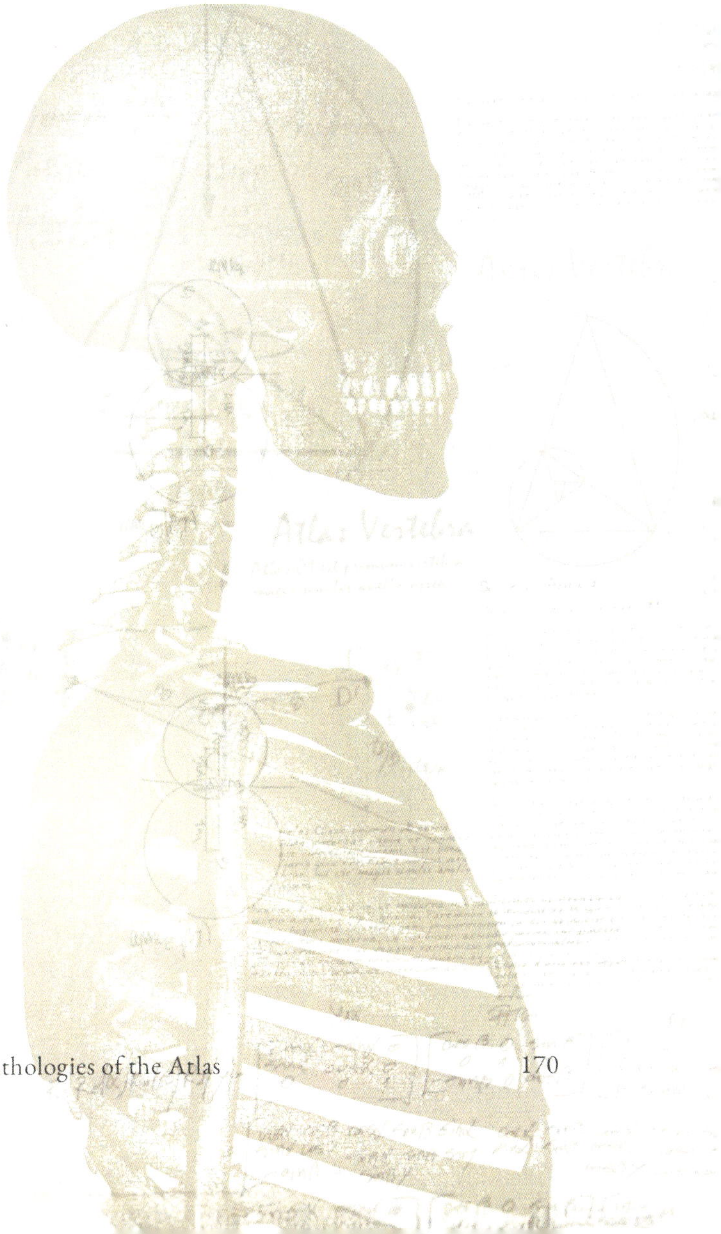

Chapter 2

Causes of Problems

Causes of Problems

In the realm of healthcare, exploring the causes of problems stands as a pivotal step towards finding effective solutions and achieving optimal health and well-being. Every health condition, regardless of its nature, stems from various factors that intertwine and influence our overall state. In this chapter, we will delve into six key areas crucial for understanding the causes of problems.

Firstly, we will explore risk factors that may serve as potential triggers for health issues. Subsequently, we will turn our attention to the intricate interplay between genetics and the environment, considering how inherited factors and life circumstances shape our health destiny.

Psychological factors also hold paramount importance in our health. We will uncover how our emotional and mental well-being can impact the physical state of our bodies, and vice versa.

We must not overlook the physical causes of problems. Injuries, illnesses, and abnormalities can significantly affect our health, as well as poor habits and irregularities in diet and lifestyle.

Social and cultural factors are also integral pieces of the puzzle. Through their examination, we will grasp how our surroundings, economic opportunities, and social relationships can shape our health challenges.

Lastly, we will explore the interplay of these factors to deepen our understanding, paving the way for more effective health solutions and holistic well-being.

Traumatic Atlas Injuries

Traumatic injuries of the atlas vertebra encompass a spectrum of incidents, each presenting unique challenges and consequences. Among the primary physical causes of atlas displacement are accidents, falls, sports-related injuries, and other mishaps.

Accidents, such as motor vehicle collisions or workplace incidents, can exert significant force on the cervical spine, resulting in sudden and forceful movements that may displace the atlas vertebra. The impact of such accidents can cause ligamentous damage, fractures, or subluxations, leading to instability and misalignment of the atlas.

Similarly, falls from heights or slips can subject the cervical spine to abrupt and unnatural forces, potentially causing traumatic injuries to the atlas vertebra. Whether from a misstep on uneven terrain or a fall from a ladder, the sudden jolt to the neck can disrupt the delicate balance of the spine, predisposing the atlas to displacement.

Sports-related injuries represent another common cause of traumatic injuries to the atlas vertebra. High-impact sports, such as football, rugby, or gymnastics, pose inherent risks of collisions, falls, and abrupt movements that can affect the cervical spine. A mistimed tackle, a fall during a routine, or a collision with an opponent can all contribute to trauma to the atlas vertebra, necessitating careful evaluation and management.

Moreover, other unfortunate accidents, such as recreational mishaps or unforeseen incidents, can also result in traumatic injuries to the atlas vertebra. Whether from a slip on the ice, a household accident, or a recreational activity gone awry, the consequences of such events can have lasting effects on spinal health.

Traumatic injuries to the atlas most commonly occur during childhood, when children are learning new skills and actively exploring their world. Falls during the development of certain skills, such as biking, rollerblading, skateboarding, sledding, and skiing, are a common cause of these injuries. As children learn to balance and coordinate movements, inevitable falls can result in traumatic injuries to the neck, including the atlas vertebra.

In later adolescence, when teenagers engage in activities that require physical exertion and skill, atlas injuries may occur in the context of sports activities. In sports such as football, basketball, or gymnastics, where rapid movements and sudden impacts are common, there is a greater risk of neck injuries. Martial arts can also expose young people to the risk of atlas injuries, particularly during training or competition.

In addition to sports activities, restless adolescence and experimentation with various activities can also lead to accidents resulting in neck injuries. Jumping from heights, climbing trees, or riding fast vehicles without proper protection can expose young people to the risk of atlas vertebra injuries.

In all of these situations, it is crucial to provide children and young adults with adequate education on safety and the proper use of protective equipment. It is also important to encourage responsible behavior during activities and provide adult supervision during risky skills. Through education, attention, and preventive measures, we can reduce the risk of traumatic injuries to the atlas and ensure safe growth for children and young people. Let me note, the problem isn't the high speed, the problem is the sudden stop.

Traumatic injuries to the atlas vertebra most commonly occur in later stages of life as a result of traffic accidents. In these instances, the forces exerted on the cervical spine during high-speed collisions can lead to severe and sometimes life-altering injuries, including those affecting the atlas vertebra.

Traffic accidents, whether involving cars, motorcycles, or other vehicles, pose a significant risk of traumatic injuries to the cervical spine. The sudden impact and rapid deceleration associated with collisions can cause the neck to undergo extreme forces, resulting in fractures, dislocations, or other types of trauma to the atlas vertebra.

The severity of these injuries can vary widely, depending on factors such as the speed of the vehicles involved, the angle of impact, and the use of safety restraints. In some cases, traumatic injuries to the atlas may result in immediate symptoms, such as neck pain, stiffness, or neurological deficits. In more severe cases, these injuries can lead to long-term complications, including chronic pain, disability, and impaired mobility.

Recovery from traumatic injuries to the atlas vertebra often requires comprehensive medical intervention, including immobilization of the neck, pain management, and rehabilitation therapy. In cases of severe injury, surgical intervention may be necessary to stabilize the spine and restore function.

Preventing traumatic injuries to the atlas vertebra in traffic accidents requires a multi-faceted approach, including efforts to improve road safety, promote the use of seat belts and other safety restraints, and raise awareness about the dangers of distracted or impaired driving. By addressing these factors, we can work towards reducing the incidence of traumatic injuries to the atlas vertebra and minimizing their impact on individuals' lives.

In many of the aforementioned cases, the key cause of atlas displacement lies in the fact that attention is often directed towards pain or injuries in other parts of the body following a collision or accident. In those moments, few consider the potential consequences of head inertia during sudden jerks or impacts, which can lead to dislocation of the atlas vertebra.

Head inertia, occurring when the body abruptly stops or changes direction of movement, can induce rapid and uncontrolled movements of the neck. During collisions or accidents, when focus is often on other aspects of injury, this sudden head movement can result in the displacement of the atlas, even if no pain or discomfort is felt at that moment.

Another factor contributing to the disregard of atlas dislocation is that this type of injury often does not cause significant pain. Unlike other injuries that are immediately noticeable and painful, atlas dislocation may go unnoticed or be misconstrued as mild discomfort. As a result, the issue of atlas dislocation may be neglected or completely overlooked.

It is important to understand that even when atlas dislocation does not cause pronounced pain, it can have serious health consequences and lead to various problems, including balance disorders, neck and back pain, as well as neurological complications.

Therefore, it is crucial to raise awareness about the potential dangers of atlas dislocation, especially in situations where attention is directed towards other aspects of injury. Education about the importance of timely and adequate diagnosis and treatment of this type of injury can play a key role in preventing long-term consequences and promoting the health of the cervical spine and the overall body.

"Let every disease that afflicts the body be healed together with the mind."

(Plato)

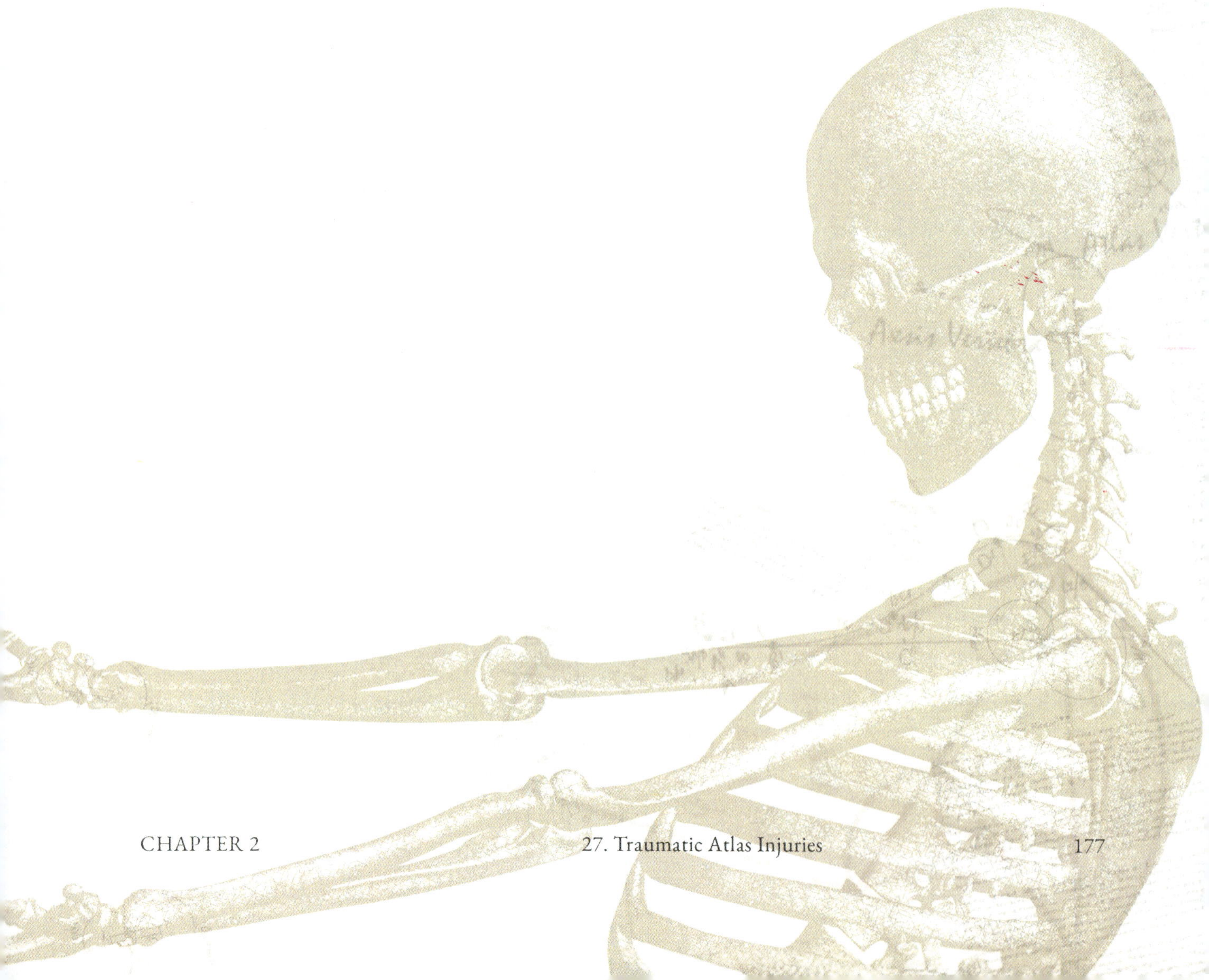

Genetics, Habits, and Health

Poor genetics, coupled with unhealthy habits and negative role models, can significantly influence not only our own health but also the health of future generations. Understanding how these factors intersect and their potential repercussions is crucial for fostering a healthier lifestyle and promoting well-being.

Genetics plays a fundamental role in shaping our predispositions and susceptibilities to various health conditions. When choosing a partner, particularly one with a promiscuous orientation and no insight into their genetic predispositions, the implications for offspring can be profound. Traits associated with promiscuity may be inherited, potentially increasing the risk of genetic disorders or health complications in the next generation.

Furthermore, environmental factors and unhealthy habits can exacerbate these genetic predispositions, leading to a myriad of health issues. For example, promoting irregularities in diet and obesity, where pressure on the spine in the abdomen area can lead to a decrease in agility and hinder previously acquired motor skills. The environment we are exposed to, coupled with our own habits, can shape our physical well-being in profound ways.

Negative role models in our environment can also exert a significant influence on our behaviors and habits. When we observe and emulate behaviors that prioritize risky activities for entertainment, such as headfirst diving or other daring stunts applauded by the crowd, we may inadvertently jeopardize our spinal health. These behaviors not only pose immediate risks but can also contribute to long-term consequences, including traumatic effects on the position of our atlas vertebra.

The consequences of these factors can be far-reaching, potentially impacting the alignment and stability of our atlas vertebra, with profound implications for our overall health and well-being. By recognizing the interplay between genetics, habits, and role models, we can take proactive steps to mitigate risks, foster healthier lifestyles, and promote a more resilient spine for ourselves and future generations.

If we delve deeper into the connection between genetics, the position of the atlas, and even the concept of telegony, we would uncover a fascinating link between HOX genes (developmental genes) and the position of the atlas vertebra in infants. HOX genes play a crucial role in the proper segmentation and formation of the body during embryonic development, including the spinal column and the positioning of vertebrae such as the atlas. Any alteration in the expression of HOX genes can lead to misalignment of the atlas, potentially affecting biomechanical stability, neural communication, and overall health later in life.

Telegony, which suggests that genetic influences from previous parental experiences can affect offspring, may further complicate this picture. For example, if parents pass on genetic predispositions for weaker atlas formation or other spinal developmental abnormalities, it could result in long-term consequences for the baby's atlas position. This interplay between genetics, atlas development, and potential influences from telegony offers a broader understanding of prenatal development and its impact on an infant's future health.

This relationship underscores the importance of both genetic inheritance and external factors in spinal development, as early atlas misalignments can have lasting effects on posture, nervous system function, and overall well-being.

High-Risk Jobs and Atlas Injuries

High-risk occupations encompass fields where workers are exposed to potentially hazardous situations and factors that can jeopardize their health and safety. These individuals often face machine vibrations, momentary lapses in traffic, or are actively engaged in activities carrying the risk of traumatic injuries, including atlas vertebra displacement.

Professional drivers and heavy machinery operators contend with daily exposure to machine vibrations transmitted to their bodies during work. Moreover, momentary lapses in traffic can lead to accidents where atlas vertebra displacement is nearly a hundred percent certain. These injuries can have serious implications for spine health and functionality. While many perceive high-speed driving as thrilling or even necessary for reaching destinations quickly, the truth is that speed itself isn't necessarily hazardous. What makes driving dangerous are the sudden and unpredictable moments, such as abrupt stops or unexpected obstacles on the road. To safeguard against these risks, it's crucial to adapt our driving to road conditions and exercise additional caution while on the road.

Builders and construction workers represent another group frequently confronted with risky working environments. Improper and frequent head positioning, without planned breaks, rest, and relaxation, can lead to lasting spinal damage. Prolonged periods of improper head positioning, where the head frequently tilts towards the ceiling or floor, can lead to displacement of the atlas vertebra and other serious neck injuries.

Professional athletes, particularly those engaged in team sports involving frequent body collisions, falls, and head jerks, as well as extreme sports like boxing, martial arts, or motorcycle riding, are also susceptible to the risk of traumatic atlas vertebra injuries. Regardless of the type of activity, such athletes often face situations that can result in serious neck and spine injuries.

These examples illustrate the complexity of high-risk occupations and the need for preventive measures to safeguard the health and safety of workers. Education, proper training, the use of appropriate protective equipment, and strict adherence to safety protocols can be crucial in reducing the risk of traumatic injuries and preserving the well-being of employees.

In addition to the risks posed by traumatic injuries, many high-risk occupations involve repetitive strain and microtraumas that can gradually affect the atlas vertebra. For example, workers who frequently carry heavy loads or engage in repetitive motions, such as lifting, pulling, or pushing, can experience cumulative damage to their neck and spine over time. Even seemingly minor movements, when repeated consistently without proper ergonomics or breaks, can lead to misalignment of the atlas and chronic neck pain.

Therefore, preventive strategies should also focus on ergonomic practices, regular physical therapy, and strengthening exercises to mitigate the long-term effects of repetitive strain in these professions.

"The greatest physician is the one who acts preventively and prevents disease before it occurs."

(Avicenna)

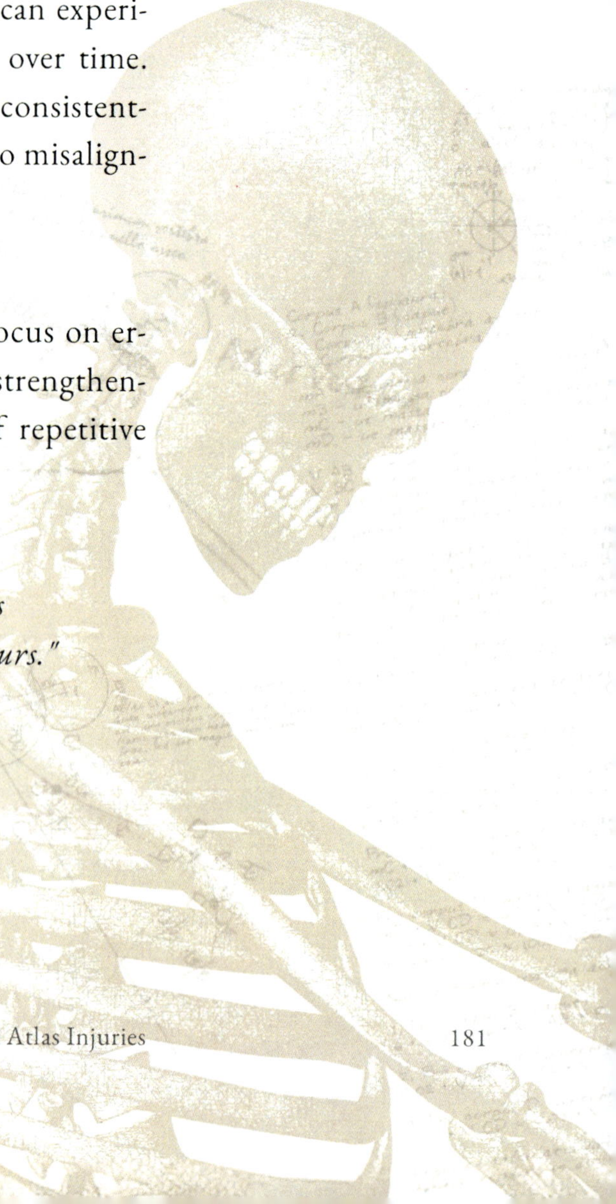

Sedentary Jobs and Atlas Dislocation

The rise of information culture has introduced social and cultural factors that condition the body to remain in a seated position. The economic opportunities and social dynamics of modern life are geared towards comfort in many sedentary occupations. There's a misconception among individuals in sedentary professions that their back pain is solely due to excessive sitting, when in fact, it often stems from issues related to the atlas vertebra.

Your back pain isn't solely due to prolonged sitting; more often, it's a result of a dislocated atlas vertebra, leading to inflammation of the neck and shoulder muscles, as well as back pain as a consequence, not the cause, of the problem. Pinched nerves in the neck area and decreased innervation of the back muscles are attributed to improper sitting. In reality, it's quite the opposite. In reality, improper sitting is often a consequence, not the cause, of a dislocated atlas vertebra.

The sedentary nature of many modern jobs has resulted in various health issues, with back pain being one of the most prevalent. However, addressing the root cause of this discomfort – often related to the alignment of the atlas vertebra – is crucial for alleviating symptoms and promoting overall well-being.

Prolonged sitting slows circulation, contributing to neck and back stiffness. Poor circulation can also cause fluid retention in the lower extremities, affecting overall health.

Recognizing the connection between sedentary occupations and atlas vertebra dislocation empowers individuals to take proactive steps in addressing the root cause of improper sitting, with the initial step being the adjustment of the atlas vertebra.

Amusement Park Safety

Amusement parks, places of excitement and adrenaline rushes, also come with potential risks and dangers. Psychological factors such as boredom and a craving for adrenaline can drive people to seek extreme entertainment and challenge physical limits. This need for excitement can sometimes lead to reckless decisions and risks that exceed safety boundaries.

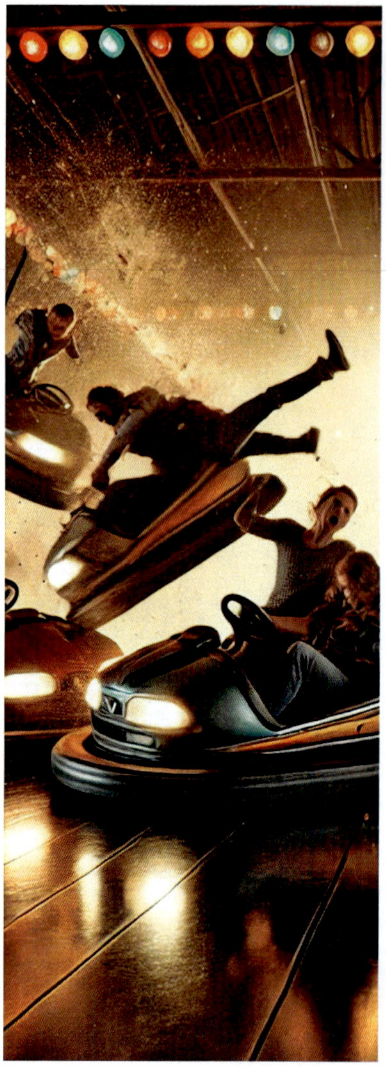

[Image 1] Bumper car crash

In amusement parks, the promotion of skills requiring exceptional physical fitness, such as horseback riding or extreme rides, can be the cause of many falls with dramatic consequences. Although these activities are often perceived as fun and thrilling, they also carry serious risks to the health and safety of participants.

The most dramatic entertainment in amusement parks may be riding small electric cars, where a collision simulation is often unavoidable [Image 1]. However, this type of entertainment can be particularly dangerous because it not only exposes participants to the risk of physical injuries but also normalizes the idea of crashes and violence, which can have negative psychological consequences.

Despite the popularity of these attractions, the question arises whether all forms of entertainment in amusement parks are truly safe and suitable for all ages. Potential risks and consequences need to be carefully considered, especially when children are involved. In many cases, injuries to other people or children in such situations are not punishable like in traffic accidents, raising further questions of responsibility and safety in amusement parks.

Therefore, it is important for legislators and regulatory bodies to carefully consider safety standards and regulations to protect visitors to amusement parks from potential injuries and risks. It is also essential to promote awareness of safety and responsible behavior to reduce the number of injuries and accidents in these popular tourist destinations. Visitor safety must be an absolute priority to ensure that amusement parks remain places of joy and excitement rather than places of danger and tragedy.

Head jerking injuries in amusement parks, such as those that can lead to atlas dislocation, are particularly insidious because they often go unnoticed and show no immediate symptoms. These injuries tend to be overlooked while their effects develop slowly and progressively. It can take years for a health issue to be diagnosed, such as scoliosis of the spine, which quietly evolves as a result of long-term misalignment of the vertebrae. Such injuries can disrupt postural balance, leading to gradual changes in posture, neck and back pain, and headaches, making them difficult to recognize and treat in their early stages.

This is why it is important to pay attention even to mild neck and head injuries that may not cause immediate discomfort, as their long-term consequences can be serious.

It is recommended to lead a calm and balanced lifestyle, avoiding amusement parks and risky behaviors, as true health and longevity stem from caring for the body and mind, rather than moments of excitement with potential long-term consequences. For this reason, choosing activities that promote long-term health is essential.

"He who walks with the wise grows wise,
but a companion of fools suffers harm."

(Proverbs 13:20)

Sleep Positions and Health

Sleep is an essential physiological need for every human being, necessary for the body and mind to recover and maintain overall health and well-being. During sleep, the body undergoes a process of regeneration, repairing damaged cells and replenishing energy reserves for the next day. However, sleep is not just a time for physical rest; it is also crucial for mental rejuvenation, information processing, and memory consolidation.

Quality sleep depends not only on the length of time spent in bed but also on other factors, including the sleeping position. While there is no universally best sleeping position, most experts agree that sleeping on the back may be most conducive to maintaining proper body alignment and reducing pressure on the spine and neck. Sleeping on the back may also decrease the risk of facial wrinkles, as the face is not pressed against a pillow during the night.

However, many people prefer sleeping on their side or stomach for greater comfort. With this choice, I agree, although I must note that the acquired habit of sleeping only on one side, without changing positions during the night, can affect the position of the atlas vertebra. While side sleeping can be particularly beneficial for those who have problems with snoring or sleep apnea, it is essential to recognize that prolonged sleeping on only one side may affect the alignment of the atlas vertebra. Sleeping on the stomach, on the other hand, can lead to unfavorable spinal and neck positions, resulting in improper body alignment and pressure on these areas of the body.

Ultimately, the choice of sleeping position is individual and may vary depending on comfort and personal needs. It is important to adjust the sleeping position to individual preferences and recognize how specific positions can affect sleep quality and overall health. Regardless of the choice, maintaining healthy sleep habits is crucial for overall health and well-being.

When viewed from the perspective of the most correct posture between the head and the atlas vertebra, and subsequently between the atlas and the axis, sleeping in a semi-seated position is considered the most ideal. In this position, the head rests on the atlas vertebra and evenly distributes its weight without creating strain, stretching, or muscle inflammation, which can occur in other sleeping positions.

This balance between the head and the atlas helps reduce tension in the neck and shoulder muscles, preventing inflammation and long-term postural issues. Unlike side, stomach, or back sleeping positions, the semi-seated position maintains the spine in a natural alignment, reducing the risk of atlas misalignment and associated problems.

This position not only alleviates neck tension but also promotes easier muscle regeneration during sleep, as the muscles are not burdened by supporting an improperly aligned head.

Ultimately, the semi-seated position is optimal for maintaining proper posture and minimizing the risk of atlas injuries, which directly improves sleep quality and overall health.

"The proper sleeping position
is the foundation of health."

(Hippocrates)

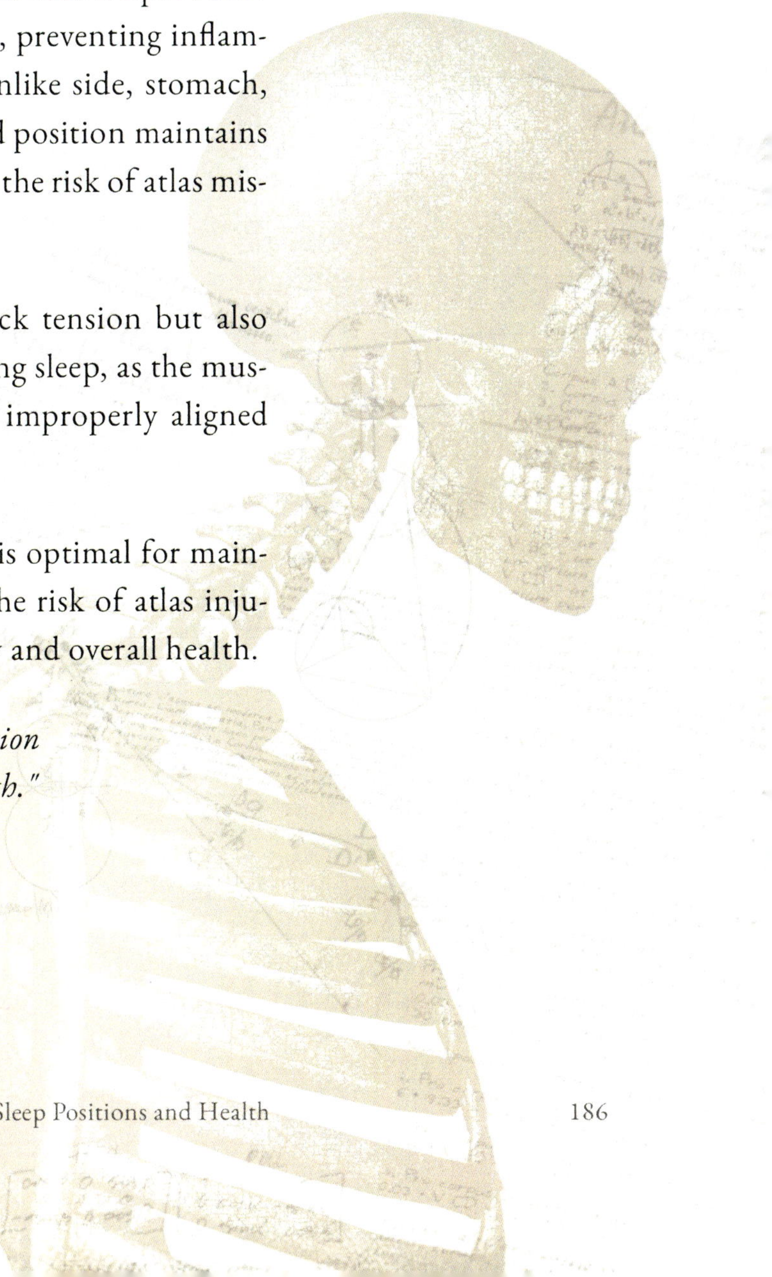

Risks of Self-Neck Massages

Self-administered neck massages with handheld devices can unintentionally pose risks, especially when delicate structures of the cervical spine are involved. Specifically, the region of the atlas vertebra, located in the cervical spine at the base of the skull, requires caution during such treatments. The risk comes from a lack of understanding of individual neck anatomy, coupled with the fact that the atlas vertebra may already be partially displaced. Massager vibrations have the potential to exacerbate this dislocation, pushing the atlas into an even more misaligned position.

Alarmingly, most manufacturers are unaware of this risk, often due to a lack of information. Additionally, many massagers are equipped with extremely strong vibrations designed for larger muscle groups, rather than the delicate and small muscles around the atlas vertebra and its supporting ligaments.

Therefore, while self-massage can provide relief, it is important to exercise caution and seek advice from qualified professionals when treating delicate areas such as the cervical spine, especially the region of the atlas vertebra. Awareness of these potential risks is crucial for preserving spine health and preventing further complications.

Self-administered head manipulation techniques, twisting, or forcefully turning the head in an attempt to relieve neck tension, may provide temporary relief by stretching the muscles or causing the release of trapped air bubbles between vertebrae. However, these methods can also lead to adverse effects, such as dislocation of the atlas vertebra and new symptoms like headaches, migraines, and disturbances in orientation and coordination.

When head manipulation is performed manually, twisting, or imprecise methods with the aim of adjusting the atlas vertebra, proper adjustment of the atlas vertebra will not be achieved. Instead, there is a risk of causing dislocation of the atlas, as adjusting the atlas requires a highly precise technique that differs from mere rotation, or twisting of the head. It's important to understand that manipulation of the head, especially in an unsupervised manner, can carry serious risks and should be approached with caution. Seeking professional guidance and treatment for neck issues is advisable to avoid potential complications and ensure proper care of the cervical spine.

In addition to the immediate risks like atlas dislocation and muscle tension, improperly performed neck massages and head manipulations can have long-term effects on overall spinal alignment and posture. Even a slight misalignment of the atlas can lead to postural issues, causing low-grade chronic pain in the back, shoulders, or hips, as the body compensates for the misalignment in the neck. If these issues are not addressed early, they can progress into more serious conditions, including altered gait, uneven pressure on spinal discs, and gradual deterioration of spinal function.

Therefore, regular monitoring of spinal health and using proper massage or manipulation techniques is crucial for maintaining long-term spinal well-being.

"Knowledge without practice is useless.
Practice without knowledge is dangerous."

(Confucius)

Preventing Atlas Misalignment

It can be concluded that awareness and education are crucial as preventive measures for both individuals and professionals, and that understanding the complex interactions between these factors can help us delve deeper into the root causes of our health issues. Recognizing how they intertwine and create intricate cause-and-effect relationships, it's evident that the causes of atlas vertebra misalignment are largely related to a restless lifestyle. Therefore, prevention should focus on avoiding risk factors and striving for a peaceful, nurturing, and fruitful life.

"For wisdom is a defence, and money is a defence: but the excellency of knowledge is, that wisdom giveth life to them that have it."

(Ecclesiastes 7:12)

Chapter 3

Atlantoaxial Subluxation and Dislocation

Atlantoaxial Subluxation

The atlas vertebra, the first cervical vertebra, plays a crucial role in supporting the head and facilitating its rotation and nodding. As part of the cervical spine, the atlas is a vital link in the mechanism of head rotation, along with the second vertebra segment, known as the axis. What makes it unique is the fact that the atlas, along with the head, rotates around the dens, a thickened projection on the second vertebra, C2, which effectively makes it part of the head rather than strictly part of the spine, as defined by traditional anatomical terms.

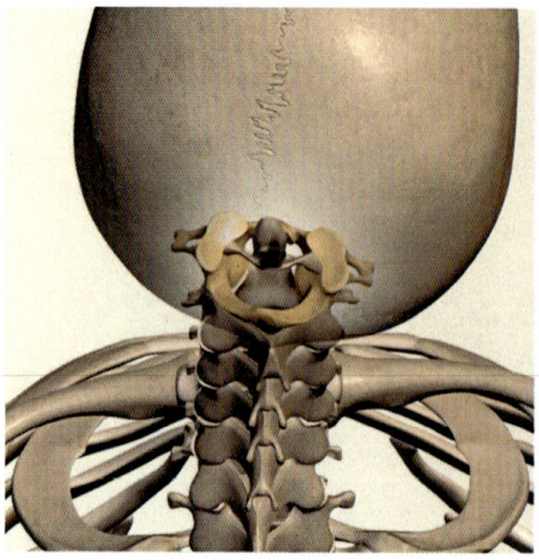

[Image 1] Head rotation mechanism

This specific anatomy implies that the dislocation or subluxation of the atlas is not merely a matter of biomechanics but also a crucial factor in maintaining proper head and neck function [Image 1]. While often considered an anatomical part of the spine, the atlas vertebra requires a special approach when it comes to manipulation and treatment, as its damage can affect the function of the entire neck and even impact neural structures [Image 2].

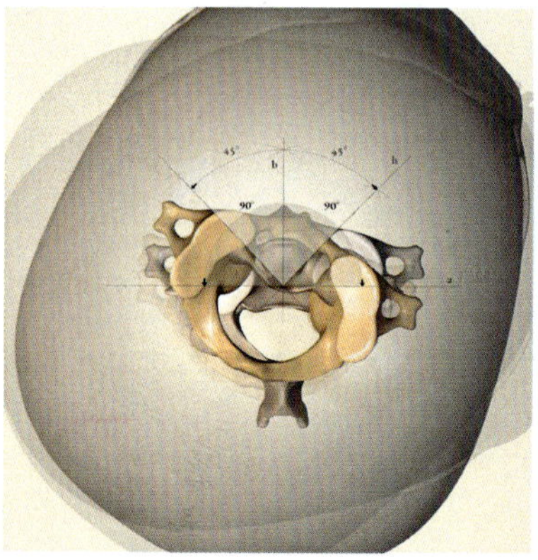

[Image 2] Head rotation around atlas

It is important to note that despite the wide application of various therapeutic approaches, chemical processes such as taking medications or supplements do not have the power to return the atlas to its correct anatomical position. Adjusting the atlas to the correct position requires careful biomechanical intervention, taking into account the complexity of anatomical structures and the functional role of this important part of the body.

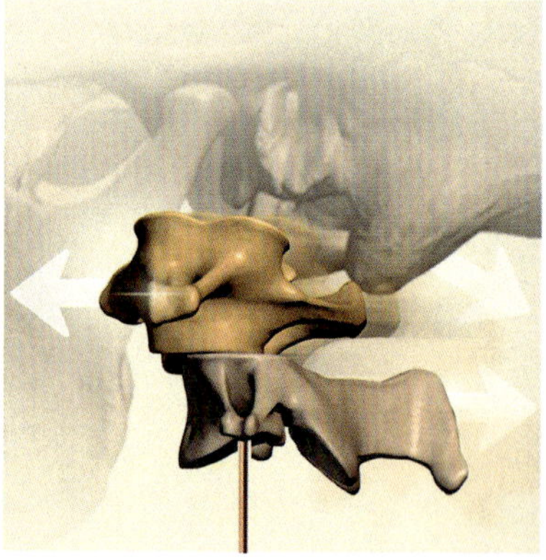

[Image 3] Atlantoaxial subluxation

Atlantoaxial subluxation is a medical term used to describe the partial or incomplete displacement of the first (atlas) and second (axis) cervical vertebrae, namely the C1 and C2 vertebrae [Image 3]. This part of the spine supports the head and facilitates its movement forward-backward (flexion and extension) and laterally (lateral flexion).

Subluxation refers to a condition where two vertebrae have partially lost their normal alignment, meaning they are not fully dislocated and remain partially in their normal position. In other words, subluxation involves a partial displacement, where the bones are not completely out of their normal positions, but are still misaligned enough to cause potential issues [Image 1].

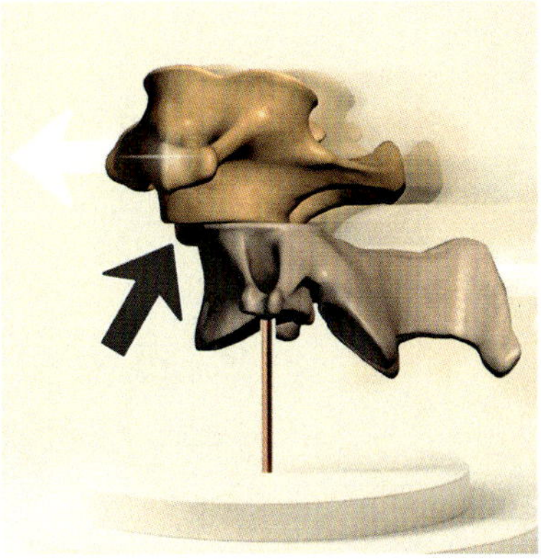

[Image 1] Subluxation is up to 2mm

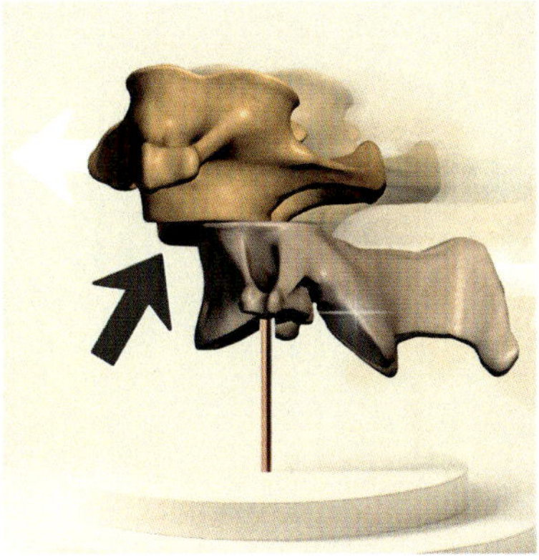

[Image 2] Dislocation is up to 4mm

When diagnosing and evaluating atlas subluxation, it's crucial to consider the subjective experience and interpretation of symptoms by the patient, as well as the clinical assessment and palpation techniques used by the doctor. Although front-facing observation of the patient provides a mirror image, the orientation used in diagnosis must align with the patient's perspective. This means that what is the left side for the patient is considered the left side of the atlas subluxation in the diagnostic context. This ensures consistency in identifying and understanding the position of the atlas vertebra, facilitating a more accurate assessment of the subluxation and proper direction of therapy for the patient.

Atlantoaxial dislocation is a serious condition characterized by complete displacement of the first cervical vertebra (atlas) in relation to the second cervical vertebra (axis), or C1 and C2 vertebrae [Image 2]. This dislocation represents a significant pathology that can be caused by trauma, congenital anomalies, inflammatory processes, or other factors.

When atlantoaxial dislocation occurs due to trauma, the normal structure and function of the atlas and axis are compromised. Symptoms of atlantoaxial dislocation can range from neck and head pain to damage to nerve structures, leading to loss of sensation and movement in the lower body. In severe cases, this dislocation can compress brain structures, leading to serious neurological deficits, such as paralysis or loss of function in certain nerve pathways, and even life-threatening conditions.

Treatment of atlantoaxial dislocation requires a multidisciplinary approach involving stabilization of the cervical spine, reduction of the dislocation, pain management, and management of any neurological complications. Additionally, careful biomechanical intervention is necessary in this case. In some cases, surgical intervention may be necessary to restore the normal position of the atlas and axis and preserve the function of the spinal column.

It is important to emphasize that atlantoaxial dislocation is a serious condition that requires urgent medical attention and expert treatment to prevent potentially serious complications and improve outcomes.

I conclude that in further writing of this chapter, I will focus on Atlantoaxial Subluxation rather than Atlantoaxial Dislocation. This decision is made because I believe Atlantoaxial Subluxation is a more prevalent occurrence that can arise from various causes, whereas Atlantoaxial Dislocation is a result of extreme traumas such as severe accidents or significant physical injuries. By focusing on Atlantoaxial Subluxation, I can delve more deeply into this more widespread phenomenon and its potential effects on patients' health and well-being.

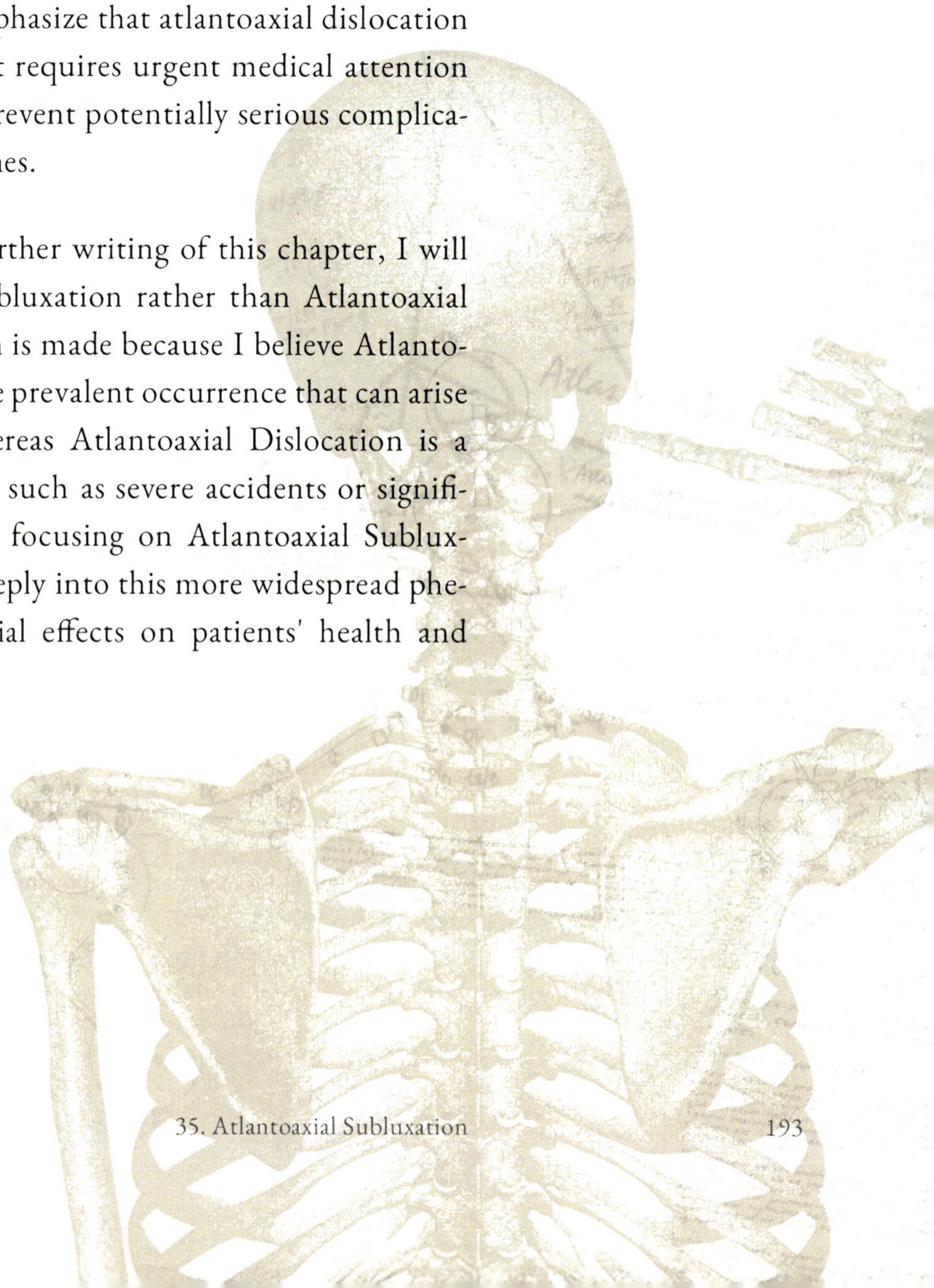

Anterior Atlas Subluxation: Causes

Anterior atlas subluxation, as a specific form of subluxation in the cervical spine, refers to a condition in which the first cervical vertebra, known as the atlas, partially shifts forward in relation to the second cervical vertebra, the axis. This type of subluxation often occurs as a result of trauma, such as a blow to the face or forehead, which can lead to destabilization of this delicate part of the spine.

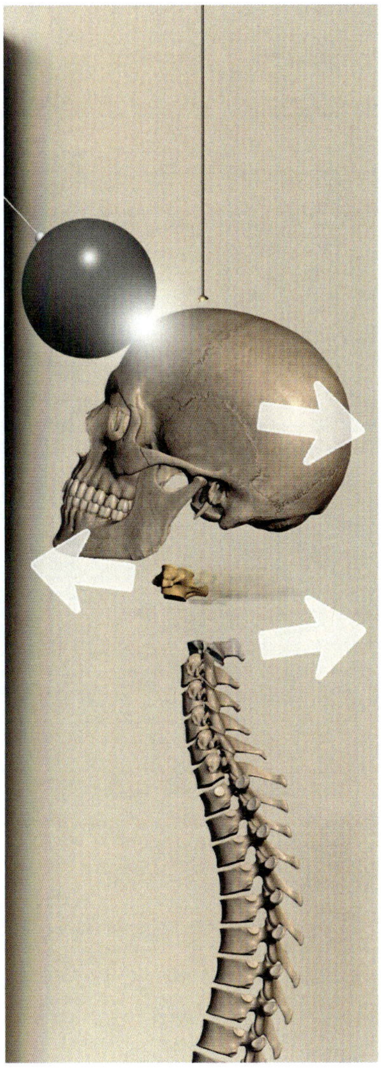

[Image 1] Subluxation mechanism

From our diagnostic experience, we have observed that impacts to the front of the head, face, or forehead often result in a tendency for the atlas to shift forward. This conclusion stems from careful observation and analysis of cases exhibiting similar patterns. When trauma occurs in these areas, the force of impact often acts in a direction that causes the atlas to shift forward, inducing anterior subluxation [Image 1]. This insight plays a crucial role in the diagnostic process as it enables us to better understand the mechanisms of injury and provide appropriate therapy to patients exposed to such situations.

Symptoms of anterior atlas subluxations can be diverse and may include neck pain, limited range of motion in the head, and possible neurological issues due to compression of nerve structures. Due to the traumatic nature of this condition, individuals who have experienced this type of injury often exhibit scars on the front of the head or face, which may indicate previous traumas.

Damage to ligaments connecting the atlas and axis, as well as pressure on the medulla oblongata and nerve structures in that area, can further complicate this subluxation. Additionally, there is a possibility of compression on blood vessels passing through the atlas region, which can cause additional problems.

Specifically, pressure on the medulla oblongata can disrupt the normal function of this vital part of the brainstem, leading to various neurological symptoms such as breathing difficulties, swallowing issues, balance problems, and cardiovascular regulation.

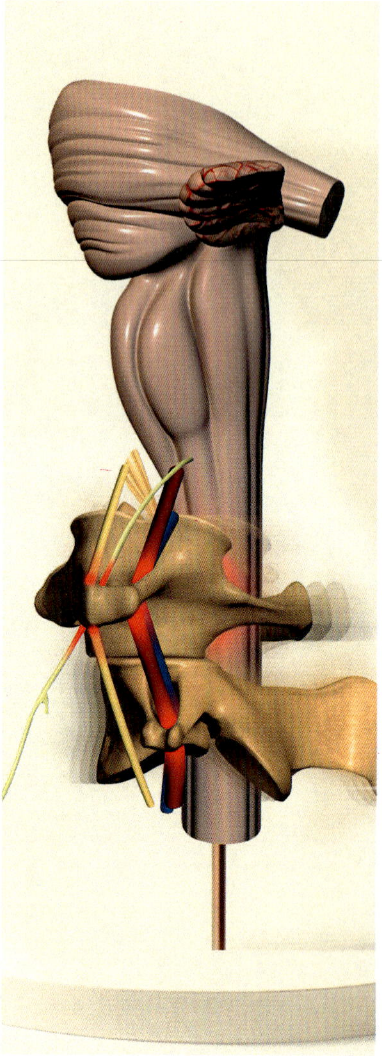

[Image 1] Compression

Furthermore, compression of nerve structures can cause pain, tingling, weakness, and loss of sensation in the neck, head, shoulders, and upper extremities [Image 1]. When blood vessels are constricted or damaged, it can result in reduced blood flow to the brain, leading to serious neurological consequences such as stroke or cerebral hypoxia.

All these complications can significantly impact the quality of life of individuals suffering from anterior atlas subluxations, underscoring the importance of recognizing this type of pathology and intervening promptly to prevent further complications.

One of the key challenges in treating anterior atlas subluxation is accurate diagnosis, as this pathology sometimes does not manifest immediately after trauma. Subtle shifts in the atlas can be difficult to detect on standard radiological imaging, making it harder to establish a correct diagnosis.

Developing specific methods for identifying these displacements, such as dynamic 3D imaging or functional MRI, can play a crucial role in precisely detecting the subluxation. Additionally, incorporating clinical assessments of symptoms such as headaches, dizziness, and balance problems can aid in the early recognition of this type of injury, allowing for quicker intervention and more effective treatment.

Clinical Impact of Atlas Subluxation

Anterior atlantoaxial subluxation can manifest with a variety of clinical symptoms and manifestations affecting different parts of the body and functions. One of the key symptoms is the straightening of the hyperlordosis, which can lead to changes in body posture and neck mobility [Image 1]. Additionally, hyperlordosis of the thoracic vertebrae, including inflammation at T2, may be observed, further affecting posture.

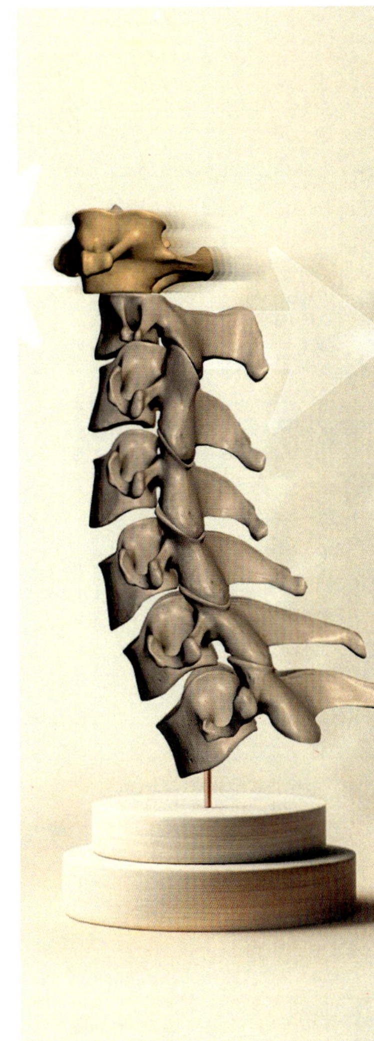

[Image 1] Hyperlordosis

Headaches and migraines are common symptoms in individuals with anterior atlantoaxial subluxation, often accompanied by nausea. Impaired coordination and orientation may be present, hindering daily activities and functionality.

Furthermore, cardiovascular symptoms such as heart arrhythmias and shallow breathing may occur, while sinus congestion can cause discomfort and respiratory issues. Blurred vision and tinnitus are also possible manifestations of anterior atlantoaxial subluxation, further impacting quality of life.

In addition to physical symptoms, anterior atlantoaxial subluxation can lead to digestive issues, dysfunction of bile function, slowed bowel peristalsis, and skin conditions. Psychological problems such as anxiety and depression may also be present, while infertility in women and complications with thyroid function can further exacerbate health issues.

The medulla oblongata is the part of the brainstem responsible for controlling vital functions of the body, such as breathing, heart activity, swallowing, and blood pressure regulation. Compression of these centers in the medulla oblongata can cause various neurological symptoms and disorders. For instance, disrupting normal breathing can lead to respiratory problems such as dyspnea (difficulty breathing) or apnea (cessation of breathing). Pressure on the center for heart activity can cause cardiac arrhythmias or other cardiovascular issues. Swallowing difficulties may result in food or liquid aspiration, leading to aspiration pneumonia or other serious complications.

Additionally, pressure on the center for blood pressure regulation can cause hypotension or hypertension, leading to dizziness, weakness, or loss of consciousness. All these complications can be severe and require urgent medical intervention to stabilize vital functions and prevent further neurological damage.

The vagus nerve is predominantly a parasympathetic nerve. It is the largest nerve of the parasympathetic nervous system and plays a key role in regulating many internal organs. If the atlas vertebra compresses the parasympathetic nerve, it can result in various negative effects on the function of organs innervated by this nerve [Image 1]. Since parasympathetic nerves are responsible for controlling relaxation and rest processes in the body, compression of the atlas vertebra can disrupt the normal function of these nerve fibers.

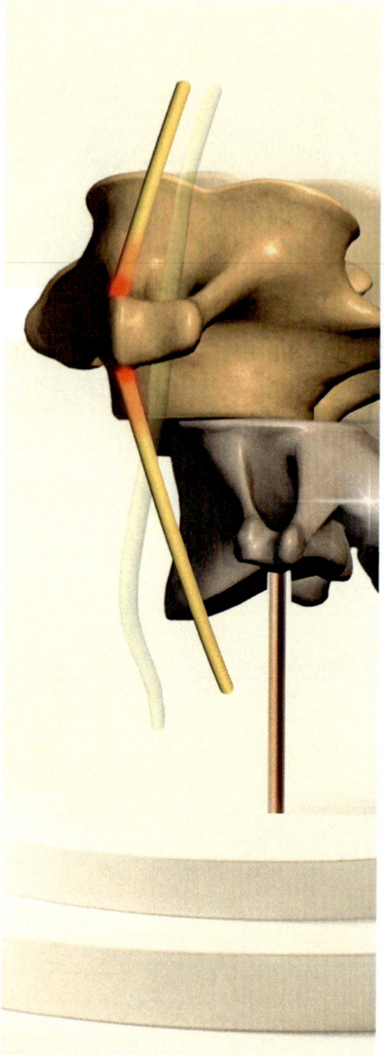

[Image 1] Vagus nerve compression

Specifically, compression of the parasympathetic nerve can lead to disturbances in the functioning of internal organs innervated by this nerve, including the heart, lungs, gastrointestinal tract, and others. This can result in changes in heart rhythm, respiratory issues, digestive disturbances, as well as other symptoms related to the parasympathetic nervous system.

Furthermore, compression of the parasympathetic nerve can affect the overall condition of the body, causing fatigue, decreased energy, and a general feeling of malaise. Therefore, it is important to recognize and treat atlas vertebra compression to prevent potential complications and preserve overall health.

In cases of anterior atlas subluxation, compression of the vertebral arteries can lead to various issues due to decreased blood flow to the brain, particularly to the posterior part encompassing the brainstem and cerebral cortex [Image 1]. This region of the brain is responsible for vital functions such as regulating breathing, heart rate, blood pressure, and various reflexes. When the vertebral arteries are constricted or damaged as a result of atlas subluxation, there may be insufficient oxygen and nutrients supplied to these parts of the brain. This can result in various neurological symptoms, including dizziness, fainting, blurred vision, loss of consciousness, or even more serious complications such as stroke or brain hypoxia. Reduced blood flow can also impair the normal functioning of the brain, leading to issues with memory, concentration, and other cognitive functions. Therefore, it is crucial to recognize and treat anterior atlas subluxation to prevent serious consequences for brain health and overall well-being.

Based on the presented facts, Anterior atlas subluxation stands out as one of the four most dangerous subluxations of the atlas, commonly diagnosed in clinical practice.

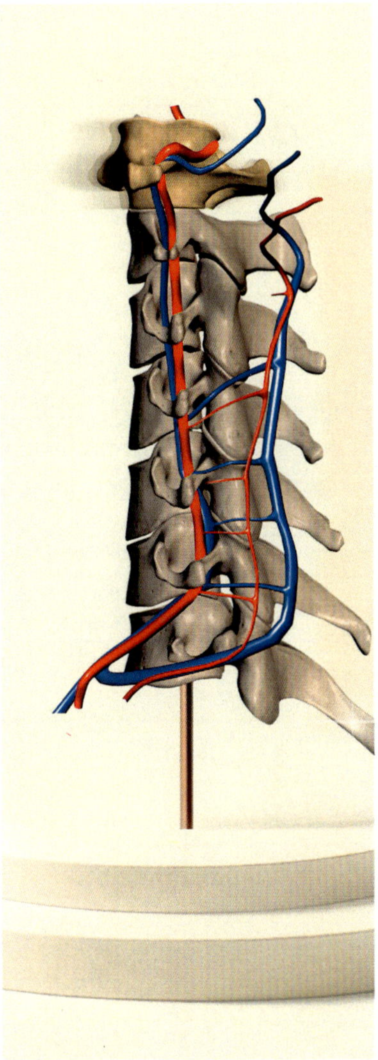

[Image 1] Vascular compression

3D Scanners for Atlas Diagnosis

The use of 3D scanners in medicine has revolutionized diagnostics and treatments, providing doctors with detailed three-dimensional information about the patient's anatomy. These sophisticated devices enable precise imaging of organs, tissues, and bones, offering clear visual representations that aid in the diagnosis of various diseases and conditions.

One of the key advantages of 3D scanners in medicine is the ability to create detailed three-dimensional models, allowing doctors to better understand the structure and condition of organs or tissues. For example, in orthopedic procedures, 3D scanners can provide accurate information about the position and shape of fractures or other bone injuries, enabling surgeons to plan and perform operations with greater precision.

Additionally, the use of 3D scanners allows for a personalized approach to treatment, as it enables doctors to tailor treatments to the specific characteristics of each patient. For instance, in aesthetic surgery, 3D scanners can provide detailed information about the structure of the face or body, allowing surgeons to plan surgeries that best suit the individual needs of the patient.

Moreover, the advancement of 3D scanning technology in medicine has led to the development of new diagnostic methods and therapies. For example, in the field of radiotherapy, 3D scanners enable precise imaging of tumors and surrounding healthy tissue, allowing doctors to adjust radiation doses and minimize harmful effects on surrounding tissue.

Overall, the use of 3D scanners in medicine brings numerous benefits, including more accurate diagnoses, personalized treatments, and improved therapy outcomes. These devices have become indispensable tools in modern medicine, providing doctors with valuable information and facilitating patient care.

Scanning the atlas vertebra with intraoral 3D scanners used for dental imaging represents the most precise technology for analyzing anterior and other subluxations of the atlas vertebra. These specialized 3D scanners, originally developed for detailed mapping of teeth and jaws, have proven to be extremely useful in medicine, particularly in diagnosing cervical spine issues.

The advantage of using these devices for atlas vertebra scanning lies in their ability to create precise three-dimensional images of this delicate part of the spine. Unlike conventional X-rays or CT scans, which provide two-dimensional images, 3D scanners offer detailed three-dimensional reconstructions, allowing physicians to analyze the structure of the atlas vertebra in detail and identify even the smallest abnormalities or subluxations.

Furthermore, employing this technology enables precise positioning and treatment planning for patients with atlas vertebra subluxations. Physicians can accurately determine the position and degree of subluxation, enabling them to tailor therapy to the individual needs of each patient. Additionally, this technology allows monitoring of treatment progress, as physicians can regularly perform precise analyses and compare images before and after treatment.

Moreover, these devices used for dental imaging are safe and non-invasive, making them suitable for patients of all ages. Patients are exposed to minimal radiation during scanning, and the procedure is quick and comfortable.

Assessing Atlas via Body Statics

Recognition of the alignment of the atlas vertebra can be crucial in diagnosing and treating various spinal issues. Experienced atlasologists can assess the position of the atlas vertebra by observing body posture, as there is a close relationship between the position of the atlas and body alignment. When the atlas is properly aligned, the overall body posture is balanced and symmetrical [Image 1]. However, any irregularity in the placement of the atlas can cause asymmetry and imbalance in body posture.

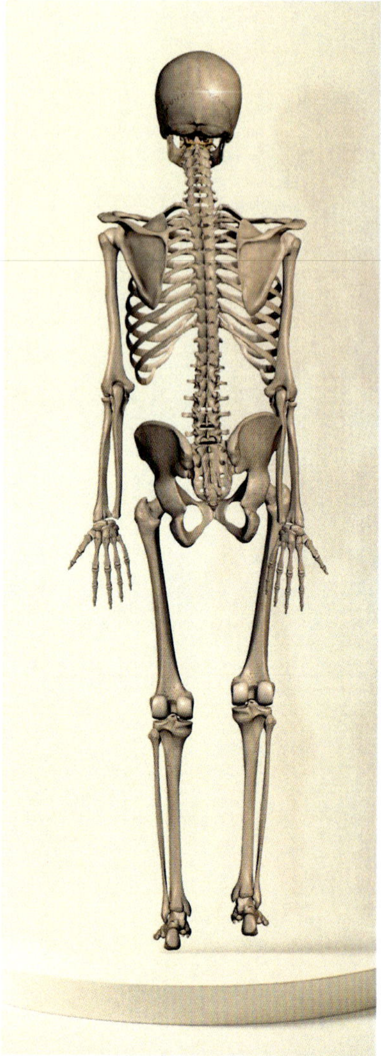

[Image 1] Postural statics

Through careful observation of body statics, an atlasologist can identify any changes in the position of the atlas and use that information for diagnosis and treatment planning. For example, if it is noticed that the head is shifted forward or backward in relation to the rest of the body, it may indicate anterior or posterior subluxation of the atlas. Similarly, lateral subluxation of the atlas can be identified through asymmetrical body alignment of the shoulders or hips.

This approach to diagnosing the position of the atlas vertebra through observation of body alignment has its advantages, especially in situations where quick recognition of problems is necessary or when there is no access to specialized imaging equipment. Additionally, this method can be useful as a complement to other diagnostic techniques, such as X-rays or magnetic resonance imaging.

In this book, various examples of observing body posture and their relationship to the position of the atlas vertebra will be detailed. Through illustrations and drawings, readers will have the opportunity to better understand how the position of the atlas affects body alignment and how this information can be useful in diagnosing and treating various spinal conditions.

Palpation for Atlas Assessment

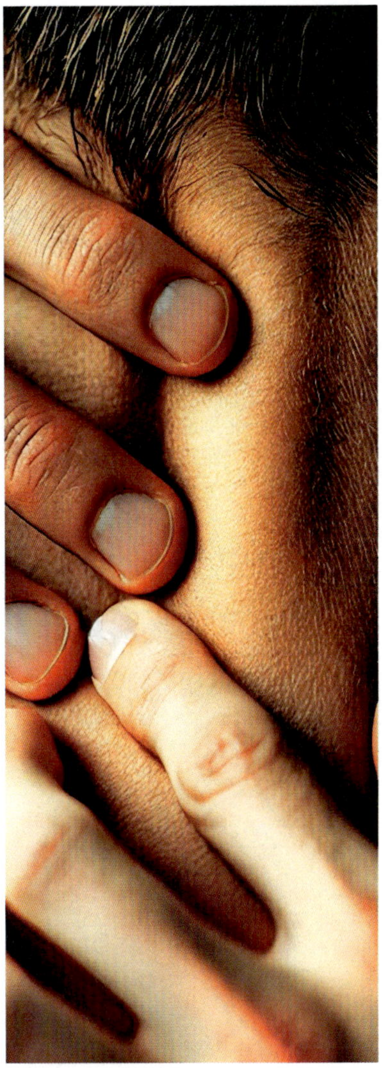

[Image 1] Palpation

This procedure is a crucial technique in medicine used to assess various parts of the body through touch. This procedure enables medical professionals to evaluate the structure, size, consistency, and sensitivity of different tissues, which can be essential for diagnosis and monitoring disease progression.

During this method, a medical expert uses their fingers and hands to feel different parts of the body, such as lymph nodes, joints, internal organs, muscles, and bones [Image 1]. This technique allows the detection of changes in tissues, such as swelling, tumors, alterations in consistency, or sensitivity, which may indicate the presence of disease or injury.

This procedure can be utilized in various medical fields, including general practice, surgery, orthopedics, gynecology, as well as in the diagnosis and monitoring of various health conditions. For example, abdominal palpation can aid in diagnosing abdominal disorders, while palpation of lymph nodes may indicate the presence of infection or cancer.

Apart from diagnostic purposes, this method can also be beneficial in therapeutic contexts, such as in physical therapy or massage. Touch can have a therapeutic effect on muscles and tissues, helping to reduce pain, improve blood circulation, and relieve tension.

It is important to note that this procedure is performed carefully and with respect for the patient, while adhering to privacy and medical standards and protocols. This technique requires practice and experience to be properly executed and interpreted, thus often serving as an indispensable tool in the diagnosis and treatment of various health conditions.

Palpation of the atlas vertebra is an important step in assessing its position and possible subluxation. Through carefully guided finger movements, we can evaluate the relationship and distance between the lateral tubercles of the atlas vertebra in relation to the mastoid process of the skull and the bones of the lower jaw [Image 1]. This technique allows us to accurately determine the degree of atlas subluxation.

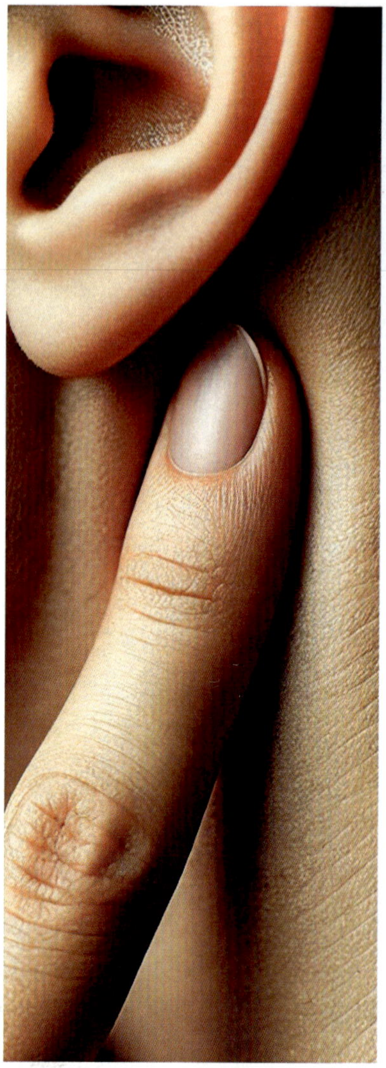

[Image 1] Position of palpation

When the lateral tubercles of the atlas vertebra are displaced relative to the mastoid process and the bones of the lower jaw, it may indicate an atlas subluxation. Changes in their position and distance can provide valuable information about the degree of atlas displacement and enable us to determine the significance of the subluxation.

This palpation technique requires precision and skill, but with proper training and experience, medical professionals can effectively use atlas vertebra palpation as part of the diagnostic process.

In addition to evaluating the relationship between the atlas and surrounding bones, palpation can also involve assessing the muscle tone and tension in the neck and shoulder area. Muscle tightness near the atlas, particularly in muscles like the trapezius and sternocleidomastoid, can indicate compensatory reactions of the body due to atlas subluxation. These muscles may become overworked and tense as they try to stabilize the head and neck in an improper position, further complicating the function and alignment of the atlas. Therefore, assessing muscle tension is crucial in the diagnostic process, as it provides additional insights into the severity of the subluxation and associated postural issues.This assessment of muscle tension can also help identify secondary problems and guide the need for specific treatments, such as massage or physical therapy, to relieve tension and restore normal atlas function.

Correcting Atlas: '*Harmonious Balance*'

Correcting anterior atlas subluxation, as well as all other atlas subluxations, can be achieved and explained through the methodology of atlas adjustment that I have developed called "Harmonious Balance" - HB. This innovative technique involves a precise and gentle approach aimed at achieving a harmonious balance in the position of the atlas vertebra.

The key characteristic of the "Harmonious Balance" method is its holistic approach, which takes into account not only the physical aspects of subluxation but also the mental-emotional and energetic factors. By carefully establishing balance between the atlas vertebra and surrounding structures, this technique aims to restore optimal function of the spinal column and the entire body.

Implementing "Harmonious Balance" requires a deep understanding of anatomy, biomechanics, and energy flow in the body. It is combined with techniques such as palpation, manipulation, and therapeutic exercises, tailored to the individual needs of each patient. Through these customized approaches, precise correction of atlas subluxation is achieved, which can result in improvement of symptoms and overall patient well-being.

"Harmonious Balance" represents a blend of scientific principles, experience, and intuitive wisdom, standing out as a holistic approach to addressing atlas subluxation issues. Through this methodology, the goal is not only to correct physical imbalances but also to support the harmonious flow of life energy and inner equilibrium.

Atlantoaxial Subluxation

Anterior subluxation of the atlas is a partial displacement of the first cervical vertebra, the atlas, relative to the second, the axis. It mainly occurs due to trauma or frontal head impact. This displacement can straighten the cervical lordosis, affecting the entire spine over time, often leading to pronounced thoracic kyphosis and straightened lumbar lordosis.

Atlas is displaced anteriorly

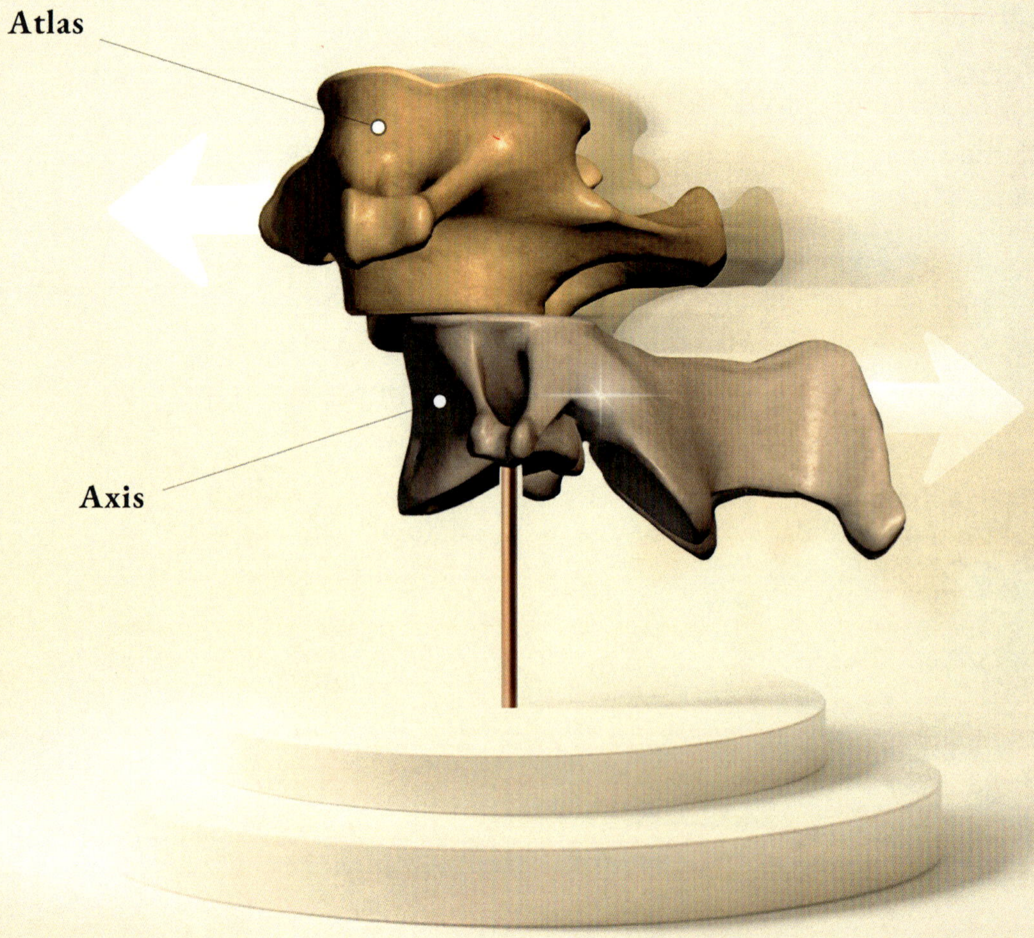

Compression of the Vagus Nerve

Atlantoaxial Subluxation compresses the Vagus Nerve, which in most cases can cause symptoms like heart arrhythmias, digestive tract problems, poor digestion, a lump-in-throat sensation, and slowed intestinal peristalsis. Restoring the atlas vertebra to its correct anatomical position immediately resolves these issues, as decompressing the Vagus Nerve is an instant process.

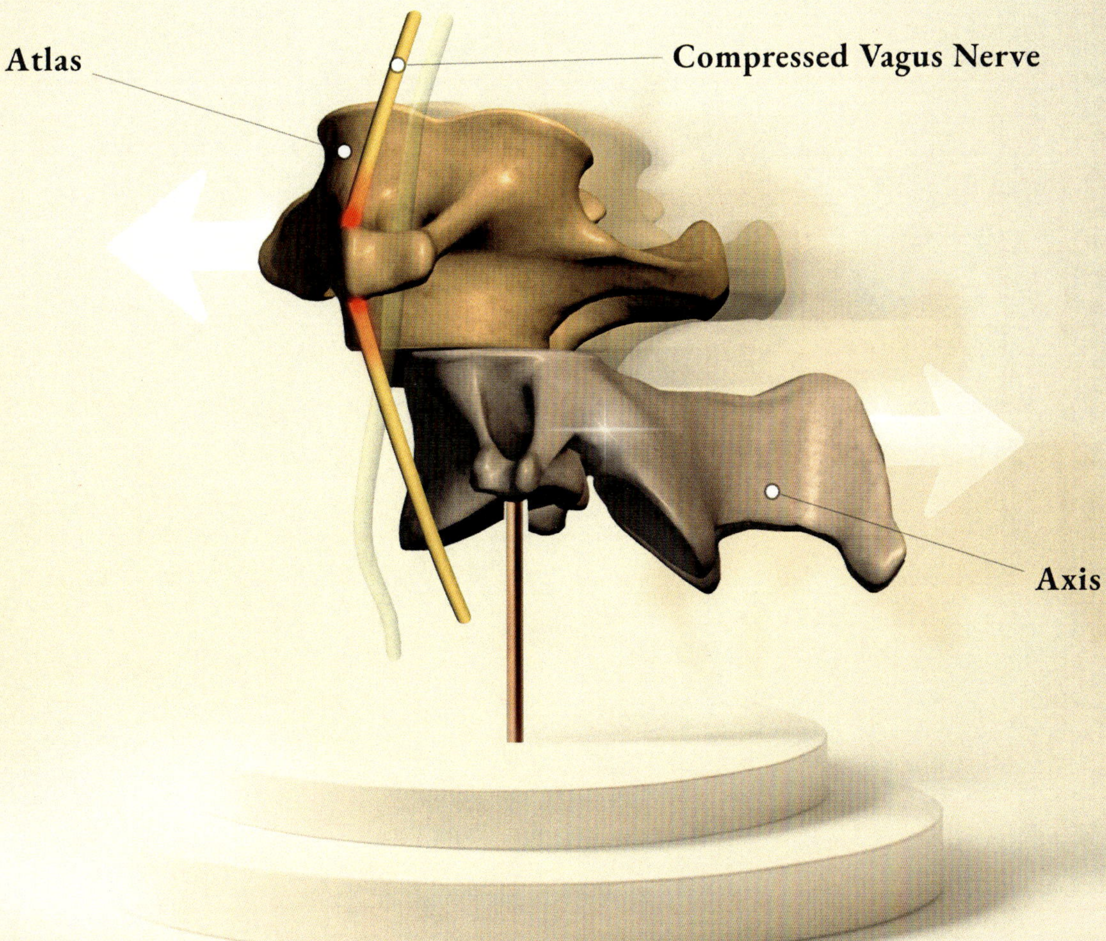

Compression of the C2 Spinal Nerve

Atlantoaxial Subluxation can cause pressure on the C2 spinal nerve. Compression of the C2 spinal nerve typically occurs at the level where the nerve exits the spinal cord between the atlas (C1) and axis (C2) vertebrae. When the C2 vertebra (axis) moves backward, opposite to the atlas, it physically presses on the root of the C2 spinal nerve, leading to compression.

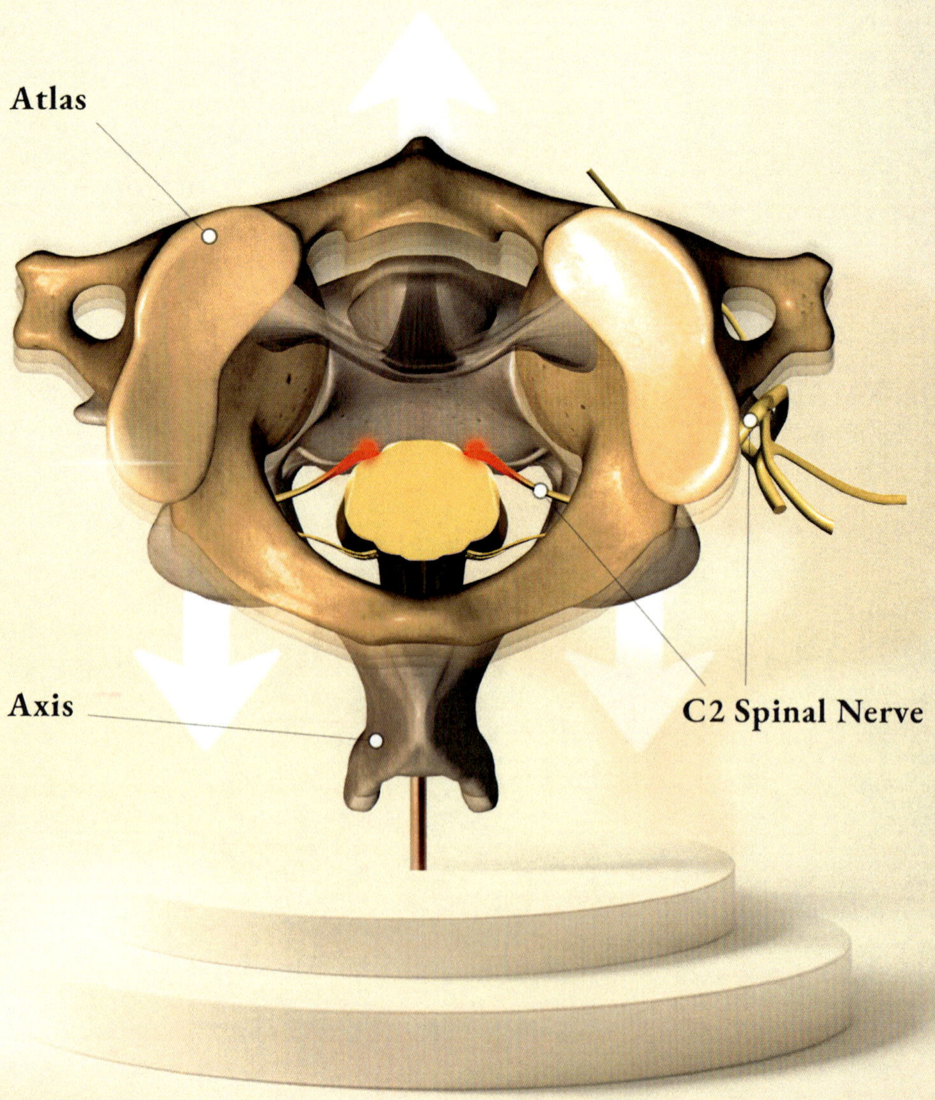

Compression of the Hypoglossal Nerve

Anterior subluxation can compress the Hypoglossal Nerve (XII cranial nerve), weakening tongue muscle control. This compression leads to unclear speech and difficulty swallowing since the tongue is crucial for these functions. Relieving the subluxation and nerve compression is essential for restoring proper muscle function and preventing complications.

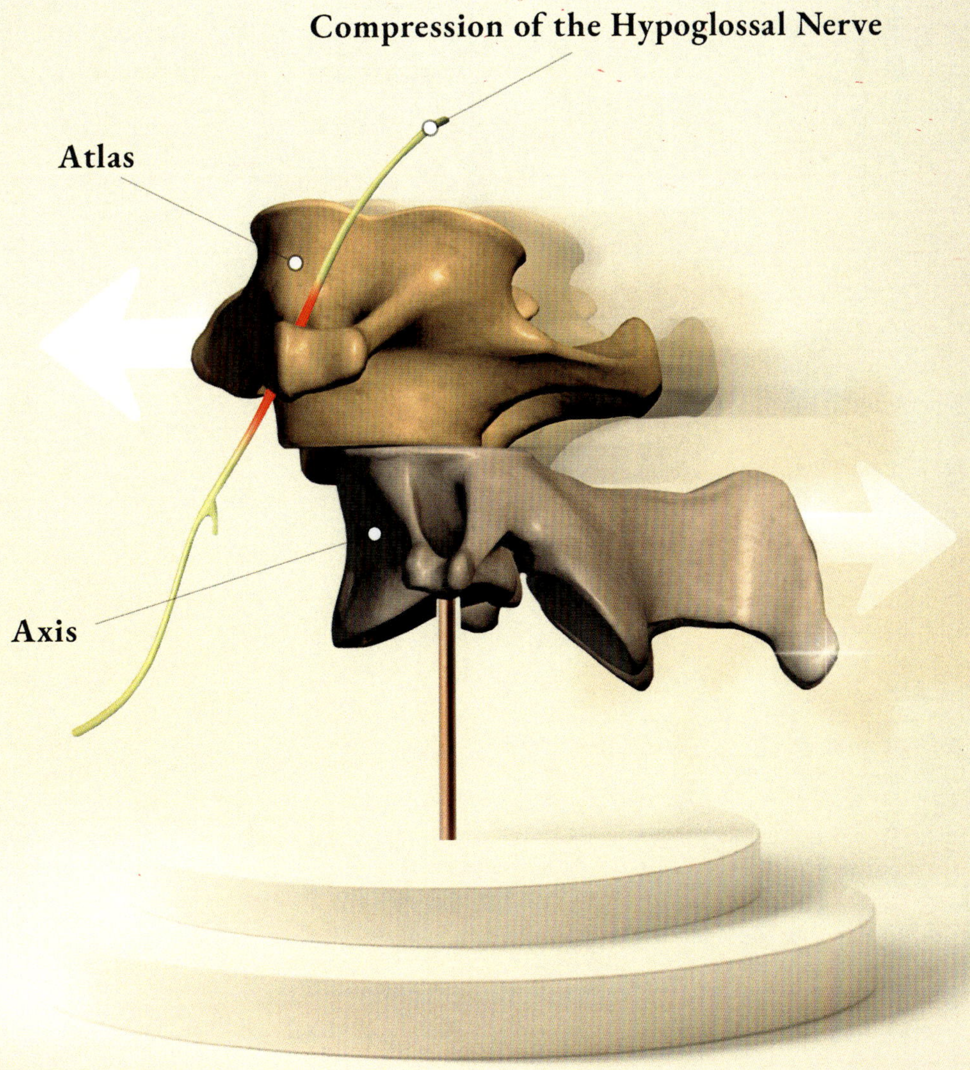

Vertebral Vein and Vertebral Artery

Anterior subluxation can compress the Hypoglossal Nerve (XII cranial nerve), weakening tongue muscle control. This compression leads to unclear speech and difficulty swallowing since the tongue is crucial for these functions. Relieving the subluxation and nerve compression is essential for restoring proper muscle function and preventing complications.

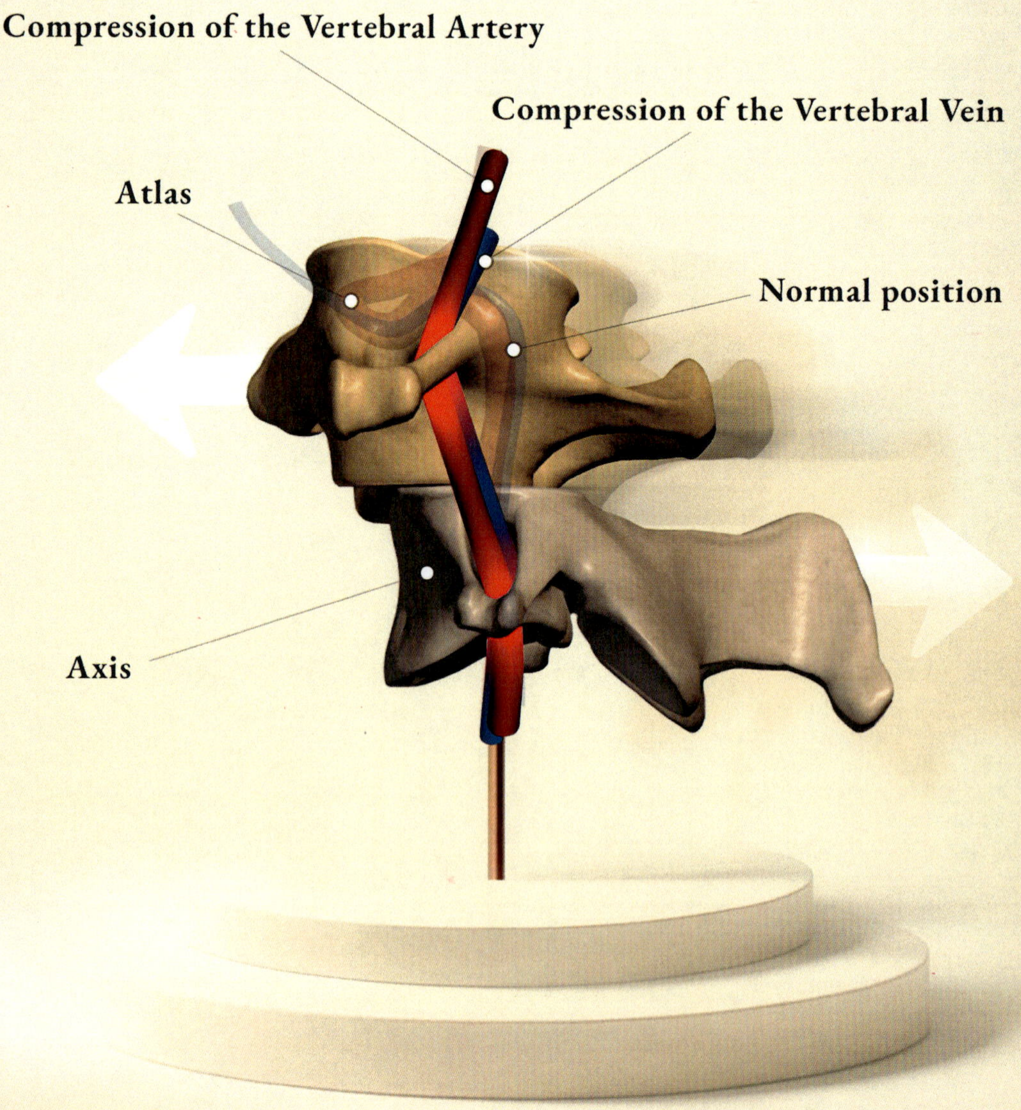

Partial Retrocollis

Partial retrocollis describes a slight backward tilt of the head that is not entirely abnormal but significant enough to cause discomfort and potential issues. This condition can be caused by various factors, including atlanto-axial subluxation, where the atlas is displaced forward and the axis vertebra is displaced backward.

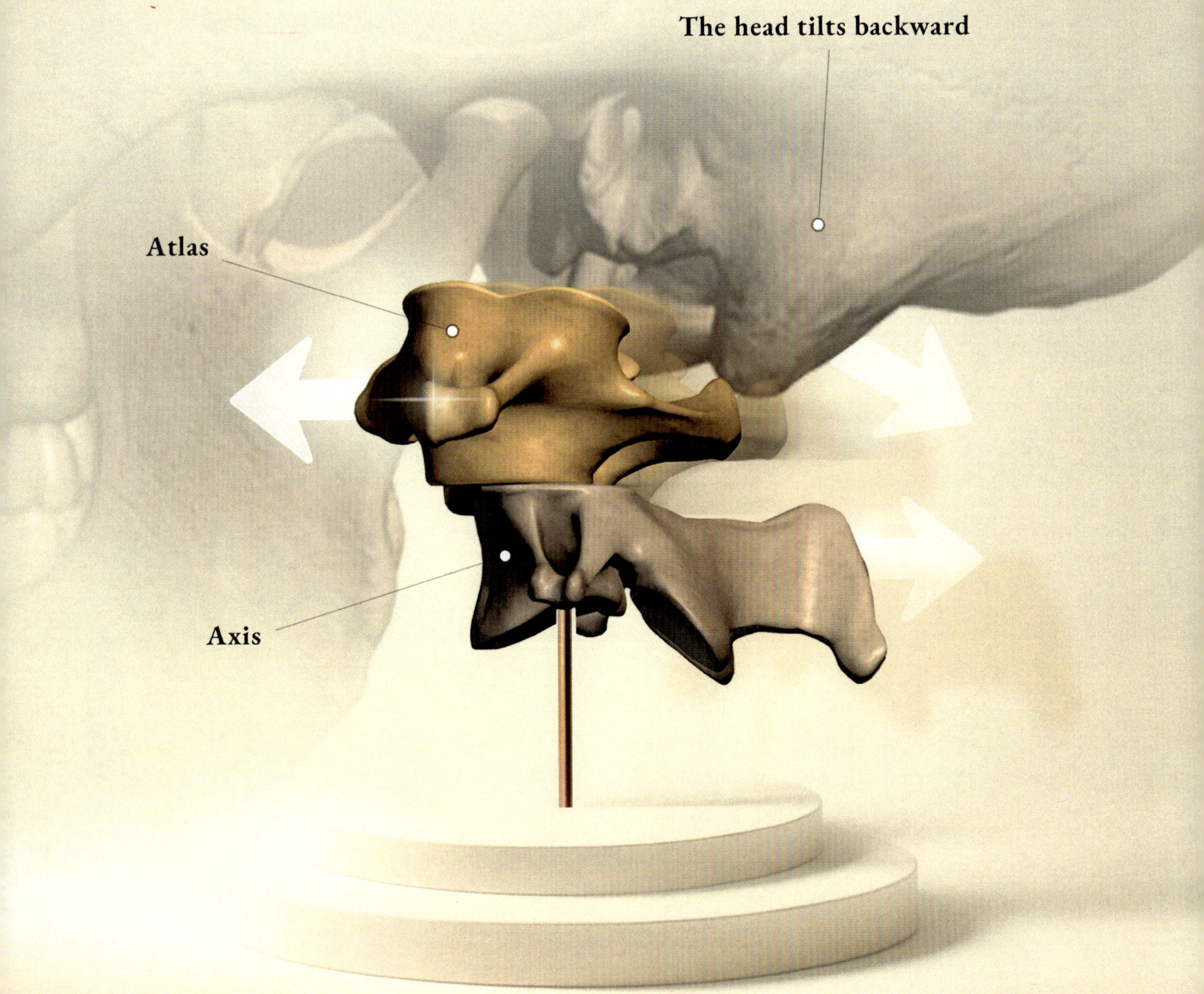

Compression in the Foramina Due to Retrocolis

Retrocolis, characterized by the backward tilt of the head, can compress nerves and blood vessels in the skull's foramina. This compression can impair cranial nerve function and restrict blood flow, leading to headaches, dizziness, facial pain, and neurological deficits. It occurs due to the forward displacement of the atlas relative to the axis in cases of anterior subluxation.

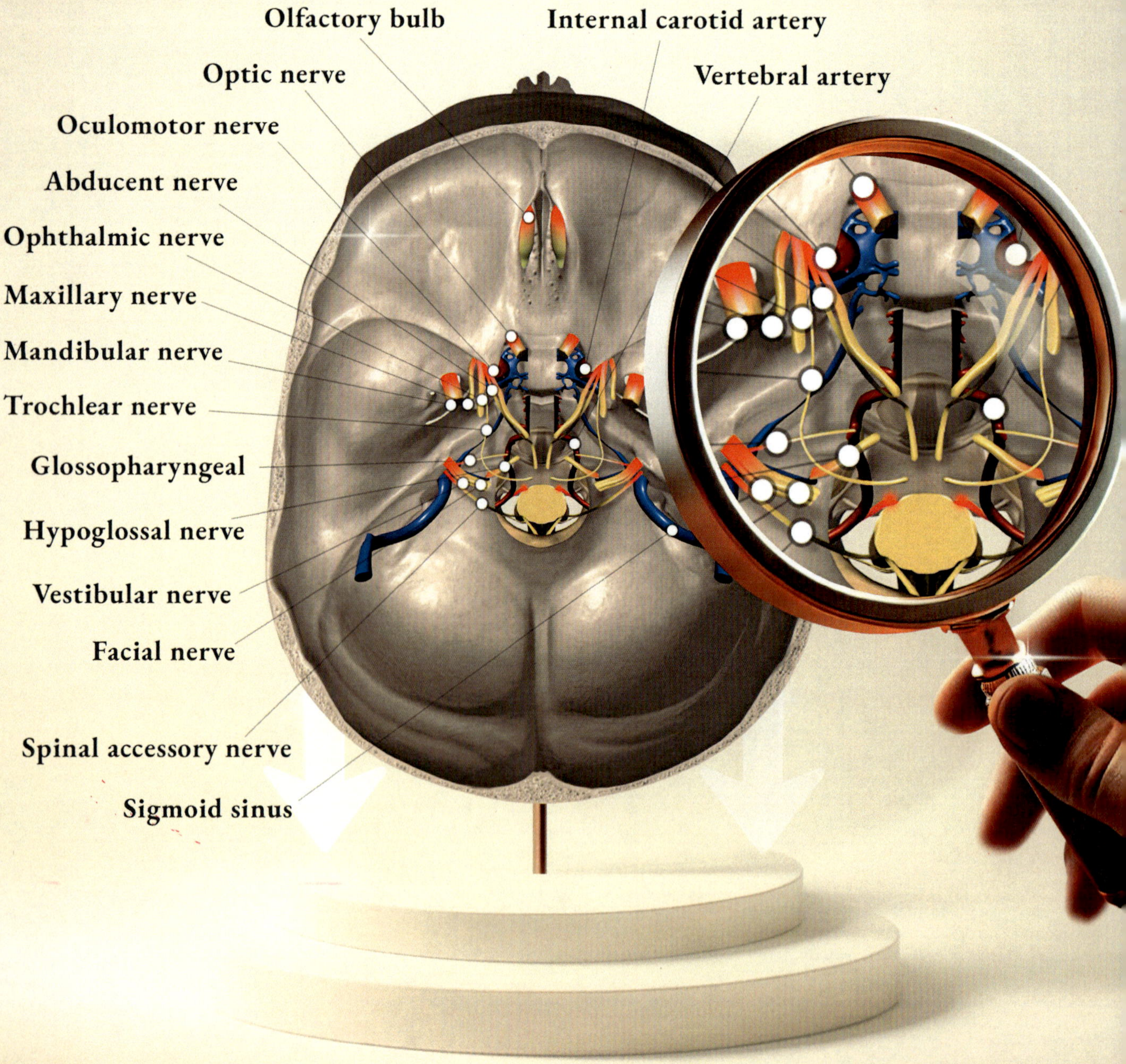

Dens Compresses the Medulla Oblongata

In the case of atlantoaxial subluxation, the Cricoform ligament is stretched, and through the Tectorial membrane, the dens of the axis compresses the anterior part of the medulla oblongata, affecting the Hypoglossal nerve (XII) and the Glossopharyngeal nerve (IX). These cranial nerves control speech, swallowing, tongue movements, and parasympathetic functions.

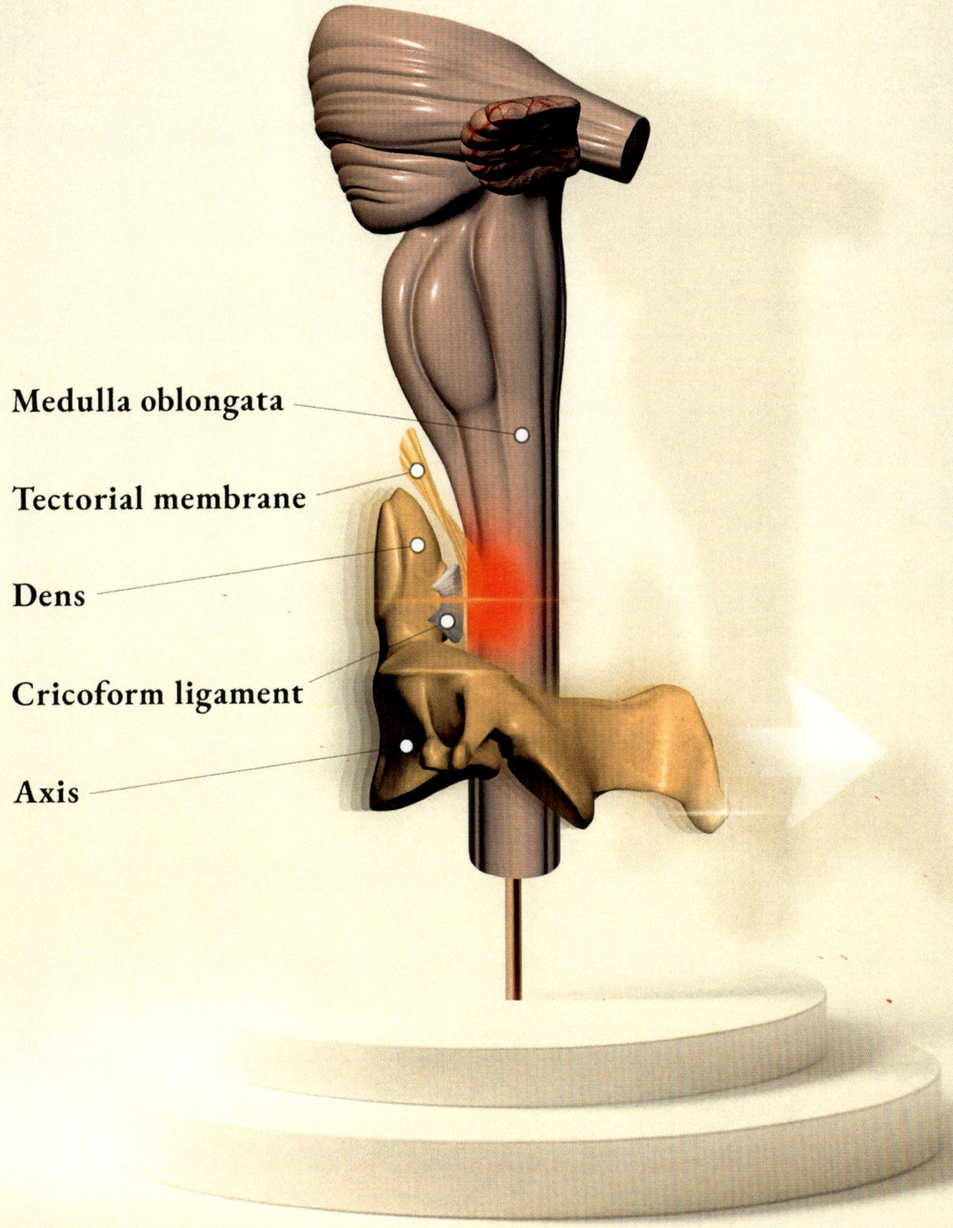

Cervical Hyperlordosis

When the atlas shifts forward, it changes the alignment of the cervical spine, causing muscle and ligament imbalance. To maintain stability, the body compensates by further curving the cervical spine, resulting in cervical hyperlordosis. Neck muscles may adjust by shortening or lengthening to stabilize the spine in this new position.

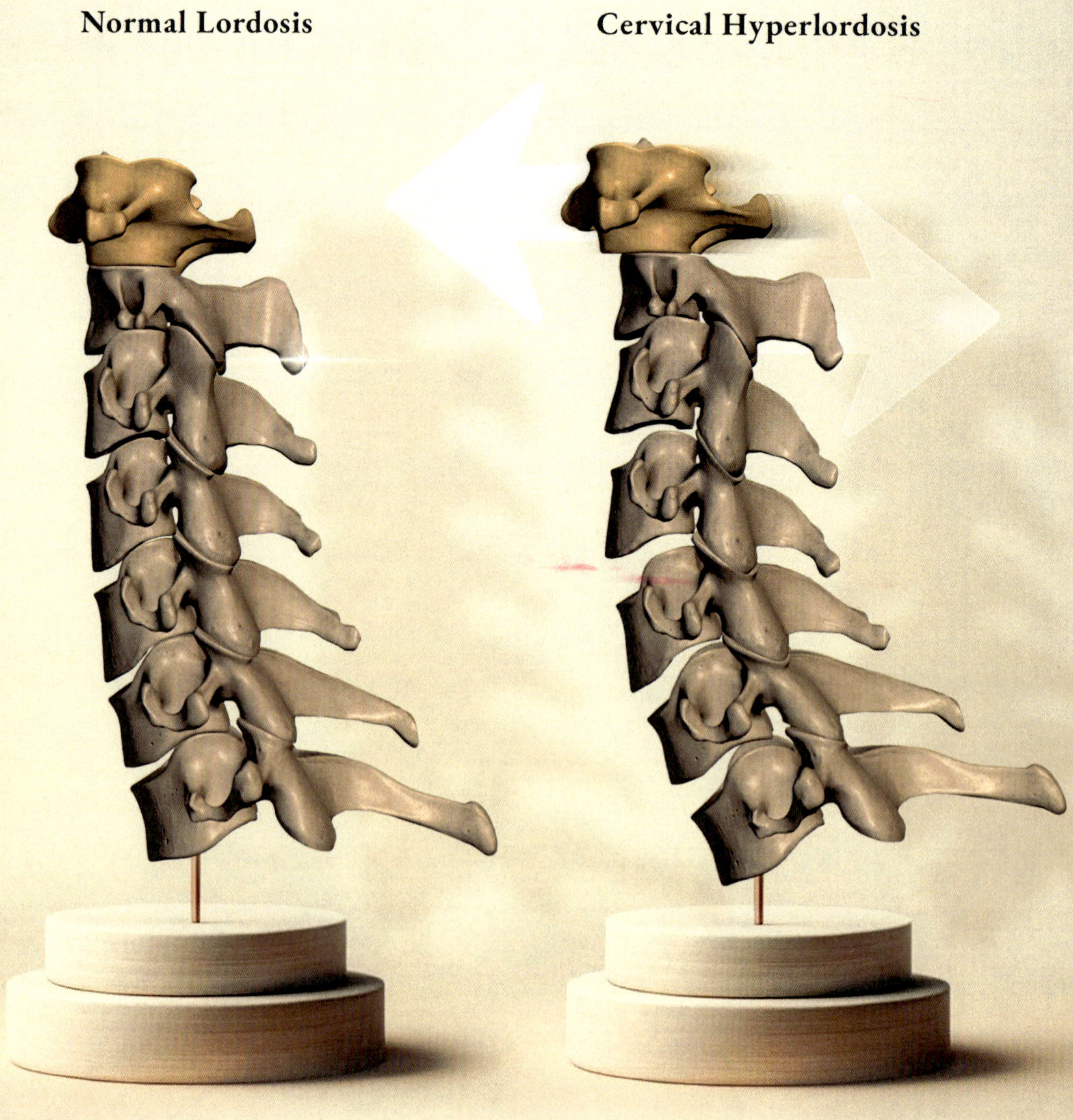

Spinal Effects of Atlantoaxial Subluxation

Atlantoaxial subluxation, which causes cervical hyperlordosis due to disrupted body mechanics and head weight, can also lead to thoracic hyperkyphosis and lumbar hyperlordosis. These compensatory changes in the thoracic and lumbar spine occur to maintain balance, often resulting in pain and reduced mobility.

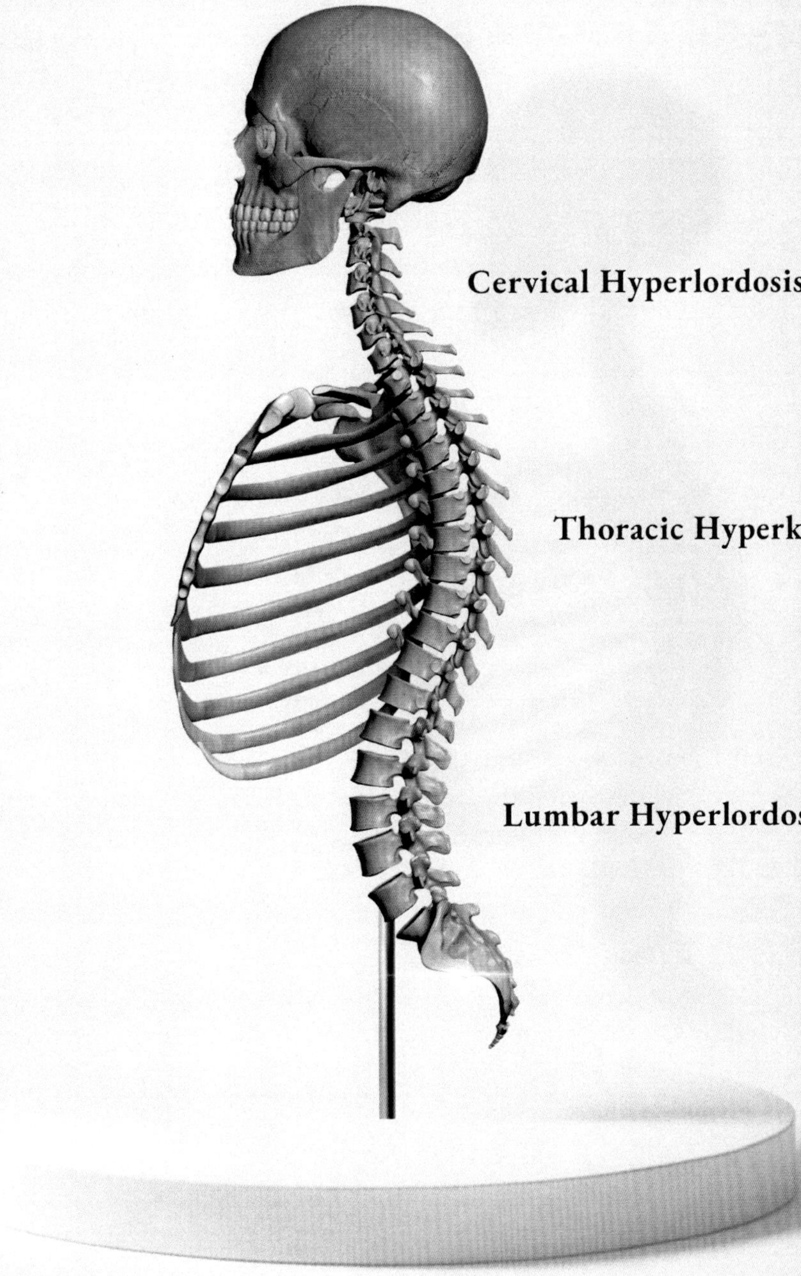

Herniated Discs

Atlantoaxial subluxation can cause cervical hyperlordosis and lumbar hyperlordosis, increasing the risk of herniated discs. Herniations most commonly occur between C5-C6 and C6-C7 in the neck, and L4-L5 and L5-S1 in the lower back, causing neck and lower back pain, and symptoms like sciatica.

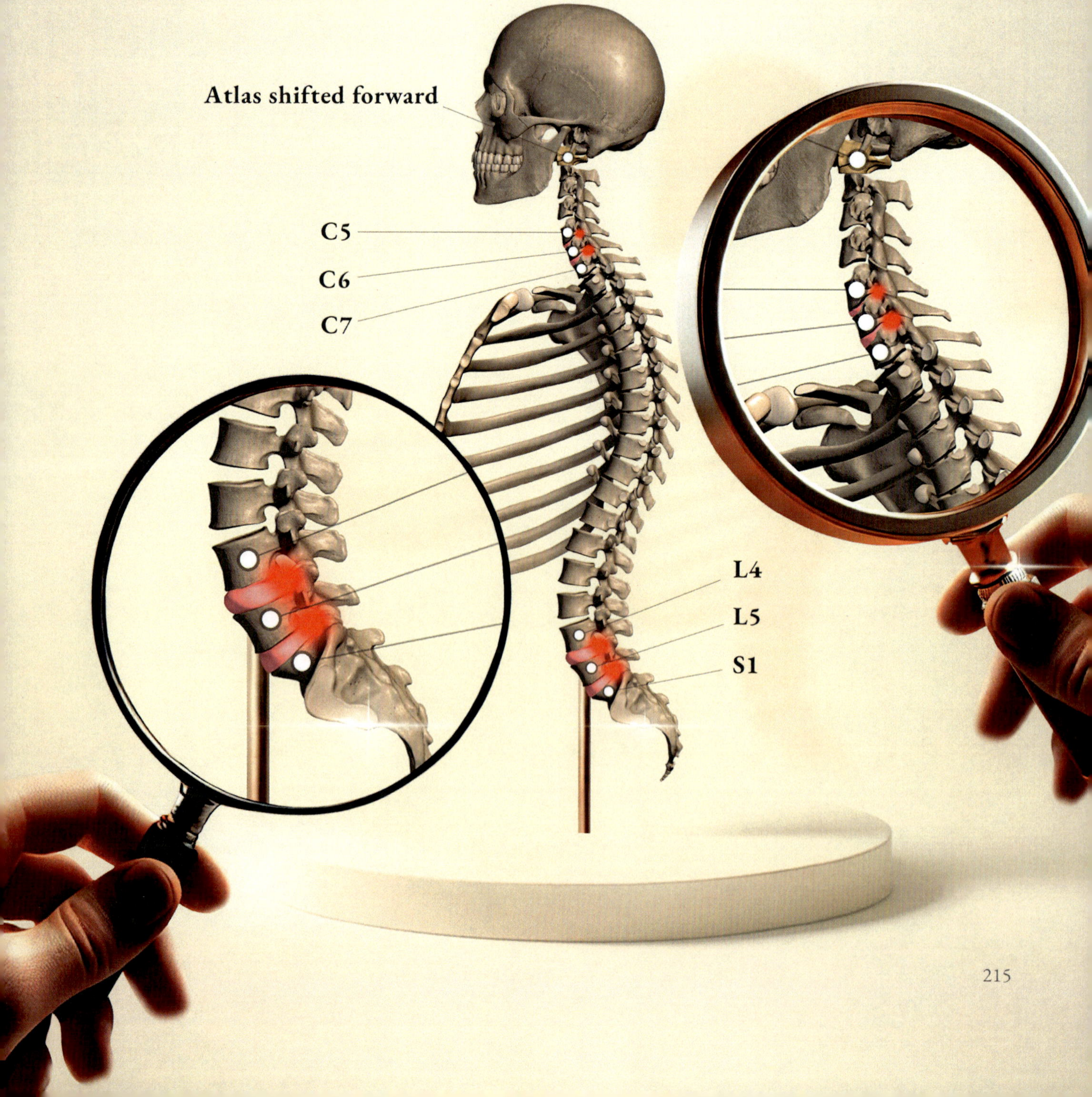

Inflamed Neck Muscles

In atlantoaxial subluxation, where the atlas shifts forward, several neck muscles become strained and inflamed. These include the suboccipital muscles, sternocleidomastoid, levator scapulae, paravertebral muscles, and upper trapezius. These muscles strain to stabilize the cervical spine, leading to tension and inflammation.

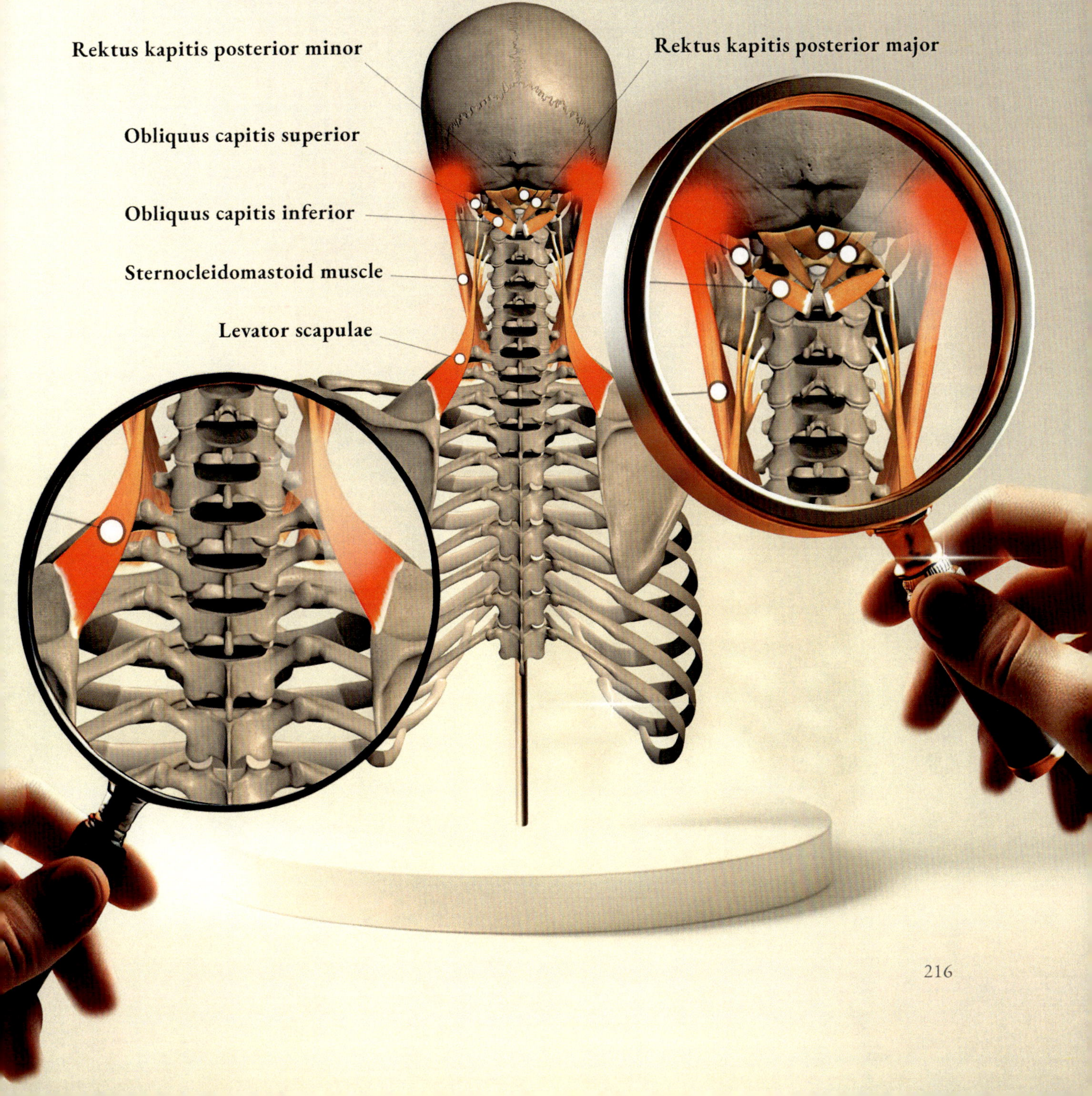

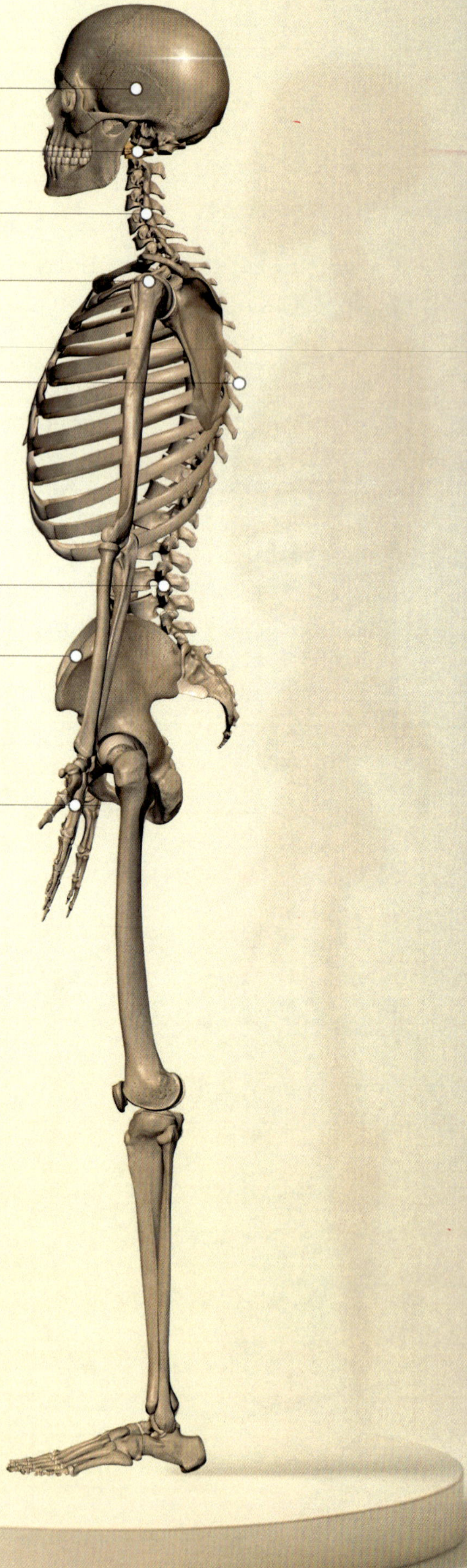

Body Posture

Atlantoaxial subluxation of the atlas disrupts body posture, as the forward shift of the atlas changes the alignment of the cervical spine. This can cause cervical hyperlordosis, thoracic hyperkyphosis, and lumbar hyperlordosis. Such spinal curvature changes lead to pain and reduced mobility.

Chapter 4

Posterior Atlas Subluxation

Posterior Atlas Subluxation

Posterior subluxation, as a specific form of subluxation in the cervical spine, represents a condition in which the first cervical vertebra, known as the atlas, partially shifts backward in relation to the second cervical vertebra, the axis [Image 1]. This type of subluxation often occurs due to trauma, inflammation, or factors affecting the stability of the cervical spine.

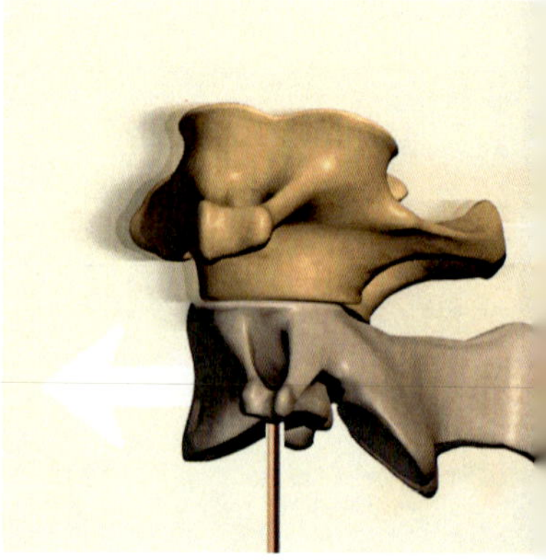

[Image 1] Posterior subluxation

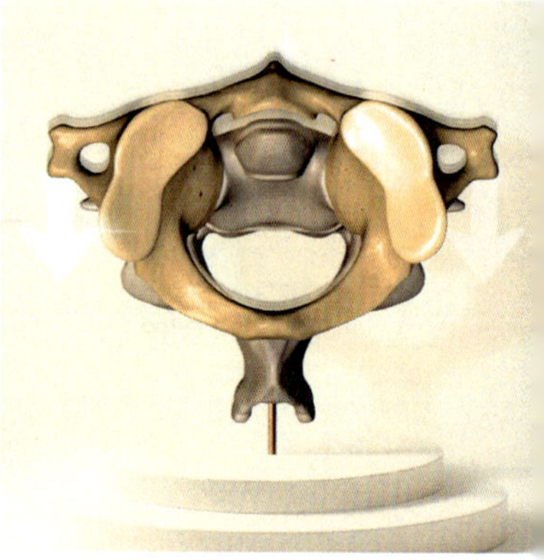

[Image 2] Top view

Characteristic of posterior subluxation of the atlas is the backward displacement of the atlas, which can lead to various symptoms in patients. Among the most common symptoms are neck pain, a sense of restricted head movement, and potential compression of nerve structures that can result in neurological issues. These symptoms can significantly impact patients' daily activities and quality of life.

In the case of posterior atlas subluxation, compression of nerve structures and blood vessels occurs near this part of the spinal column. Specifically, pressure on structures such as spinal nerves, vertebral arteries and veins, as well as surrounding soft tissues, can lead to various neurological and vascular complications [Image 2].

Posterior subluxation is the rarest type, typically occurs in uncommon situations involving impacts to the back of the head and neck. Unlike anterior subluxations caused by frontal impacts, posterior subluxations are less frequently observed due to the lower incidence of trauma to the occipital region and upper back. Because of this, posterior subluxations are relatively uncommon in clinical practice, often arising from specific injury mechanisms like high-impact trauma or unusual force distribution, making them more challenging to diagnose and manage compared to other misalignments. Posterior subluxations are uncommon, complicating diagnosis and treatment due to subtle symptoms and specific injuries.

Causes and Impact of Posterior Subluxation

Posterior atlas subluxation often arises from specific yet less common situations that generate powerful forces directed towards the front of the chest and the occiput. Blows to the chest can cause posterior atlas subluxation, especially if the impact disrupts the atlas's position relative to the axis. Furthermore, a posterior atlantoaxial subluxation (Atlas and axis) can stem from typical scenarios where impacts are directed to the occipital region of the head, which may result from accidental falls, sports injuries, or other incidental events.

Traffic accidents often play a role in the occurrence of posterior atlantoaxial subluxations, particularly in cases of unexpected frontal collisions, impacts to the chest, or excessive strain on seat belts. When a vehicle is suddenly struck from the front, the head can jerk forward abruptly, exerting significant forces that may cause the atlas to shift backward in relation to the axis.

These particular circumstances generate rare but potentially serious situations that can lead to atlas subluxation. Understanding these causes is crucial for identifying and promptly treating posterior subluxations, enabling effective therapy and rehabilitation for patients exposed to such traumatic events.

A posterior atlantoaxial subluxation is considered the rarest among its counterparts, mainly because it occurs in uncommon circumstances. It typically manifests following impacts to the back of the head or chest, situations that are relatively infrequent compared to other types of trauma.

In posterior atlas subluxations, the atlas moves backward, typically from impacts to the back of the head or thorax during sudden head jerks, like in accidents or sports injuries.

Clinical Features of Posterior Subluxation

Posterior subluxation of the atlas, although rare, can cause various clinical characteristics and symptoms that affect the overall spine structure. When this type of subluxation occurs, changes in the normal curves of the spine can be observed, including cervical kyphosis, thoracic lordosis, and lumbar kyphosis.

A kyphotic deformity of the cervical vertebrae may result from changes in the position of the atlas and axis due to the posterior subluxations. This change in the curvature of the cervical spine can cause pain, a feeling of tension, and restricted movement in the neck.

Additionally, kyphosis of the cervical vertebrae resulting from posterior atlas subluxations can contribute to shoulder girdle pain, along with feelings of tension and heaviness in the shoulders. This altered curvature of the cervical spine can lead to muscle tension and discomfort in the chest area, further impacting the mobility and functionality of the upper body. Patients may find it difficult to perform overhead movements or maintain proper posture due to symptoms related to cervical spine kyphosis. Therefore, addressing and correcting the posterior subluxation of the atlas is important not only for proper spine alignment but also for alleviating associated discomfort in the shoulders and chest.

On the other hand, thoracic lordosis, a natural curve of the spine that exhibits convex curvature forward, can also be affected by posterior subluxation of the atlas. This change can cause discomfort in the upper back, reduced mobility, and possible dysfunction of internal organs.

Furthermore, the alteration in the curvature of the thoracic spine, characterized by lordosis resulting from posterior subluxations of the atlas, can lead to changes in the shape of the rib cage. This abnormal curvature can create biomechanical imbalances, placing excessive stress on the muscles surrounding the thoracic region. As a consequence, chronic inflammation may develop in the chest muscles, contributing to discomfort and restricted mobility. Individuals with thoracic lordosis may experience persistent soreness, stiffness, or even localized tenderness in the muscles of the chest wall. Addressing the underlying cause of this postural distortion, such as correcting the posterior subluxation of the atlas, is crucial for alleviating these symptoms and restoring optimal thoracic spine function.

Neurovascular symptoms can also be a significant part of the clinical presentation of posterior atlas subluxation. The backward displacement of the atlas can compress or irritate surrounding nerve structures, such as the vertebral arteries or cranial nerves, leading to various symptoms. For example, pressure on the vertebral arteries can reduce blood flow to the brain, potentially causing symptoms such as dizziness, blurred vision, fainting, or a feeling of instability. Additionally, pressure on the nerves exiting from the cervical spine can cause pain, tingling, or weakness in the upper extremities, as well as headaches or migraines.Furthermore, posterior atlas subluxation can negatively affect the function of the vagus nerve, leading to symptoms such as digestive issues, heart rate irregularities, and even changes in anxiety levels. These symptoms, which involve the autonomic nervous system, may be less immediately apparent but are very serious in the long term, highlighting the need for prompt diagnosis and treatment.This neurovascular component makes the clinical presentation of posterior subluxation even more complex, indicating the potential for systemic consequences that extend beyond the biomechanical dysfunction itself.

Diagnosing and Treating Posterior Subluxations

Diagnostic approaches for identifying posterior atlas subluxations and therapeutic strategies and treatments for them are parallel to those applied in the case of anterior atlas subluxation. Starting with the diagnostic approach, advanced imaging technologies such as 3D scanners are used, providing detailed insights into the structure and position of the atlas vertebra. Following this, the statics of the patient's body are carefully analyzed to identify any shifts and imbalances in the cervical spine.

Palpation also plays a crucial role in the diagnostic process, allowing physicians to assess the position of the atlas vertebra and identify any subluxations. The combination of these methods enables precise and comprehensive diagnosis of posterior atlas subluxations.

After diagnosis, the "Harmonious Balance" (HB) method is implemented, focusing on precisely adjusting the atlas vertebra to restore optimal spine and nervous system function. This therapeutic technique is tailored to the individual needs of each patient, offering a personalized and effective approach to treating posterior atlas subluxations.

In addition to diagnosis and primary therapy, monitoring progress and rehabilitation are vital for successful treatment of posterior atlas subluxations. Regular follow-up exams ensure atlas stability and optimal spinal alignment, along with reevaluating body statics and symptoms for long-term success.

Incorporating targeted neck and spinal exercises can help maintain atlas stability and prevent reoccurrence. Physical therapy strengthens cervical support, maintaining postural balance and reducing pain. These strategies enhance treatment outcomes and ensure long-term atlas stability.

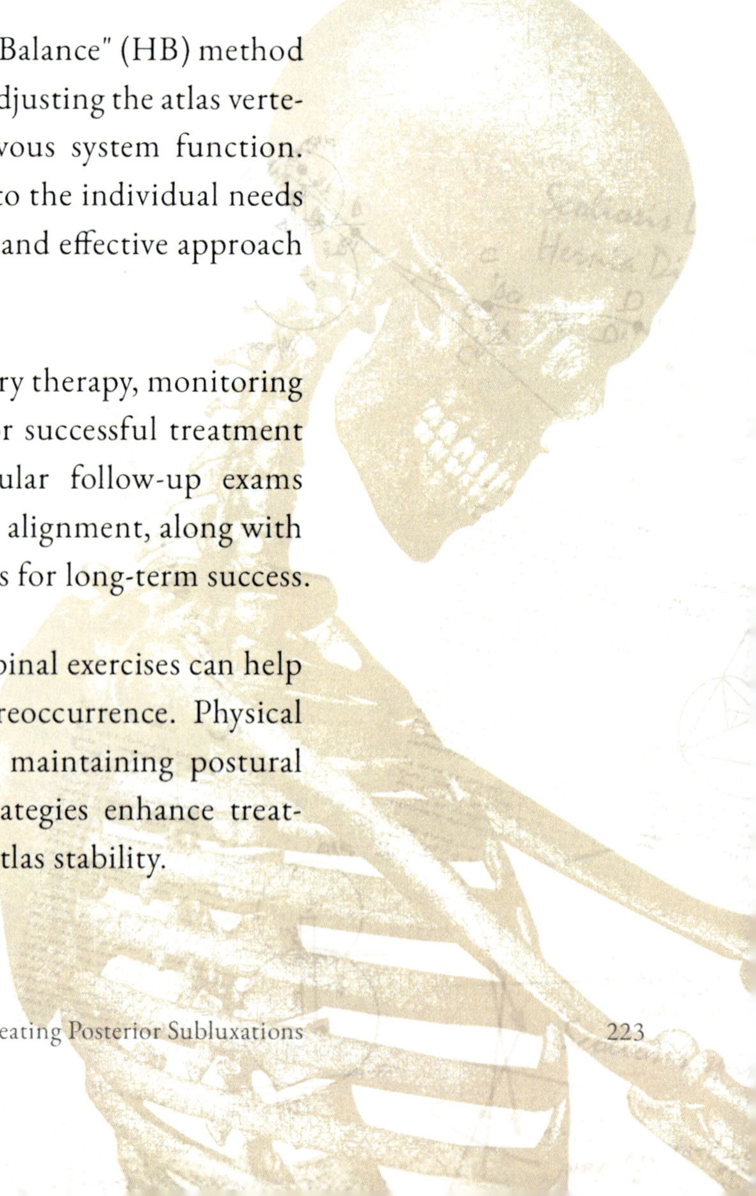

Posterior Subluxation of the Atlas

Posterior subluxation of the atlas is characterized by the backward displacement of the atlas relative to the axis. This type of subluxation often occurs due to trauma or physical impact to the back of the head or neck. As a result, it can compress nerve structures and blood vessels, leading to symptoms such as neck pain, headaches, dizziness, and neurological deficits.

Atlas is displaced posteriorly

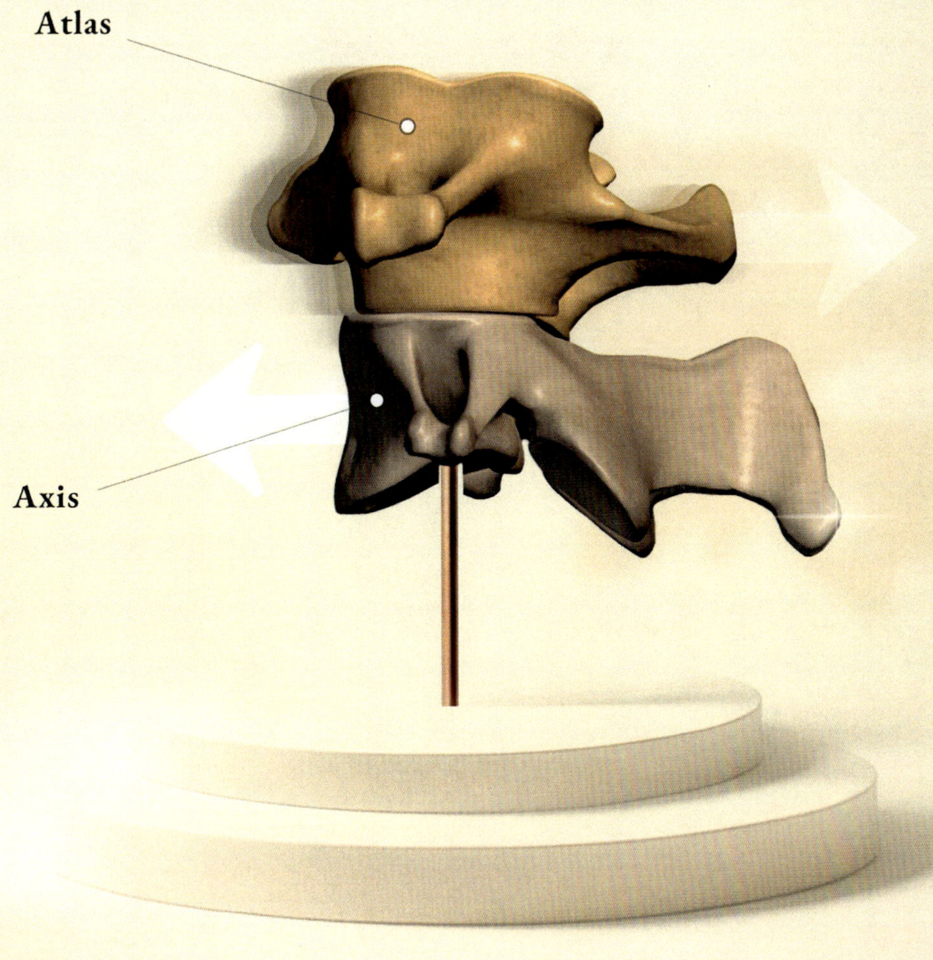

Posterior Subluxation: 2 to 4 Millimeters

The backward displacement of the atlas (posterior subluxation) can be limited by anatomical structures, especially the dens of the axis, which acts as a barrier. Generally, the atlas can move backward by a few millimeters before the dens of the axis restricts further movement. Typical backward displacement of the atlas in subluxation can be between 2 to 4 millimeters.

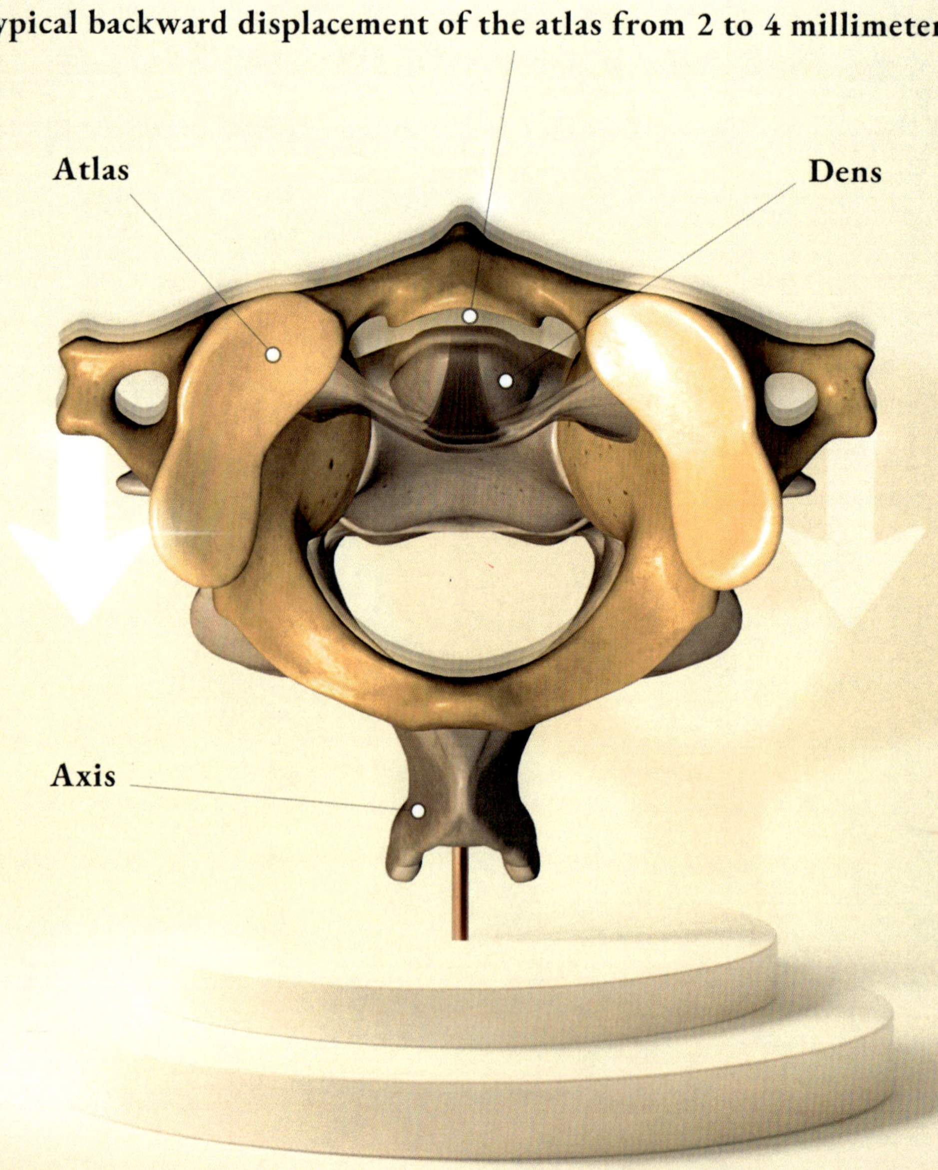

Loss of Cervical Lordosis

When the atlas vertebra shifts backward relative to the axis and the head, it can cause a condition known as loss of cervical lordosis. This results in the straightening of the cervical spine's natural curve, with the atlas leaning forward due to the head's weight. This leads to cervical kyphosis, altered alignment, muscle tension, nerve compression, and postural changes.

Normal Lordosis **Loss of cervical lordosis**

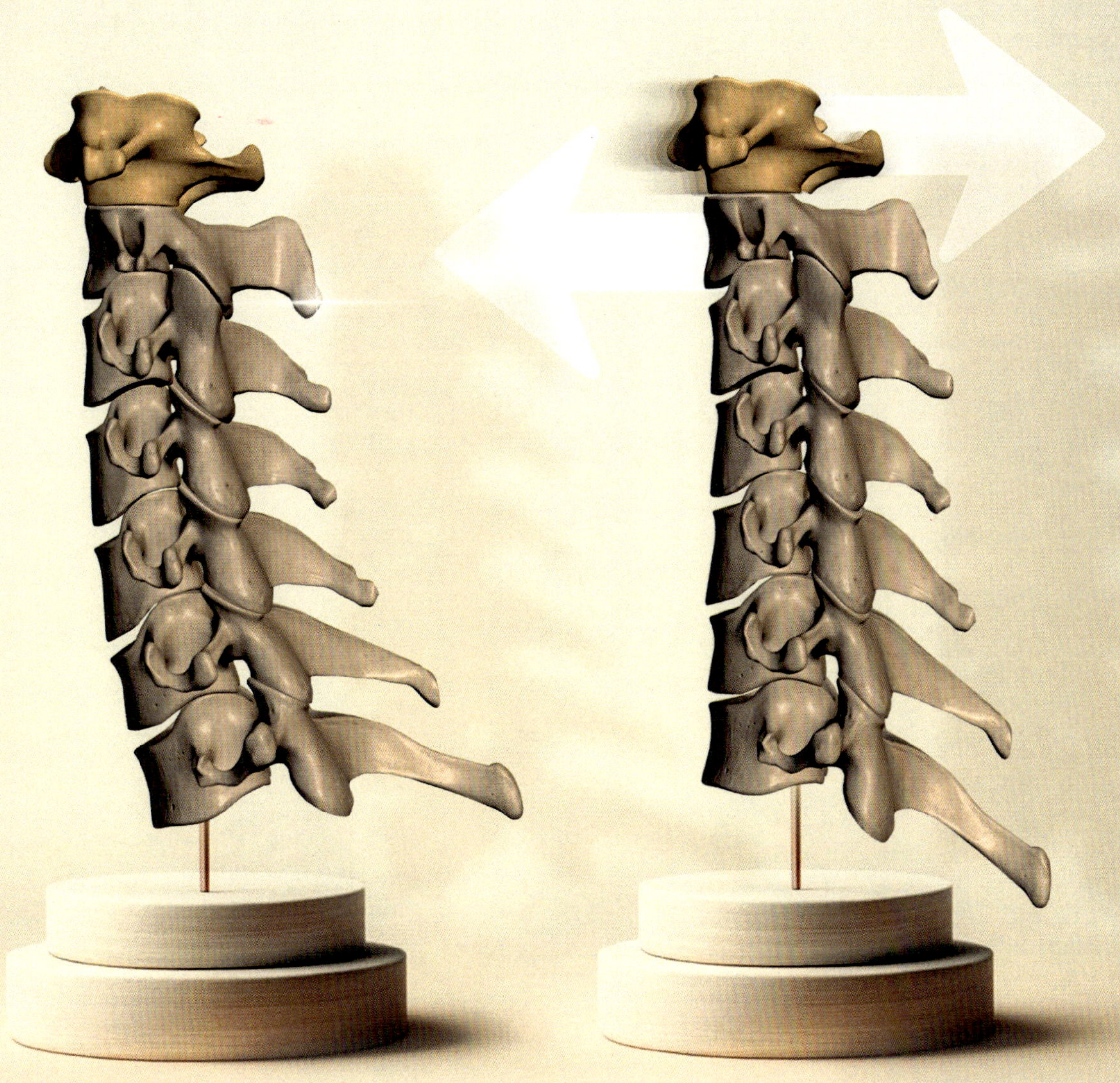

Compression of Spinal Nerves

When the atlas shifts backward relative to the axis and the head, the first, second, and third cervical nerve roots (C1, C2, C3) can be subjected to pressure. These nerve roots continue as the suboccipital nerve (C1), greater occipital nerve (C2), and third occipital nerve (C3). Compression of these nerve roots can cause neck pain, headaches, dizziness, and numbness.

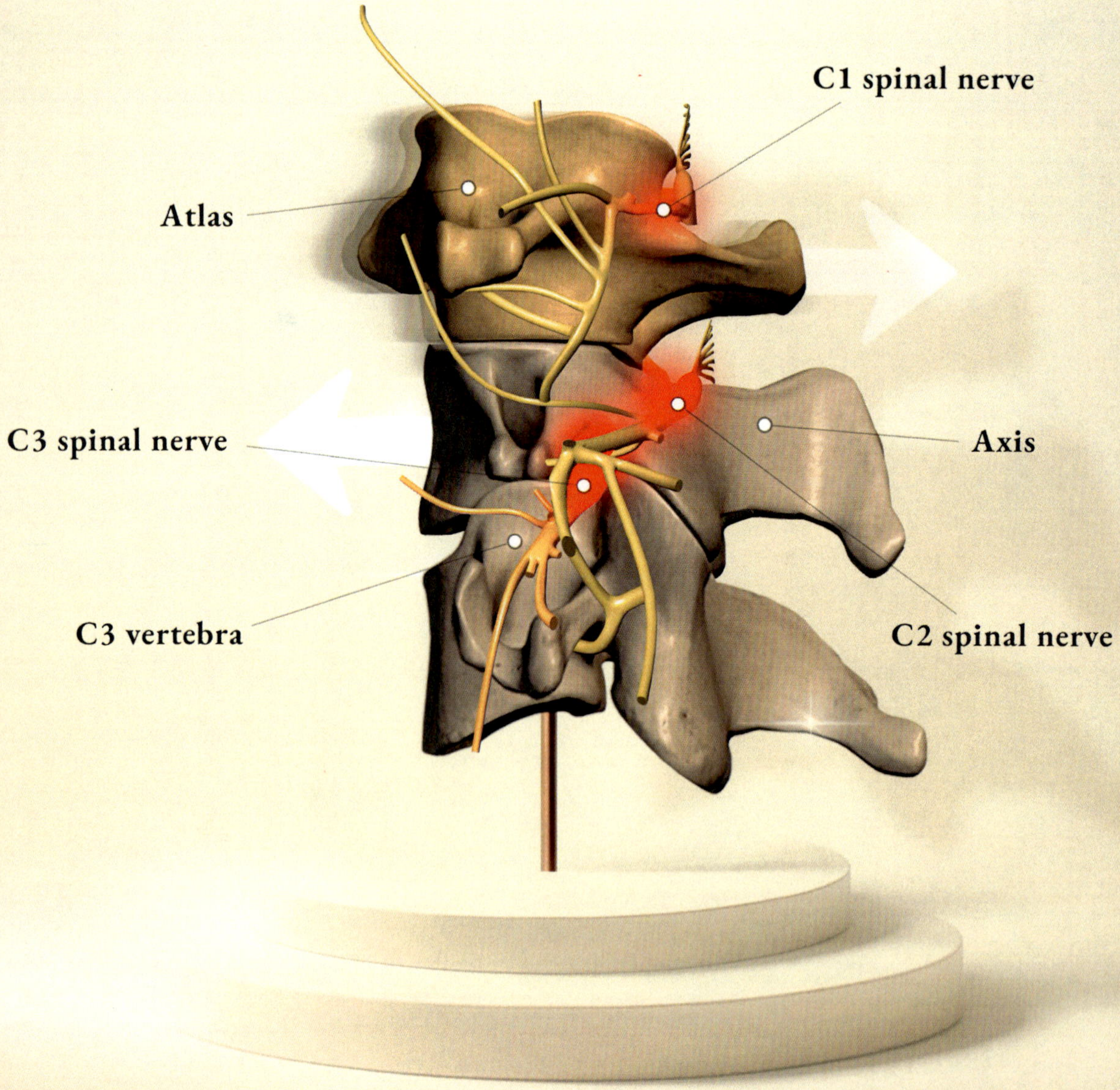

Compression of Vertebral Arteries

During the correction of cervical lordosis, the vertebral arteries, which pass through the cervical vertebrae, can become compressed. This can reduce blood flow to the brain, leading to symptoms like dizziness, headaches, blurred vision, and balance problems. Compression can worsen due to additional pressure from vertebral displacement or muscle tension.

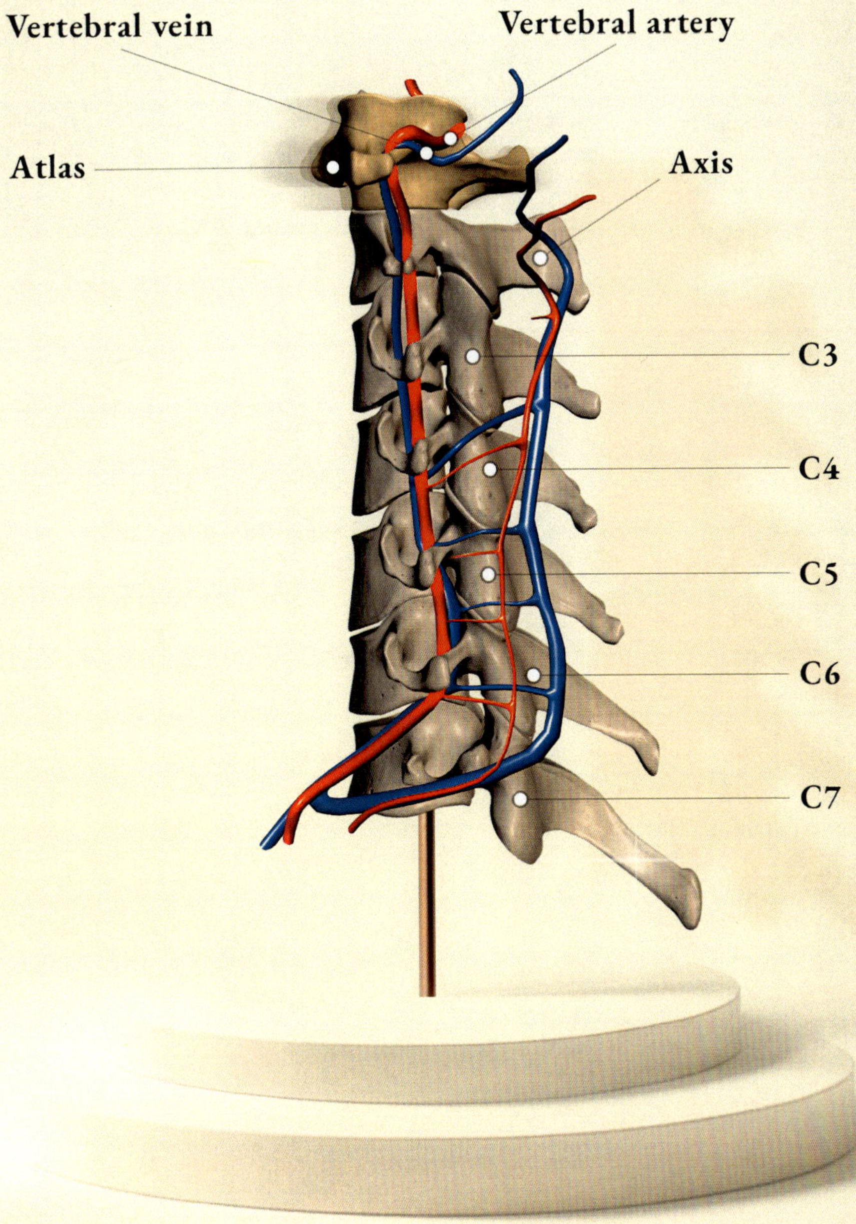

Head Positioning

Posterior subluxation of the atlas straightens cervical lordosis and moves the head forward, tilting it downward. As subluxation progresses, the atlas tilts further, leading to cervical vertebral kyphosis and a more forward head posture. This misalignment worsens the forward tilt, disrupting the cervical spine's natural curve and causing postural and neurological issues.

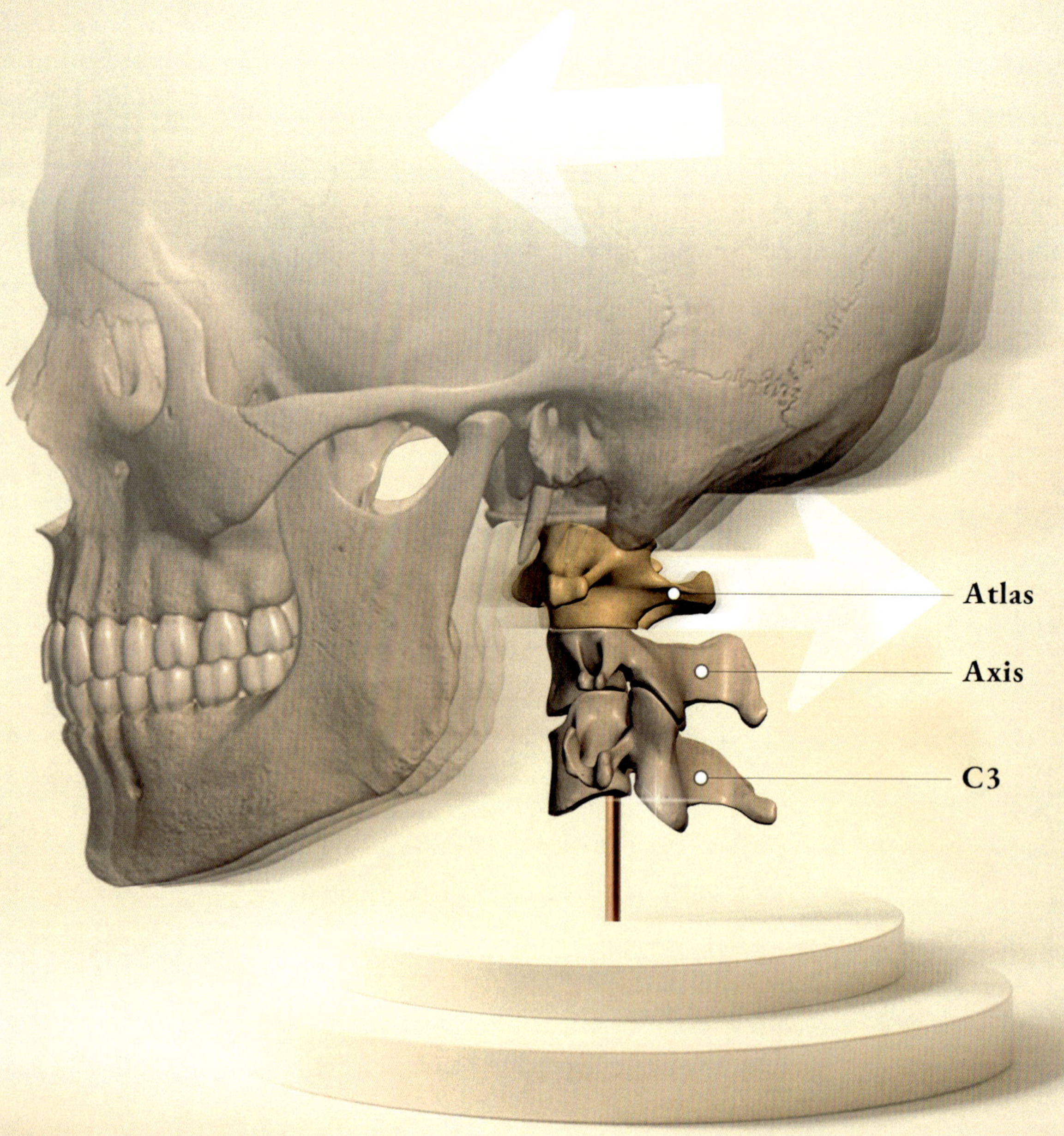

Muscles Affected by Posterior Atlas Subluxation

Muscle groups such as the suboccipital muscles, sternocleidomastoid, levator scapulae, paravertebral muscles, trapezius, and shoulder girdle muscles are most affected by stretching and inflammation. These muscles attempt to compensate for disrupted posture and stabilize the cervical spine, leading to tension, inflammation, pain, and limited mobility.

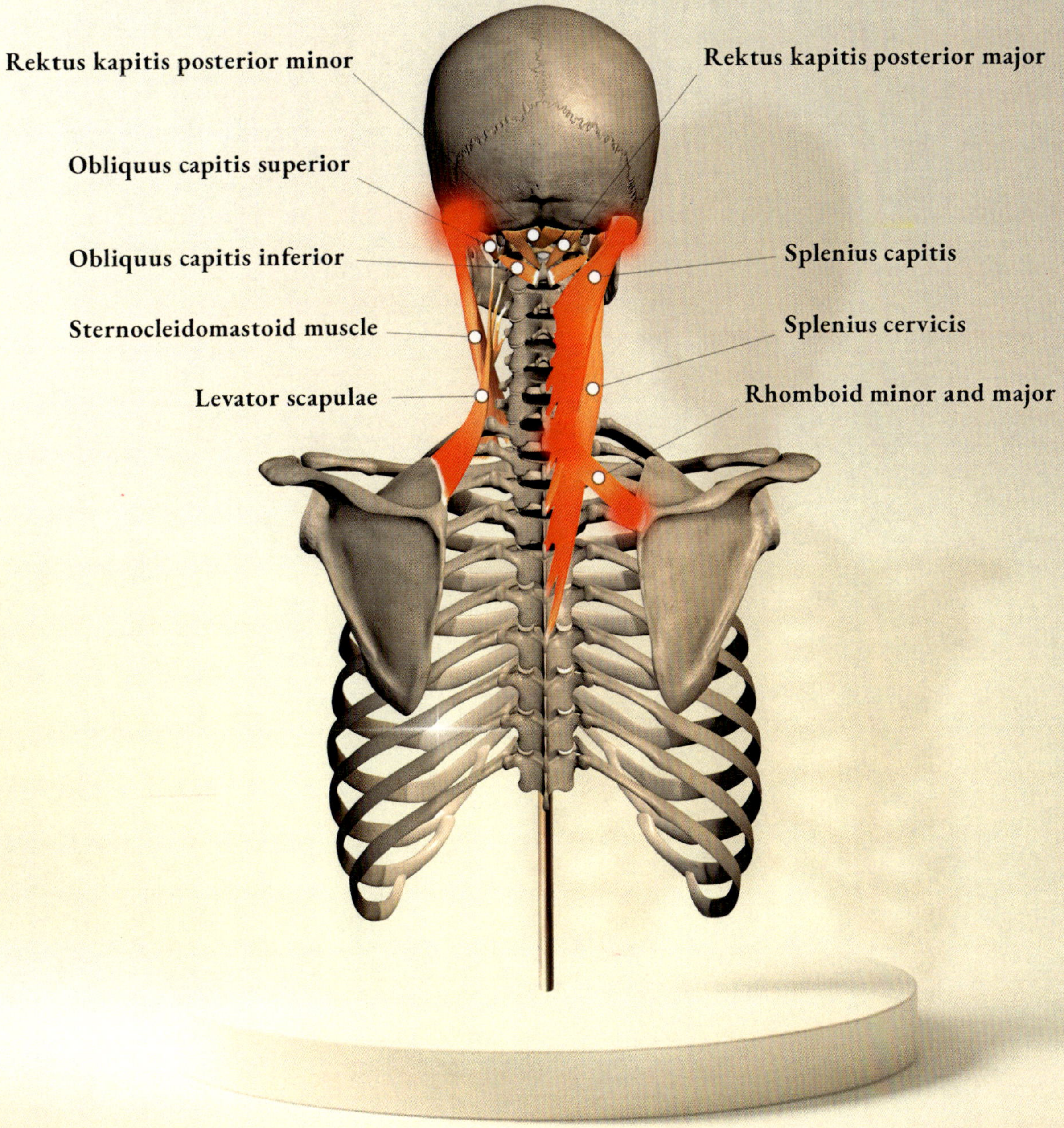

Trapezius Inflammation from Atlas Subluxation

In posterior atlas subluxation, the upper trapezius muscle often becomes inflamed due to abnormal posture from straightened cervical lordosis and forward head tilt. Overcompensation to stabilize the head and neck leads to tension, fatigue, and inflammation. Symptoms include neck, shoulder, and upper back pain, tension headaches, and reduced mobility.

Trigger points of the trapezius muscle

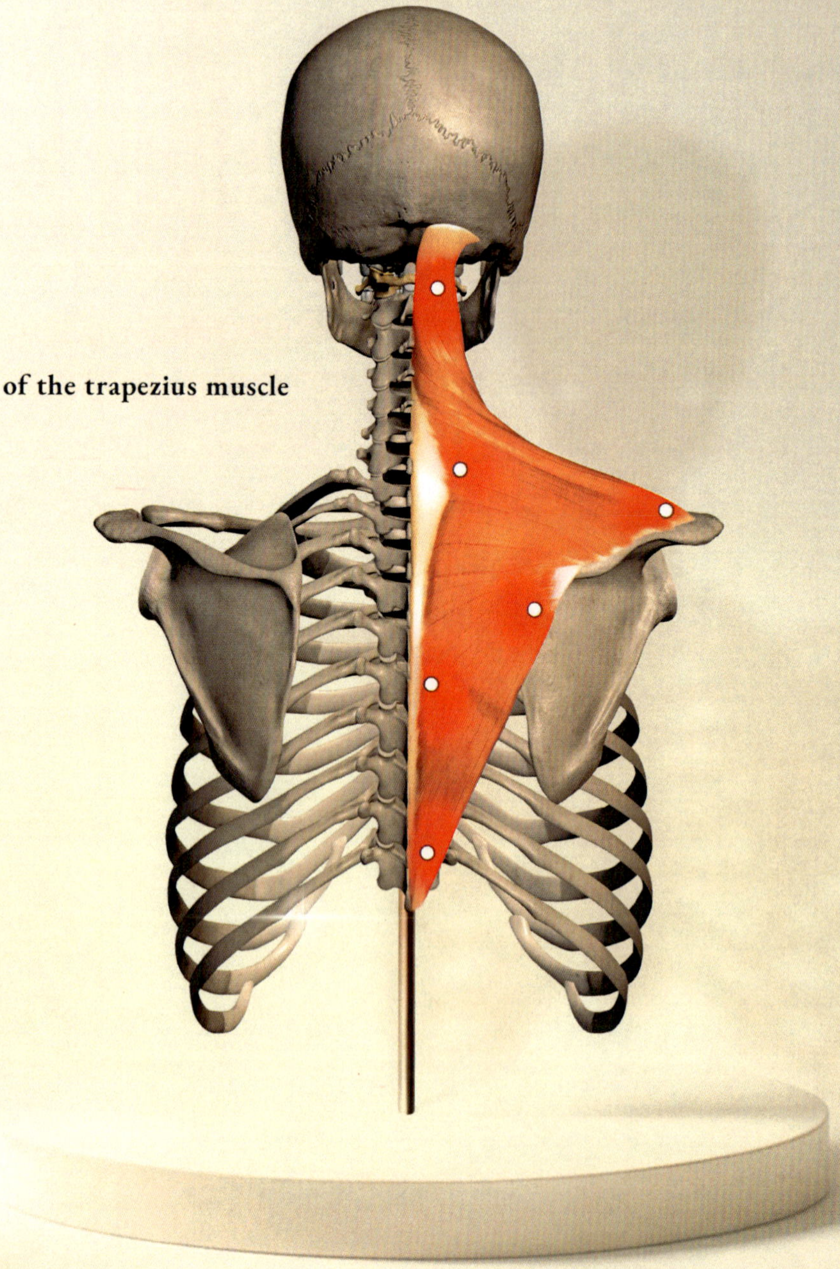

Disorientation and Coordination Disorder

Posterior atlas subluxation, the eighth cranial vestibulocochlear nerve can become compressed in the short canal of the temporal bone, called the internal acoustic meatus. This nerve transmits impulses from the inner ear to the brain, providing balance (vestibular) and hearing (cochlear) functions. These issues arise because posterior subluxation can alter cervical spine alignment and tension, putting pressure on the vestibulocochlear nerve. Lying on the back, when the pillow pushes the relaxed head, can cause and worsen dizziness and disturbances in orientation and coordination.

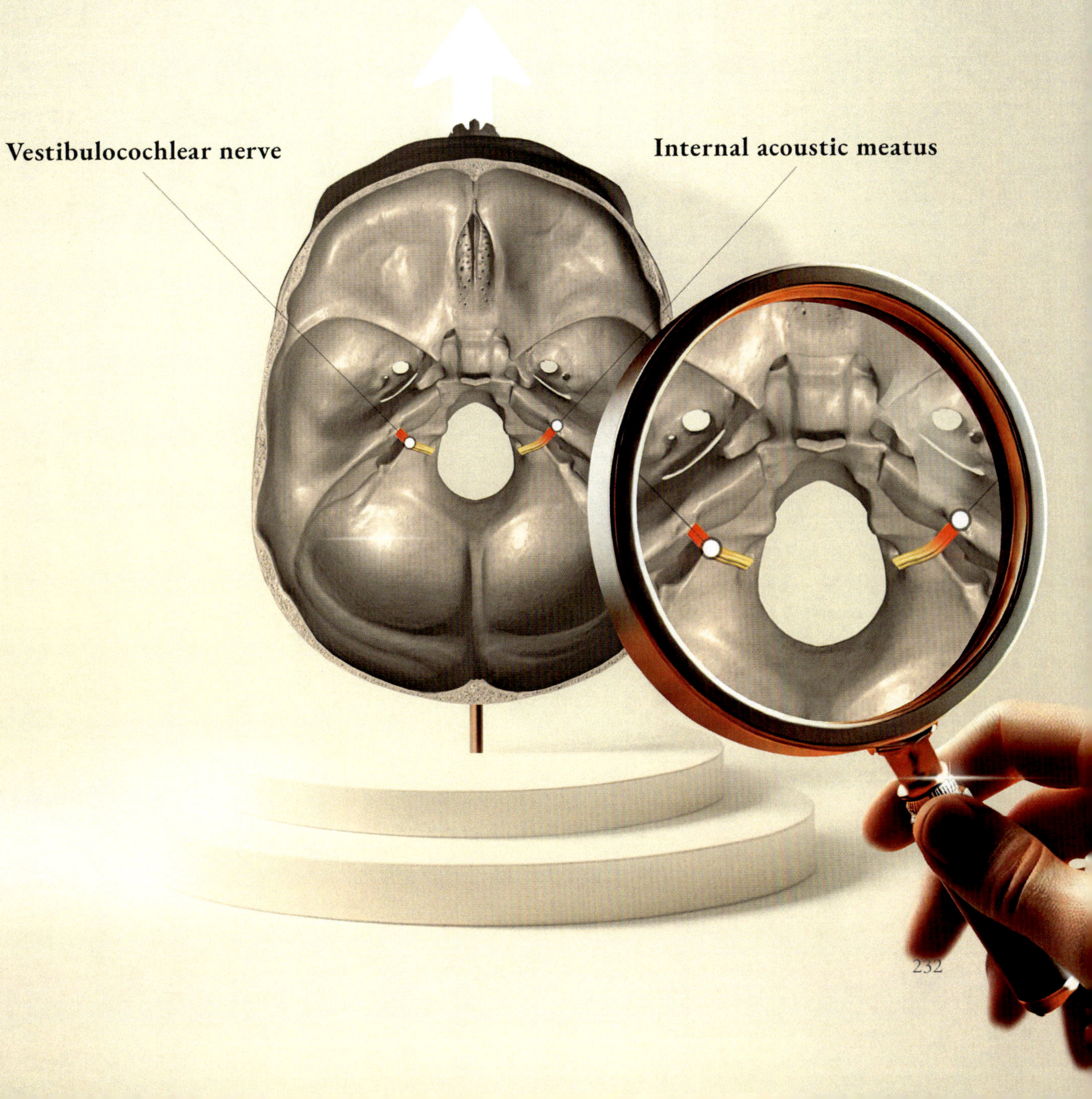

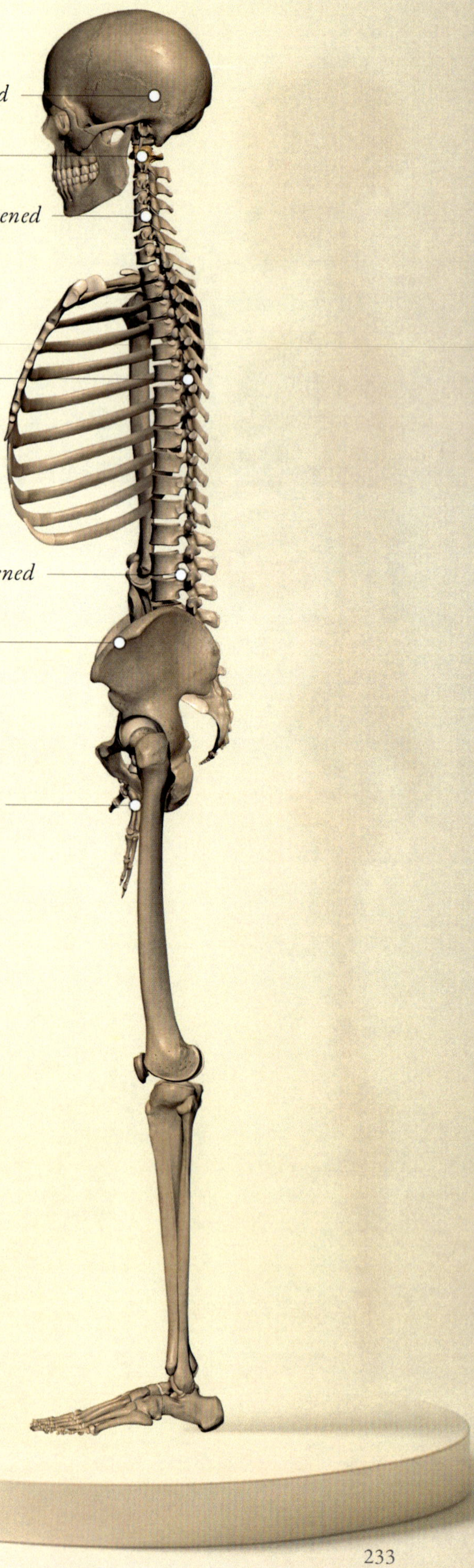

Body Posture

Posterior subluxation of the atlas affects body posture by shifting the atlas backward, altering the alignment of the cervical spine. This can result in straightened cervical lordosis, straightened thoracic kyphosis, and straightened lumbar lordosis. These changes in spinal curvature can lead to pain and limited mobility.

Chapter 5

Lateral Atlas Subluxation

Lateral Atlas Subluxation

Lateral subluxation of the atlas often occurs as a result of trauma, with traffic accidents being the most common form of such trauma. In these situations, the impacts typically involve the lateral and frontal parts of the head, though rarely at a perfect angle. It's noteworthy that direct, perpendicular impacts to the head are less common, as the head tends to be slightly rotated during such events. This rotational aspect of the head during impact can contribute to lateral displacement of the atlas vertebra.

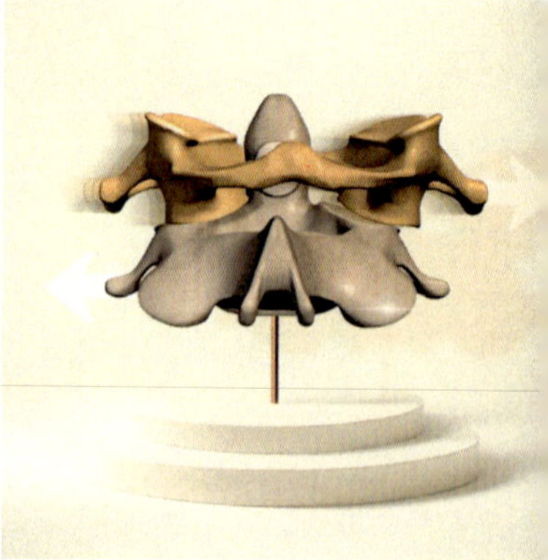

[Image 1] Right lateral subluxation

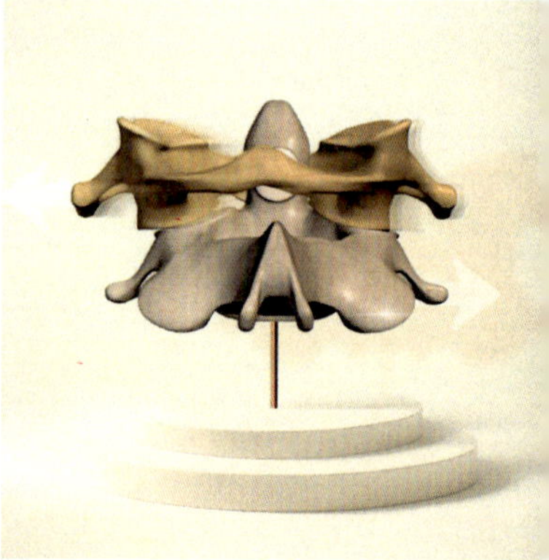

[Image 2] Left lateral subluxation

Inflammation or improper vertebral alignment, often resulting from poor posture, most commonly arises as a consequence of the habit of sleeping on one side of the body. This poor habit can lead to an imbalance in the spine's alignment, which in turn can cause the vertebrae to shift and create tension in the muscles. It's important to pay attention to sleeping habits and adopt positions that support the natural curvature of the spine to avoid potential posture and spinal issues.

It is of utmost importance to accurately diagnose whether the lateral subluxation of the atlas is on the right or left side, as these two distinct subluxations result in different symptoms and health issues. Identifying the specific side of the subluxation allows for targeted treatment and management strategies tailored to the individual's condition, ensuring optimal outcomes and relief from symptoms. Therefore, a precise diagnosis is crucial for developing an effective treatment plan and addressing the underlying cause of the lateral subluxation.

Lateral subluxation of the atlas to the right is often more prevalent and pronounced [Image 1], with lesser implications for the patient's health compared to lateral subluxation of the atlas to the left [Image 2]. This observation is commonly noted in clinical practice, where asymmetries in spinal alignment are frequently encountered. The biomechanical factors contributing to this phenomenon may involve habitual patterns of movement, postural imbalances, or previous traumas affecting the spine. Despite being more common, right-sided lateral subluxation of the atlas tends to exhibit milder symptoms and is typically easier to address through therapeutic interventions. Conversely, left-sided lateral subluxation may present with more significant health concerns and may require more comprehensive management strategies to alleviate associated discomfort and restore optimal spinal function.

Lateral atlas subluxation not only affects spinal alignment but also leads to muscle compensation on both sides of the neck and shoulders. When the atlas is displaced laterally, the muscles on one side of the neck may become overstretched, while those on the opposite side can become tight and overworked in an attempt to stabilize the head and neck. This muscle imbalance can contribute to further misalignment and may exacerbate symptoms such as neck pain, shoulder tension, and headaches. Over time, these muscular compensations can create a feedback loop, where muscle tension reinforces the subluxation, making it more difficult to correct without targeted therapeutic interventions. Addressing muscle imbalances through physical therapy or specific exercises can be crucial in complementing the realignment of the atlas and preventing future subluxations.

Additionally, nerve compression can also be a consequence of lateral atlas subluxation. The displacement of the atlas can put pressure on nearby nerve structures, potentially leading to symptoms such as tingling, numbness, or weakness in the arms and shoulders. These neurological symptoms indicate the importance of timely diagnosis and treatment to prevent long-term nerve damage.

Causes of Lateral Atlas Subluxation

The most dramatic factors leading to lateral subluxations of the atlas are traumas or impacts to the left and right temporal region and impacts to the left and right shoulder girdle. These impacts can result from various events, including traffic accidents, sports injuries, or accidents. When the body experiences trauma or a strong impact, it can lead to a dislocation of the atlas, i.e., lateral subluxations of the atlas in relation to the axis. Lateral subluxations of the atlas can cause pain, limited movement, neurological issues, and other uncomfortable symptoms, making them crucial for timely diagnosis and treatment to prevent potential complications.

When an impact affects the left temporal region, the result is a subluxation of the atlas to the left, while an impact to the right temporal region causes a lateral subluxation of the atlas to the right side. In other words, in lateral subluxations of the atlas, the movement of the atlas in relation to the axis is in the direction of the impact. This principle can be explained by the law of action and reaction in physics, where force acts in the opposite direction of the impact. These impacts can be extremely harmful and lead to serious health issues, highlighting the importance of identifying and treating atlas subluxations to prevent potential complications.

Although ligaments play a crucial role in maintaining a strong connection between the atlas and the skull, even minimal movement of the atlas can have serious consequences for the spine. One of the main causes of developing scoliosis is precisely this process. When even a slight shift of the atlas occurs, it can result in uneven distribution of the weight of the head onto the spine. Over time, this irregular pressure can lead to gradual deformation of the spinal column in the form of scoliosis.

It is essential to understand that even minor shifts of the atlas can have a significant impact on the spinal structure. This pressure not only induces changes in the position of the vertebrae but can also cause rotation and bending of the spinal column, gradually leading to the formation of scoliosis. These processes typically unfold over an extended period but can result in serious spinal and posture issues if not recognized and treated promptly.

In addition to traumatic causes, degenerative changes in the cervical vertebrae and joints can also play a significant role in contributing to lateral atlas subluxation. As the body ages, the joints and ligaments that stabilize the atlas become less elastic and more prone to wear and tear. These degenerative changes, which may include arthritis or degeneration of intervertebral discs, can weaken the structure of the cervical spine and lead to atlas displacement. This is especially common in older individuals or those suffering from chronic neck and spine problems. The weakening of connective tissues can make lateral atlas displacement easier, even without obvious trauma, resulting in pain, stiffness, and restricted mobility. Additionally, asymmetrical activities and improper movements, such as prolonged incorrect sitting, carrying heavy bags on one side, or repetitive head movements in the same direction, can gradually contribute to lateral atlas subluxation. These factors can cause postural imbalances and overstrain one side of the neck and spine, increasing the risk of atlas subluxation.

Overall, the causes of lateral subluxation may be a combination of trauma, degenerative changes, and postural habits, highlighting the need for a comprehensive approach to diagnosis and prevention of this type of injury.

Action and Reaction in Lateral Subluxation

The law of action and reaction can be applied to explain why lateral subluxation of the atlas occurs when sleeping on one's side. According to this law, when one body exerts a force on another body, the second body will react with a force of equal magnitude but opposite direction. In other words, the force acting on one body creates an equal and opposite force on the other body.

As previously mentioned, the atlas vertebra is part of the skull, as it rotates together with the head around the dens of the axis vertebra. When a force is exerted on the head, it is transmitted to the ligaments connecting the atlas vertebra to the skull. As a reaction, equal and opposite forces act on the pillow, causing the atlas to shift to the right if the force action is on the right side of the face.

When we sleep, the muscles of the neck relax as the body enters a state of deep relaxation. This relaxation of the neck muscles is part of the natural sleep process, where muscle tone gradually decreases to allow the body to rest and rejuvenate. The muscles of the neck, including those that support the atlas vertebra, become less active and more relaxed during sleep, allowing the head and neck to naturally adjust to the body's position during rest. The relaxation of the neck muscles enables the gradual displacement of the atlas vertebra, even during deep sleep, potentially compressing nerves and blood vessels, leading to uncomfortable reactions that may awaken us.

During lateral subluxation of the atlas, pressure on the vagus nerve can lead to disturbances in heart function, resulting in unpleasant reactions during sleep, particularly towards dawn. The vagus nerve is responsible for regulating the heart rhythm and other vital functions, so compression of this nerve can cause heart arrhythmias, including accelerated or decelerated heart rate and other pulse irregularities. These changes may be sufficient to awaken a person from sleep and induce feelings of discomfort or anxiety.

Secondly, the displacement of the atlas can exert pressure on the blood vessels that supply the brain with blood, leading to temporary reduction in blood flow to cerebral structures. This can result in cerebral hypoxia and cause sudden changes in sleep quality, including awakening before dawn, feelings of disorientation or dizziness, as well as increased nervousness or discomfort during sleep.

In the medulla oblongata, which is part of the brainstem, contains vital centers that regulate numerous body functions. These centers are responsible for specific bodily functions and control various aspects of the nervous system. On the left side of the medulla oblongata are centers that regulate functions more dominant on the left side of the body, such as speech control and motor functions of the left side of the body. These centers are particularly important for individuals who are left-handed, as the left hemisphere of the brain is usually dominant for speech and other cognitive functions.

On the other hand, on the right side of the medulla oblongata are centers that regulate functions more dominant on the right side of the body, such as motor functions of the right side of the body and sensory signals from the left side of the body. These centers are responsible for coordinating movements and sensations on the right side of the body, playing a crucial role in maintaining balance and motor skills. The precise functioning of these centers enables efficient body function and coordination of movements throughout the body.

In conclusion, it can be observed that poor and long-term sleeping habits may induce lateral dislocation of the atlas, leading to symptoms during sleep due to the compression of blood vessels, the vagus nerve, and centers within the medulla oblongata. These findings underscore the importance of maintaining proper sleeping positions to preserve optimal spine health and overall nervous system function.

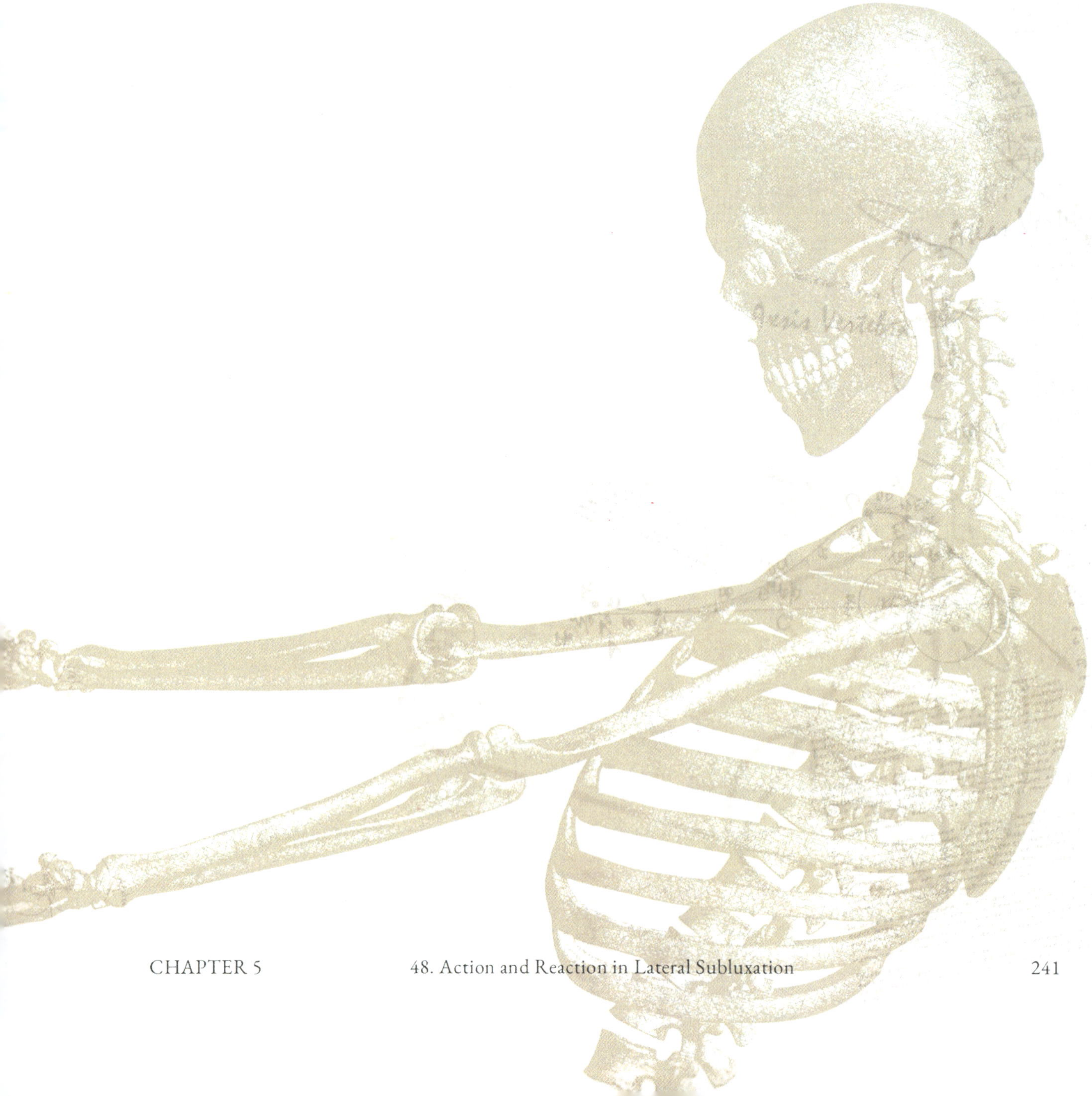

Equation

1

If we have four bodies: **Body A** (sphere), **Body B** (head), **Body C** (atlas vertebra), and **Body D** (axis vertebra), where **Body B** (head) and **Body C** (atlas vertebra) are connected by less elastic ligaments, and **Body C** (atlas vertebra) and **Body D** (axis vertebra) are connected by more elastic ligaments, with a ligament connecting **Body C** (atlas vertebra) to **Body D** (axis vertebra) around the dens of **Body D** (axis vertebra), will **Body C** (atlas vertebra) tend to move in the direction from which the impact and force of **Body A** (sphere) come, if **Body A** (sphere) hits **Body B** (head)?

1. **Body A** (sphere)
2. **Body B** (head)
3. **Body C** (atlas vertebra)
4. **Body D** (axis vertebra)

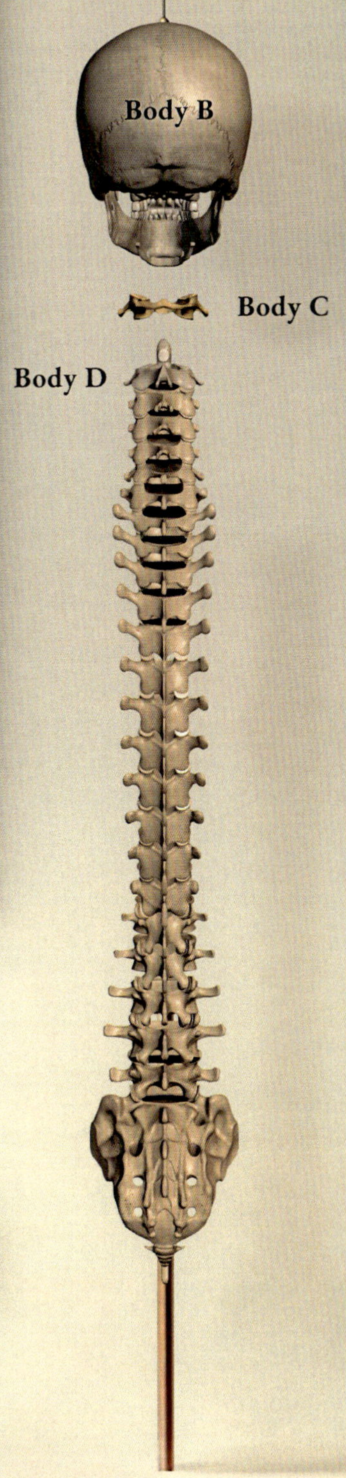

Defining the Problem

In this part of the task, we define the interaction problem between four bodies: sphere, head, atlas vertebra, and axis vertebra. We describe ligament connections of different elasticity and ask if the atlas vertebra (**Body C**) will move in the direction of the sphere's (**Body A**) impact if it hits the head (**Body B**).

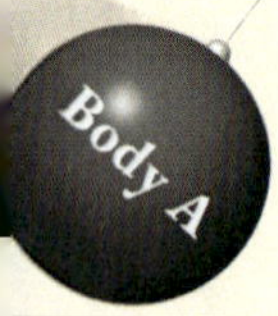

Setup

2

To determine the movement of **Body C** after **Body A** hits **Body B**, we need to consider the mechanics of the system and the effects of the elastic ligaments.

Let's denote certain variables:

m_A - as the mass of **Body A** (sphere),
m_B - as the mass of **Body B** (head),
m_C - as the mass of **Body C** (atlas vertebra),
m_D - as the mass of **Body D** (axis vertebra).

V_{AB} - as the velocity of **Body B** (head) after the impact,
V_{BC} - as the velocity of **Body C** (atlas vertebra) after force transmission via the ligament between **Bodies B** and **C**,
V_{CD} - as the velocity of **Body D** (axis vertebra) after force transmission via the ligament between **Bodies C** and **D**,

F_{AB} - as the force **Body A** (sphere) applies to **Body B** (head),
F_{BC} - as the force **Body B** (head) applies to **Body C** (atlas vertebra) via the ligament between **Bodies B** and **C**,
F_{CD} - as the force **Body C** (atlas vertebra) applies to **Body D** (axis vertebra) via the ligament between **Bodies C** and **D**.

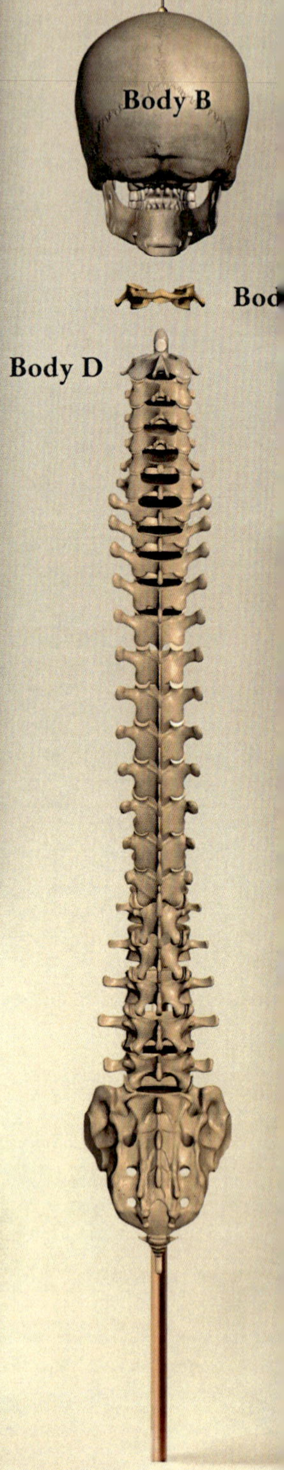

Variables and Setup

In this part of the task, we define variables and set the basic framework for the calculation. This includes the masses of the bodies (sphere, head, atlas vertebra, and axis vertebra), the speeds of the bodies after impact, and the forces acting between them through the ligaments.

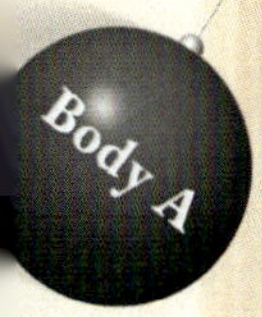

Using the laws of conservation of momentum, we can write: **3**

1. For **Body B** (head): $m_B \cdot V_{AB} = m_B \cdot V'_{AB} + F_{BC} \cdot t$
2. For **Body C** (atlas vertebra): $m_C \cdot V_{BC} = m_C \cdot V'_{BC} + F_{CD} \cdot t$
3. For **Body D** (axis vertebra): $m_D \cdot V_{CD} = m_D \cdot V'_{CD}$

Here, V'_{AB}, V'_{BC} and V'_{CD} are the velocities of **Bodies B**, **C**, and **D** after the force application, and t is the duration of the force application.

To solve these equations, we need to know specific values for the masses, velocities, and forces, as well as to assume the shape and properties of the ligaments to calculate the forces F_{BC} and F_{CD} acting on **Body C** and **Body D**.

Assigning Values

1. Force = 50 kg
2. Mass of the head = 6 kg
3. Mass of the atlas = 20 grams
4. Mass of the axis = 30 grams

To solve the system of equations, we need to use certain unit conversions, as the masses are expressed in kilograms, while the standard system uses grams (g). Additionally, we apply the law of conservation of momentum, assuming there are no external forces acting on the system.

First, convert masses to kilograms:

1. Mass of the head $m_B = 6$ kg
2. Mass of the atlas $m_C = 20$ g $= 0.02$ kg
3. Mass of the axis $m_D = 30$ g $= 0.03$ kg

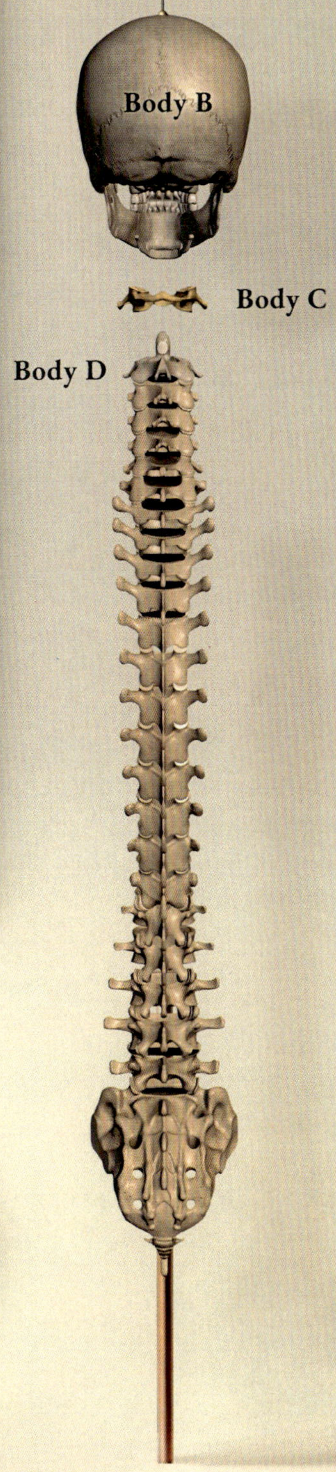

Momentum Equations

In this part of the task, we use the laws of conservation of momentum to write equations for bodies **B**, **C**, and **D**. To solve these equations, we need specific values for masses, velocities, and forces. We assume the shape and properties of the ligaments to calculate the forces F_{BC} and F_{CD}.

Now we can use the law of conservation of momentum for each body:

4

1. For **Body B** (head):

$m_B \cdot V_{AB} = m_B \cdot V'_{AB} + F_{BC} \cdot t$

$6 \cdot V_{AB} = 6 \cdot V'_{AB} + F_{BC} \cdot t$

2. For **Body C** (atlas vertebra):

$m_C \cdot V_{BC} = m_C \cdot V'_{BC} + F_{CD} \cdot t$

$0.02 \cdot V_{BC} = 0.02 \cdot V'_{BC} + F_{CD} \cdot t$

3. For **Body D** (axis vertebra):

$m_D \cdot V_{CD} = m_D \cdot V'_{CD}$

$0.03 \cdot V_{CD} = 0.03 \cdot V'_{CD}$

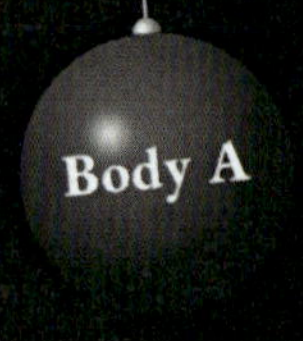

We note that we are missing the value for the force F_{BC}, which can be calculated using the mass of the head and the speed after the impact, as well as the force F_{CD}, which can be calculated using the mass of the atlas and the speed after the impact. The speeds after the impact can be expressed using the impulse, which is the product of the force and the duration of the force application.

After solving the system of equations and calculating the speeds, we can determine the movement of the atlas and axis vertebrae.

Momentum Laws

Using the conservation of momentum for each body, we write equations for bodies **B**, **C**, and **D**, using their masses and velocities before and after the impact. To solve these equations, we need to calculate the forces F_{BC} and F_{CD} using the impulse, which is the product of force and the duration of the force application.

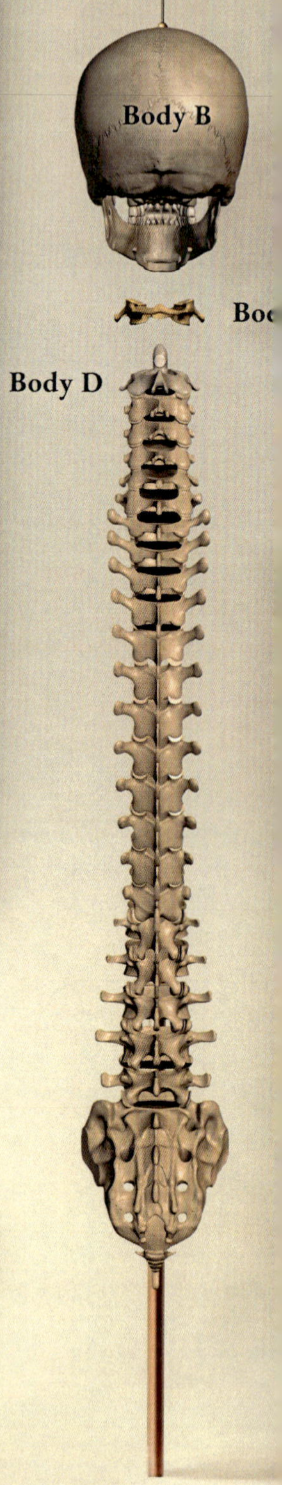

Assigning More Values: 5

5. Speed of the sphere = 30 km/h

To solve the system of equations and determine the movement of the atlas and axis vertebrae, we first need to calculate the forces acting between **Body B** and **Body C** (F_{BC}) and between **Body C** and **Body D** (F_{CD}). Thus, we need the speed of **Body B** after the impact.

Given that the speed of the sphere V_{AB} = 30 km/h, it needs to be converted to meters per second (m/s), as the other quantities are expressed in **SI units**.

$30 \text{ km/h} = 30 \text{ X } 1000/3600 \text{ m/s} \sim 8.33 \text{ m/s}$

Now we can solve the system of equations:

1. For **Body B** (head):
$6 \cdot 8.33 = 6 \cdot V'_{AB} + F_{BC} \cdot t$

2. For **Body C** (atlas vertebra):
$0.02 \cdot V_{BC} = 0.02 \cdot V'_{BC} + F_{CD} \cdot t$

3. For **Body D** (axis vertebra):
$0.03 \cdot V_{CD} = 0.03 \cdot V'_{CD}$

It is also necessary to calculate the impulse needed to transmit the force from **Body B** to **Body C** and from **Body C** to **Body D**. The impulse is calculated as the product of the force and the duration of the force application. To obtain the force value, we need to know the duration of the force application.

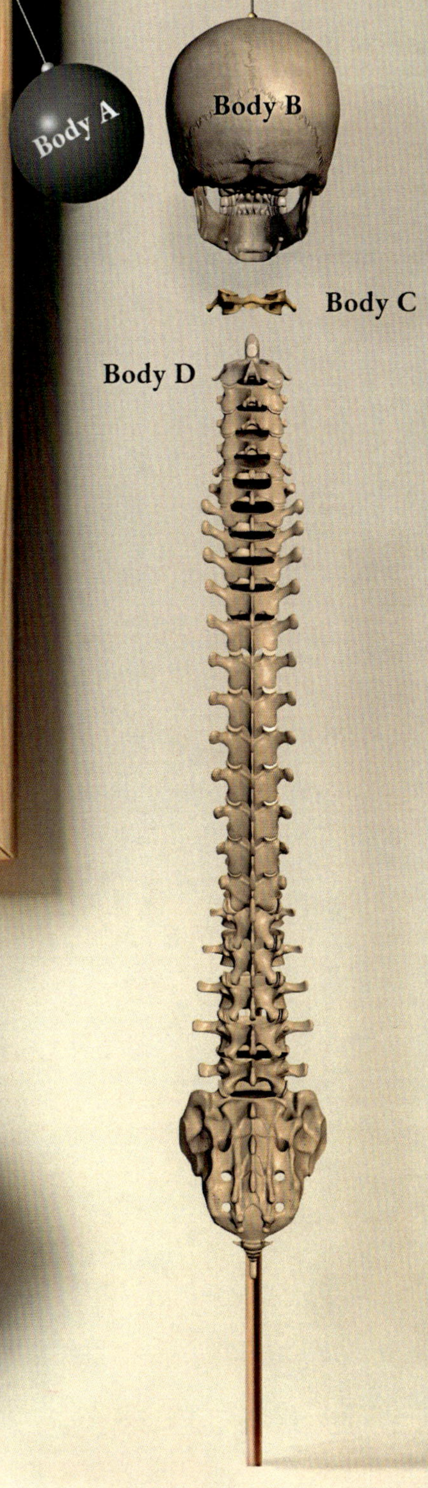

Assigning More Values

In this part, we assign additional values for the speed of the sphere and convert it to **SI units**. We then use these values to solve the system of equations for bodies **B**, **C**, and **D**.

Additionally, it is necessary to calculate the impulse required to transfer force between the bodies.

Assigning More Values (6)

6. Duration of the force application is ***1 second***

Now that we have the value of the force application time t = 1 second, we can calculate the impulse transmitted to **Bodies B**, **C**, and **D** during the impact. The impulse is the product of the force and the duration of the force application.

Using the formula: Impulse = F • t

Where:

1. F - is the force
2. t - is the duration of the force application

First, we will calculate the impulse transmitted to **Body B**, which will allow us to calculate the speed of **Body B** after the impact. Then, using that speed, we can calculate the forces F_{BC} and F_{CD}.

1. Impulse on **Body B**:
Impulse B = $F_{AB} \cdot t$

In this case, F_{AB} = 50 kg (the force is known to be 50 kg) and t = 1s, so:
Impulse B = 50 x 1= 50 kg • m/s

Now, using the definition of impulse as the change in momentum, we can calculate the speed of **Body B** after the impact, assuming that the initial speed of **Body B** before the impact was zero. According to the law of conservation of momentum, the impulse received by **Body B** will be equal to the change in momentum of that body.

Impulse B = $m_B \cdot V'_{AB} - m_B \cdot V_{AB}$

Calculating Impulse

In this part of the task, we determine the duration of the force application and use this value to calculate the impulse transmitted to bodies **B**, **C**, and **D** during the impact.

By using the impulse, we can calculate the speed of **Body B** after the impact and the forces F_{BC} and F_{CD}.

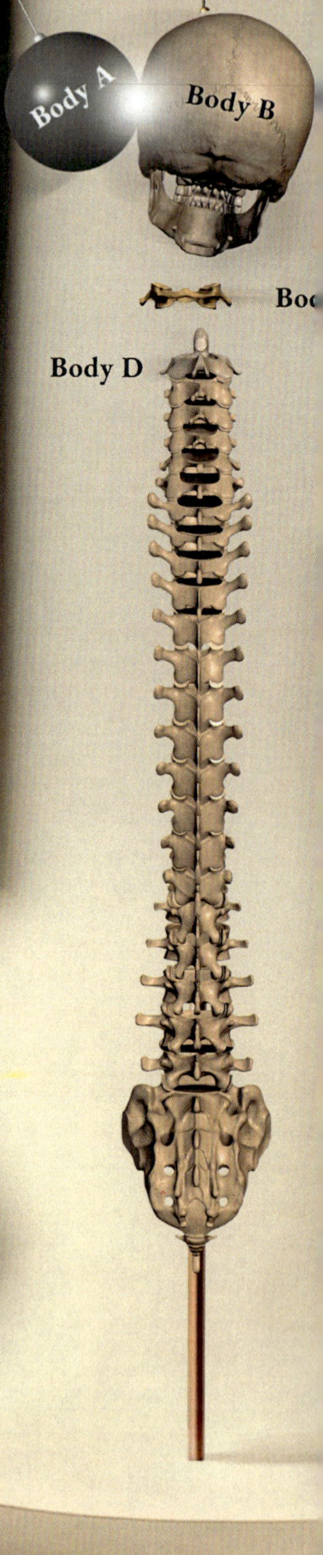

Where:

7

1. m_B - is the mass of **Body B**
2. V_{AB} - is the speed of **Body B** before the impact (zero)
3. V'_{AB} - is the speed of **Body B** after the impact

Using this, we can calculate the speed of **Body B** after the impact. After that, we can further calculate the forces F_{BC} and F_{CD}.

To determine the speed of **Body B** after the impact, using the law of conservation of momentum. Before the impact, the speed of **Body B** is zero, so the change in momentum is equal to the impulse received by **Body B** during the impact. This can be expressed as:

Impulse B = $m_B \cdot V'_{AB} - m_B \cdot V_{AB}$

Where:

1. m_B = 6 kg (mass of **Body B**)
2. V_{AB} = 0 m/s (initial speed of **Body B**)
3. V'_{AB} - is the speed of **Body B** after the impact, which needs to be calc lated

Using the impulse value we already calculated (50 kg·m/s), we can calculate the speed of **Body B** after the impact:

$50\ kg \cdot m/s = 6\ kg \cdot V_{AB} \cdot 6\ kg \cdot 0\ m/s$

$50\ kg \cdot m/s = 6\ kg \cdot V'_{AB}$

$V'_{AB} = 50\ kg \cdot m/s\ /\ 6\ kg$

$V'_{AB} \sim 8.33\ m/s$

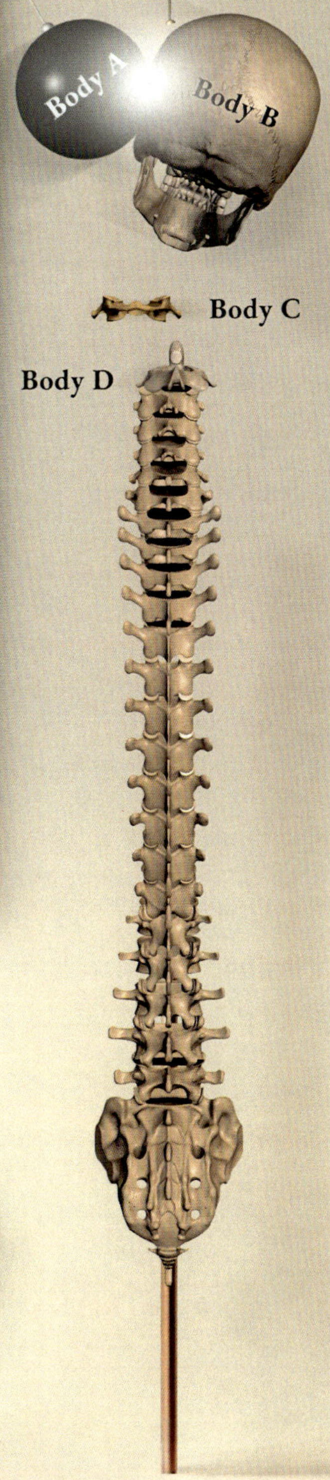

Speed After Impact

In this part of the task, we use the law of conservation of momentum to calculate the speed of **Body B** after the impact.

Before the impact, the speed of **Body B** is zero, so the change in momentum is equal to the impulse that **Body B** receives during the impact.

Now that we know the speed of ***Body B*** *after the impact, we can calculate the forces* F_{BC} *and* F_{CD}*, using the law of conservation of momentum.*

8

Where:

Now that we know the speed of **Body B** after the impact (V'_{AB} ~ 8.33 m/s), we can calculate the forces F_{BC} and F_{CD}, using the law of conservation of momentum.

First, we will calculate the impulse transferred to **Body B** during the impact. Impulse is equal to the product of force and the duration of the force application:

Impulse B = $F_{AB} \cdot t = 50\ N \cdot 1\ s = 50\ kg \cdot m/s$

Now, according to the law of conservation of momentum, the impulse received by **Body B** during the impact will be equal to the change in momentum of that body:

Impulse B = $m_B \cdot V'_{AB} - m_B \cdot V_{AB}$

Where:

1. m_B = 6 kg is the mass of **Body B**
2. V_{AB} = 0 m/s is the initial speed of **Body B**
3. V'_{AB} - is the speed of **Body B** after the impact, which needs to be calculated

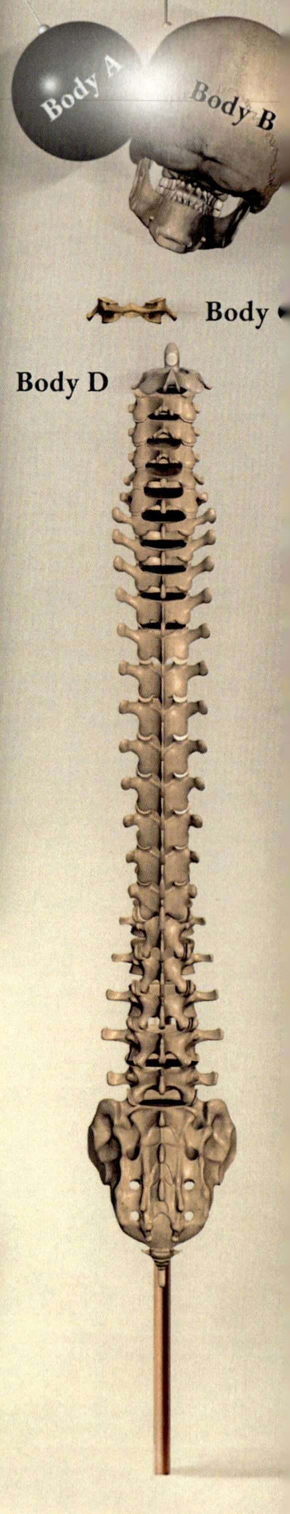

Calculating Forces

Now that we know the speed of **Body B** after the impact, we can calculate the forces F_{BC} and F_{CD} using the law of conservation of momentum. First, we will calculate the impulse transferred to **Body B** during the impact, which is equal to the product of the force and the duration of the force application.

We can now solve this equation for F_{BC}.

9

Next, let's calculate the force F_{CD}. According to the law of conservation of momentum, we can write:

Impulse C = $m_C \cdot V'_{BC} - m_C \cdot V_{BC}$

Where:

1. $m_C = 0.02$ kg is the mass of **Body C**
2. $V_{BC} = 0$ m/s is the initial speed of **Body C**
3. V'_{BC} - is the speed of **Body C** after the impact

We can now solve this equation for F_{CD}.

Now we will solve the equation for the force F_{BC}:

Impulse B = $m_B \cdot V'_{AB} - m_B \cdot V_{AB}$

$50\ kg \cdot m/s = 6\ kg \cdot V'_{AB} - 6\ kg \cdot 0\ m/s$

$50\ kg \cdot m/s = 6\ kg \cdot V'_{AB}$

$V'_{AB} = 50\ kg \cdot m/s / 6\ kg$

$V'_{AB} = 8.33\ m/s$

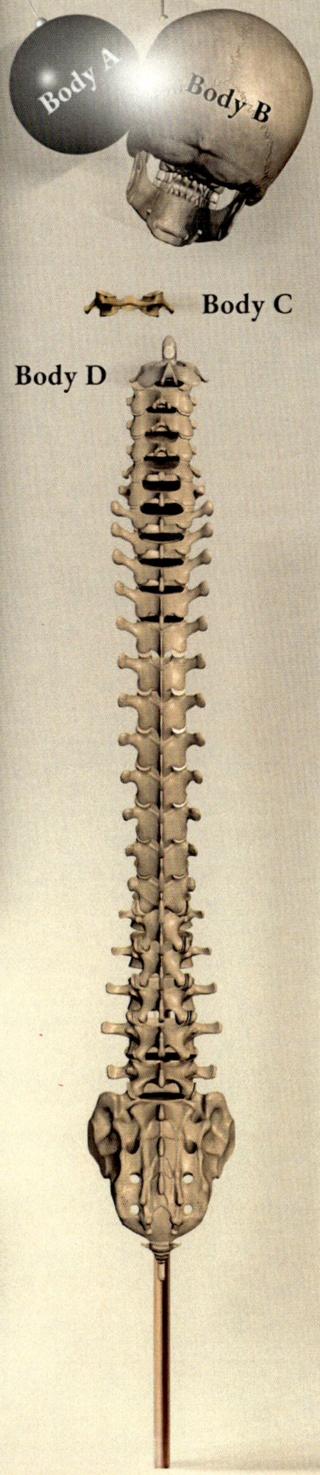

Normal Aspect

In this part, we solve the equations for the forces F_{BC} and F_{CD} using the law of conservation of momentum. We calculate the impulse for bodies **B** and **C** and use these values to determine the forces acting on the atlas and axis vertebrae, ensuring accurate results based on the impulses calculated.

10

Now that we have the speed of **Body B** after the impact, we can calculate the impulse acting on **Body C**, using the law of conservation of momentum:

Impulse C $= m_C \cdot V'_{BC} - m_C \cdot V_{BC}$

Impulse C $= 0.02\ \text{kg} \cdot V'_{BC} - 0.02\ \text{kg} \cdot 0\ \text{m/s}$

Now we can calculate the impulse **Impulse C** which is equal to the impulse received by **Body C** during the impact. Then, we can calculate the speed of **Body C** after the impact, and subsequently the force $\boldsymbol{F_{CD}}$.

Given that the initial speed of **Body C** ($\boldsymbol{V_{BC}} = 0$ m/s) before the impact, the impulse received by **Body C** during the impact will be equal to the change in momentum of that body. Thus,

Impulse C $= m_C \cdot V'_{BC}$

$50\ \text{kg} \cdot \text{m/s} = 0.02\ \text{kg} \cdot V'_{BC}$

Now we can calculate the speed of **Body C** after the impact:

$V'_{BC} = 50\ \text{kg} \cdot \text{m/s} \ / \ 0.02\ \text{kg}$

$V'_{BC} = 2500\ \text{m/s}$

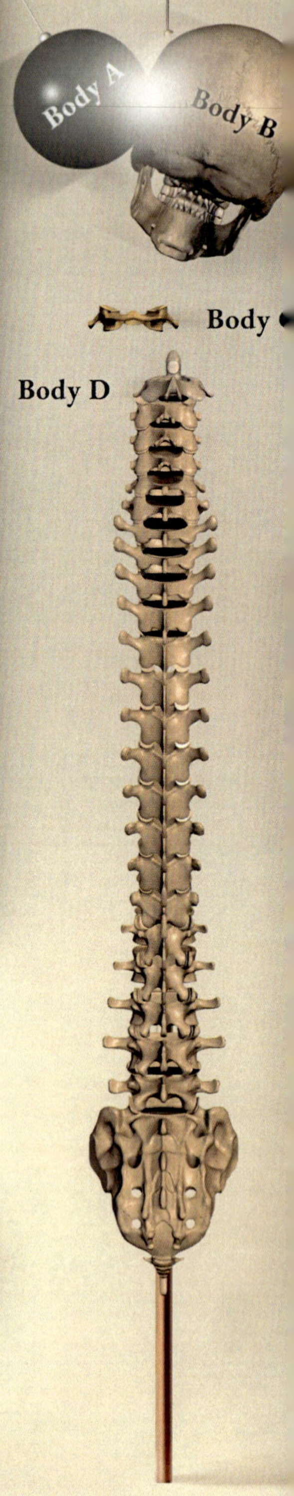

Impulse for Body C

Now that we know the speed of **Body B** after the impact, we can calculate the impulse acting on **Body C** using the law of conservation of momentum.

Then, we calculate the speed of **Body C** after the impact and the corresponding force $\boldsymbol{F_{CD}}$.

11

Now that we know the speed of **Body C** after the impact, we can calculate the force:

Impulse C = $m_C \cdot V'_{BC} - m_C \cdot V_{BC}$

Impulse C = $m_C \cdot V'_{BC}$

$F_{CD} \cdot t = m_C \cdot V'_{BC}$

Now we can calculate the force F_{CD}:

$F_{CD} = m_C \cdot V'_{BC} \,/\, t$

$F_{CD} = 0.02\ \text{kg} \cdot 2500\ \text{m/s} \,/\, 1\ \text{s}$

$F_{CD} = 50\ \text{kg} \cdot \text{m/s} \,/\, 1\text{s}$

$F_{CD} = 50\ \text{N}$

Thus, the force F_{CD} that **Body C** exerts on **Body D** via the ligament between **Bodies C** and **D** is 50 N.

We have calculated the forces F_{BC} and F_{CD}, and determined the speeds after the impact for **Bodies B** and **C**. Based on the calculated force and speed values, we can conclude the direction in which the atlas (**Body C**) will move after the impact.

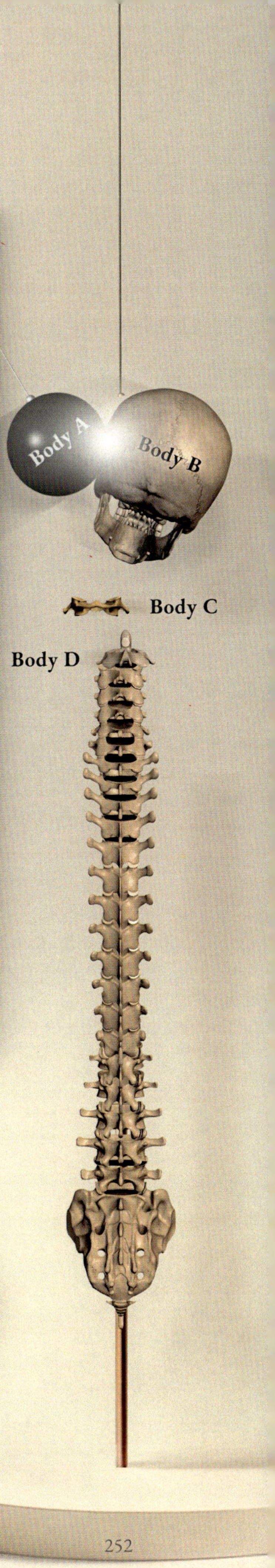

Calculating Force F_{CD}

Now that we know the speed of **Body C** after the impact, we can calculate the force F_{CD}.

After calculating the forces F_{BC} and F_{CD} and the speeds of the bodies after the impact, we can conclude the direction in which the atlas (**Body C**) will move after the impact.

Conclusion

12

From this task, it is evident that the atlas vertebra moves in the direction from which the sphere impacts the head. How and why does this happen?

The force F_{BC} acts on **Body C** from **Body B** (head) towards **Body C**. Since this force is directed towards **Body C**, it will cause an acceleration of **Body C** in the same direction, i.e., in the direction of the impact.

The force F_{CD} acts on **Body C** from **Body D** (axis vertebra) towards **Body C**. This force also acts towards **Body C**, which will also cause an acceleration of **Body C** in the same direction, i.e., in the direction of the impact.

Therefore, based on the calculated forces, we can conclude that the atlas (**Body C**) will tend to move in the direction from which the impact and force of **Body A** (sphere) come.

How:
When the sphere (**Body A**) hits the head (**Body B**), **it generates a force that is transmitted through the head to the atlas vertebra** (**Body C**). This force is carried through the ligaments connecting the bodies.

Why:
The forces F_{BC} and F_{CD} act on **Body C**, causing it to accelerate in the direction of the impact. According to the conservation of momentum, the momentum from the sphere is transferred through the head and ligaments to the atlas vertebra. This transfer of **momentum** results in the atlas vertebra moving in the direction from which the sphere came.

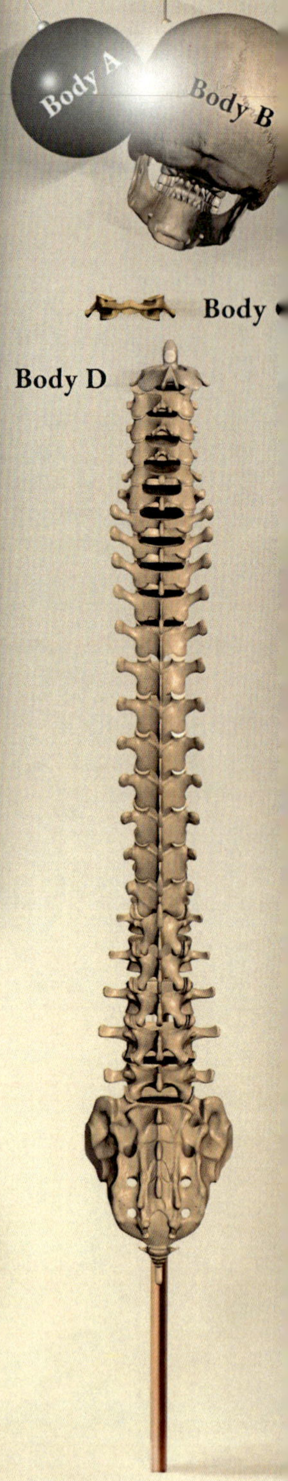

Conclusion

Based on the calculated values of forces and speeds, we can determine the direction in which the atlas (**Body C**) will move after the impact.

The forces F_{BC} and F_{CD} act on **Body C**, causing it to accelerate in the direction of the impact.

Cervical Spine Scoliosis

Cervical spine scoliosis represents a curvature of the cervical spine characterized by lateral bending Predlažem da umetnete slike na sledećim mestima [Image 1]. While scoliosis is more commonly associated with the thoracic and lumbar regions, deformities in the cervical spine can have significant implications for health and functionality.

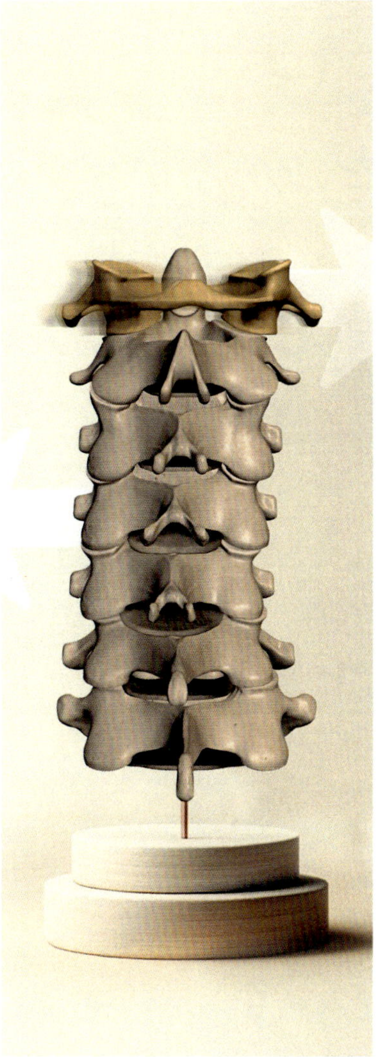

[Image 1] Cervical spine scoliosis

The primary causes of cervical spine scoliosis are typically linked to structural changes, such as irregularities in vertebral formation or uneven distribution of loads on the cervical spine. This imbalance can lead to lateral bending of the cervical vertebrae, resulting in the appearance of scoliosis.

Symptoms of cervical spine scoliosis can vary depending on the degree of deformity and individual factors. These may include neck pain, stiffness, limited range of motion, headaches, and balance issues. These symptoms can vary in severity and can impact daily activities and quality of life.

Treatment for cervical spine scoliosis typically involves a combination of conservative therapeutic methods and, in rare cases, surgical interventions. Conservative therapies may include physical therapy, wearing orthopedic supports, neck muscle strengthening exercises, and maintaining proper posture. Surgical procedures are reserved for severe cases when conservative methods fail to yield satisfactory results or when the deformity significantly affects the patient's health and functionality.

Timely diagnosis of cervical spine scoliosis is crucial, and initiating appropriate treatment is essential to prevent complications and improve the quality of life for patients facing this condition. Regular check-ups and collaboration with specialists are crucial for effectively managing this deformity.

Cervical Scoliosis Symptoms and Treatment

Scoliosis of the cervical vertebrae can be accompanied by various symptoms, including neck and shoulder pain, as well as a feeling of burden on the shoulders. These symptoms may result from the irregular curvature of the spine, leading to an imbalance in the load on the muscles and ligaments in the neck region.

Neck pain is common in individuals with cervical vertebral scoliosis, as the irregular curvature of the spine can cause tension and irritation of the muscles and ligaments. Additionally, the uneven loading on the muscles of the neck and shoulders can lead to the onset of pain in these areas.

The sensation of burden on the shoulders may also be present in individuals with cervical vertebral scoliosis due to increased strain on the shoulder muscles and ligaments. The irregular curvature of the spine can disrupt the balance of the muscles supporting the shoulders, resulting in a feeling of heaviness or discomfort in the shoulders.

It is important to note that the symptoms of cervical vertebral scoliosis may vary depending on the degree of deformity and individual factors. In some individuals, symptoms may be mild and intermittent, while in others, they may be more pronounced and continuous.

Treatment for neck and shoulder pain from cervical scoliosis typically involves a combination of physical therapy, neck and shoulder exercises, orthopedic supports, and posture techniques. However, by focusing on all methods aimed at treating the consequences, we cannot address the root cause of the problem, *and the primary cause of cervical vertebral scoliosis is the misaligned atlas vertebra.*

Managing Dyspraxia

Disruption in coordination and orientation can significantly impact an individual's daily life, affecting their ability to perform tasks efficiently and navigate their surroundings effectively. This condition, often referred to as dyspraxia or developmental coordination disorder (DCD), manifests as difficulties in planning and executing movements, resulting in clumsiness, awkwardness, and a lack of fluidity in physical actions.

People with dyspraxia may struggle with various motor skills, including both fine and gross motor coordination. Simple activities such as tying shoelaces, buttoning shirts, or catching a ball can pose significant challenges, leading to frustration and a sense of inadequacy. In addition to motor difficulties, individuals with dyspraxia may also experience challenges in spatial awareness, balance, and spatial organization, making tasks like navigating crowded spaces or following directions particularly challenging.

The causes of dyspraxia are not fully understood by conventional medicine but are believed to involve a combination of genetic, neurological, and environmental factors. Structural differences or abnormalities in the brain, particularly in regions responsible for motor control and coordination, may contribute to the development of dyspraxia. Additionally, environmental factors such as prenatal exposure to toxins or maternal health during pregnancy may play a role in increasing the risk of dyspraxia.

Despite dyspraxia's challenges, individuals can manage symptoms and improve coordination through targeted therapies. Occupational therapy, physiotherapy, and speech therapy can all be beneficial in addressing specific motor difficulties and enhancing overall functioning.

Additionally, strategies such as breaking tasks down into smaller steps, providing visual cues and prompts, and practicing activities in a structured and supportive environment can help individuals with dyspraxia develop coping mechanisms and improve their independence.

It is essential for individuals with dyspraxia to receive early intervention and ongoing support to address their coordination and orientation difficulties effectively. With patience, understanding, and the right support network in place, individuals with dyspraxia can learn to navigate the world more confidently and lead fulfilling lives despite the challenges they may face.

Despite these facts, which are already well-known in conventional medicine, in this book, you will learn the true cause of dyspraxia. Not only that, but you will also discover which nerve, specifically its compression, is the cause of this problem the cranial nerve that emerges from the medulla oblongata. While the diagnosis itself is important, it does not necessarily offer a solution to the root cause of the problem. However, through the method of atlas vertebra adjustment, this dyspraxia diagnosis becomes a thing of the past, as it is now the experience of thousands of patients with this diagnosis.

Diagnoses often overlook body statics, especially the position of the head. A twisted and displaced head position compresses nerve pathways, particularly the cranial nerves passing through the foramina, leading to symptoms like coordination issues, dizziness, and other neurological problems. This pressure can result in loss of function or reduced signaling through cranial nerves, worsening the clinical picture. Unfortunately, standard diagnoses often ignore mechanical factors like head and atlas misalignment, potentially causing the issue.

Arrhythmias and Tachycardia

Arrhythmias and tachycardia, characterized by irregular heartbeats or a rapid heart rate, can have serious implications for health and lead to various complications. Tachycardia involves the heart beating faster than the normal rhythm, while arrhythmias refer to irregularities in the heart's rhythm.

Several factors can contribute to the development of arrhythmias and tachycardia, including heart diseases, high blood pressure, metabolic disorders, stress, anxiety, stimulants such as caffeine or nicotine, and certain medications. In many cases, these disorders may be temporary and transient, but in some situations, they can become chronic and require medical intervention.

Symptoms of arrhythmias and tachycardia can vary but often include rapid or irregular pulse, palpitations, dizziness, shortness of breath, chest pain, or fainting. These symptoms can be distressing and alarming, especially when they occur suddenly or unexpectedly.

Diagnosing arrhythmias and tachycardia typically involves medical assessment, an electrocardiogram (EKG), and other diagnostic tests to determine the cause and severity of the problem. Based on the results of diagnostic tests, the doctor may recommend appropriate treatment, which may include medications, lifestyle changes such as dietary modifications and exercise, or other therapeutic methods.

It is crucial to treat arrhythmias and tachycardia promptly and adequately to reduce the risk of complications such as heart attack, stroke, or cardiac arrest. Regular medical checkups and monitoring of heart rhythm can be crucial for maintaining heart health and preventing serious issues in the future.

Managing Gallbladder Issues

The gallbladder, that small yet crucial organ in our body, often goes unnoticed until it starts causing issues. When everything is functioning as it should, the gallbladder acts as a silent and unobtrusive ally in the process of digestion. However, when complications arise, their impact can be painful and serious.

One of the most common complications associated with gallbladder function is the formation of gallstones. These small, hard clusters can form in the gallbladder and block the flow of bile. The result can be sudden, intense pain in the upper right abdomen, known as biliary colic. Besides pain, these stones can also cause other problems such as inflammation of the gallbladder or even blockage of the bile ducts, requiring urgent medical intervention.

Another common complication related to the gallbladder is gallbladder dyskinesia. This condition is characterized by a disorder of gallbladder movement, which can lead to irregular bile release. The consequence of this can be chronic discomfort or pain in the upper abdomen, especially after meals.

In addition to stone formation and dyskinesia, the gallbladder can be susceptible to other complications such as inflammation, infections, or even tumors. These issues can be serious and require careful monitoring and treatment by medical professionals.

It is important to note that complications with gallbladder function can affect not only physical but also emotional and mental health. The pain and discomfort resulting from these conditions can be extremely stressful and draining for the patient.

Managing complications with gallbladder function requires a comprehensive approach that may include medication, dietary changes, and even surgical interventions in certain cases. Regular medical check-ups and monitoring of symptoms are crucial for detecting and managing these complications in a timely manner.

Ultimately, it's important to remember that gallbladder health is not something to be taken for granted. Listening to the signals our body sends and taking care of the overall health of the digestive system can help prevent or manage complications related to gallbladder function, ensuring a better quality of life and well-being.

Managing complications with gallbladder function requires a comprehensive approach that may include medication, dietary changes, and even surgical interventions in certain cases. Regular medical check-ups and monitoring of symptoms are crucial for detecting and managing these complications in a timely manner.

Ultimately, it's important to remember that gallbladder health is not something to be taken for granted. Listening to the signals our body sends and taking care of the overall health of the digestive system can help prevent or manage complications related to gallbladder function, ensuring a better quality of life and well-being.

By treating the underlying cause, such as atlas misalignment, the body can begin to heal naturally without the need for invasive procedures. This approach not only resolves the immediate symptoms but also restores overall balance and long-term health.

Pelvic Dislocation Recovery

Pelvic dislocation, although rare, can have a profound and serious impact on a person's life. The pelvis, that structural marvel of the body which bears the weight of our trunk, provides the foundation for movement, stability, and support to our body. When a dislocation occurs, that foundation is shaken, leaving the individual facing challenges they may never have encountered before.

Pelvic dislocation is not just a physical problem; it often has emotional and psychological consequences as well. A person may feel a loss of control over their body, fear of further movement, or even fear of returning to normal life. This can lead to feelings of helplessness, frustration, and depression.

However, despite the challenges, pelvic dislocation can also be a path to discovering strength and resilience that the person may not have known they possessed. Through the recovery process, an individual can learn to appreciate their body in an entirely new way, becoming aware of their strength and ability to overcome challenges.

Recovery from pelvic dislocation requires patience, dedication, and support from both the medical team and family and friends. Physical therapy, medical care, and psychological support can be crucial in the healing process and returning to normal life.

Although pelvic dislocation can be extremely difficult and demanding, it can also be an opportunity for personal growth and development. Through grappling with their challenges, an individual can become stronger, braver, and with a deeper understanding of their body and mind.

Ultimately, pelvic dislocation may be a formidable obstacle on life's journey, but it can also be an opportunity for personal growth and development. Through support, perseverance, and self-confidence, an individual can overcome these challenges and rediscover strength and joy in their body and life.

Simply knowing the root cause of pelvic dislocation is already a positive step toward recovery. Twisting of the spine, scoliosis, and other spinal issues are directly linked to pelvic bone dislocation, unless caused by physical trauma to the pelvis itself. After the atlas is adjusted, which is the underlying cause of the dislocated pelvis, recovery and the return of the pelvis to its correct anatomical position often happen instantly, right after the treatment. This occurs due to a domino effect, where the corrected position of the atlas transfers to the rest of the spinal vertebrae, forcing the pelvis to follow this realignment process.

Correcting atlas misalignment not only alleviates chronic back pain and hip discomfort but also improves posture and gait. The adjustment restores balance to the musculoskeletal system, enhancing mobility and reducing tension in muscles and ligaments. Many patients experience increased confidence and well-being once their body is realigned, while the long-term benefits of atlas correction positively impact overall spinal health and quality of life.

In more severe and advanced stages of atlas, spine, and pelvic dislocation, the process of returning the vertebrae and pelvis to their proper positions may take longer, but with consistent treatment, gradual realignment and recovery are achievable. Consistency is crucial for long-term success. With guidance and persistence, patients can achieve lasting relief.

Leg Cramps: Self-Care

Leg cramps, those unexpected spasms that seize our muscles, can be a frustrating and sometimes painful experience. Often occurring at the most inconvenient times, like in the middle of the night or during exercise, leg cramps can leave us feeling helpless and uncomfortable. But beyond the physical discomfort, leg cramps can also teach us valuable lessons about listening to our bodies and taking care of ourselves.

At their core, leg cramps are a reminder that our bodies are intricate and interconnected systems that require proper care and attention. They can be a signal that something is amiss, whether it's dehydration, electrolyte imbalance, muscle fatigue, or even underlying health conditions. Instead of brushing them off as mere inconveniences, leg cramps encourage us to pause and reflect on our lifestyle choices and habits.

Moreover, leg cramps can serve as a humbling reminder of our own vulnerability. In the midst of our busy lives, it's easy to overlook the signals our bodies send us until they forcefully demand our attention. Leg cramps force us to slow down, to acknowledge our limitations, and to practice self-compassion as we navigate discomfort and pain.

Yet, amidst the frustration and discomfort, there's also opportunity for growth. As we learn to manage and prevent leg cramps, we become more attuned to our bodies' needs and more proactive in our self-care routines. Whether it's staying hydrated, stretching regularly, or adjusting our exercise regimen, we gain a deeper understanding of what it means to nurture our physical well-being.

Furthermore, experiencing leg cramps can foster empathy and connection with others. Sharing our experiences and remedies with friends and loved ones creates a sense of solidarity in facing common challenges. It reminds us that we're not alone in our struggles and that there's strength in community and support.

In the end, leg cramps, while uncomfortable, can be powerful teachers if we're willing to listen. They prompt us to tune into our bodies, to prioritize self-care, and to cultivate resilience in the face of adversity. So, the next time a leg cramp strikes, instead of cursing its inconvenience, perhaps we can greet it as a gentle reminder to slow down, listen, and care for ourselves a little more deeply.

Leg cramps, though seemingly a muscle issue, often have a deeper cause rooted in problems with the nerves that innervate those muscles. When nerves are temporarily compressed in the neck or pelvic area, it disrupts the normal flow of impulses through the nerve pathways. This disruption can shock the nerves, resulting in muscle dysfunction—most commonly in the form of sudden cramping and pain.

This dysfunction in nerve signaling can be caused by misalignment of the vertebrae, particularly the atlas or pelvis, which can put pressure on surrounding nerve structures. When nerves are under pressure, the electrical impulses that control muscle relaxation and contraction become disrupted, causing the muscle to spasm uncontrollably. These cramps are a direct result of this imbalance in the nervous system, explaining why typical relief methods like massage or stretching often provide only temporary relief.

Understanding that these cramps stem from nerve issues, not just muscles, offers deeper treatment insight. Relieving pressure on the neck or pelvic nerves can greatly reduce cramp frequency and intensity, restoring normal, pain-free function.

Lateral Subluxation

Lateral subluxation of the atlas most commonly occurs to the right when observed from the back of the head. Over time, this condition can lead to cervical scoliosis and a visible dislocation of the head to the left, opposite to the direction of the atlas displacement. The axis vertebra follows the head's dislocation, which can be confirmed through palpation or 3D imaging.

Atlas is displaced to the right

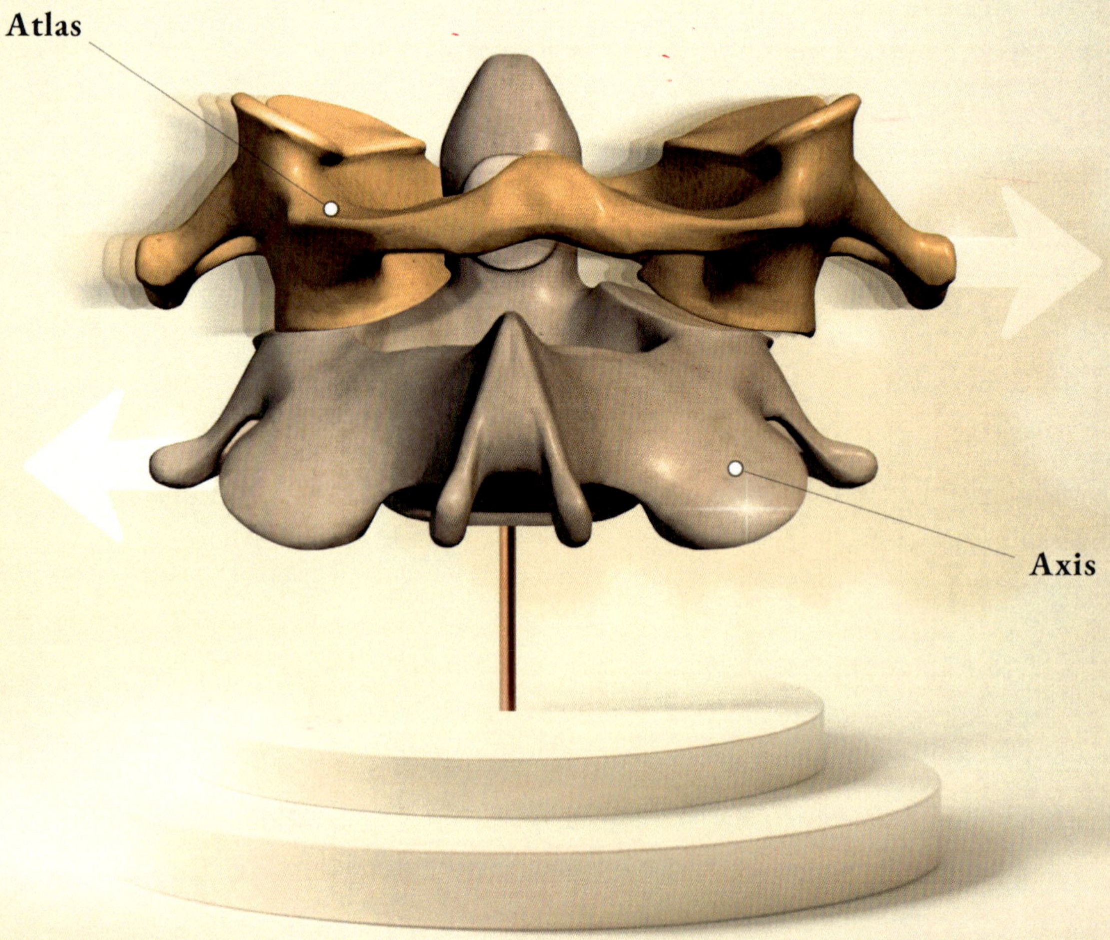

Effects of Rightward Atlas Displacement

Rightward displacement of the atlas causes asymmetry in the head and neck, often visible as tilting of the head to the opposite side to compensate for the imbalance. This displacement can exert pressure on the spinal cord and surrounding nerves, leading to pain, tingling, numbness, or weakness. The asymmetry of the atlas affects the position and function of cervical vertebrae, potentially causing problems in the cervical spine segment. It can also impact the vertebral arteries, restricting blood flow to the brain, resulting in dizziness, headaches, and balance issues.

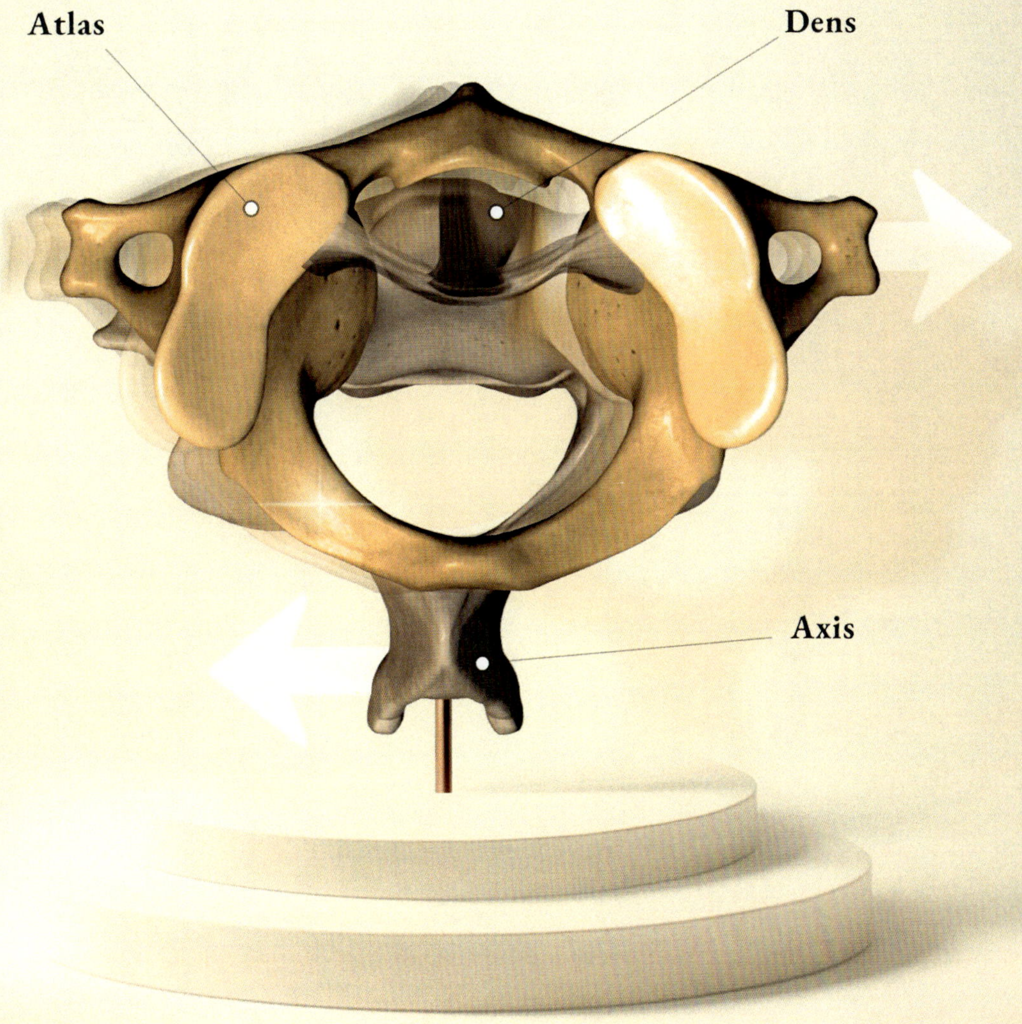

Cervical Vertebrae Scoliosis

Right lateral subluxation of the atlas can cause cervical vertebrae scoliosis, resulting in a sideways curvature of the neck. This misalignment leads to asymmetry, with the head often tilting to the left to compensate. The abnormal positioning can compress the spinal cord and nerves, causing pain, tingling, and numbness. It may restrict blood flow, causing dizziness.

Normal Lordosis **Vertebrae Scoliosis**

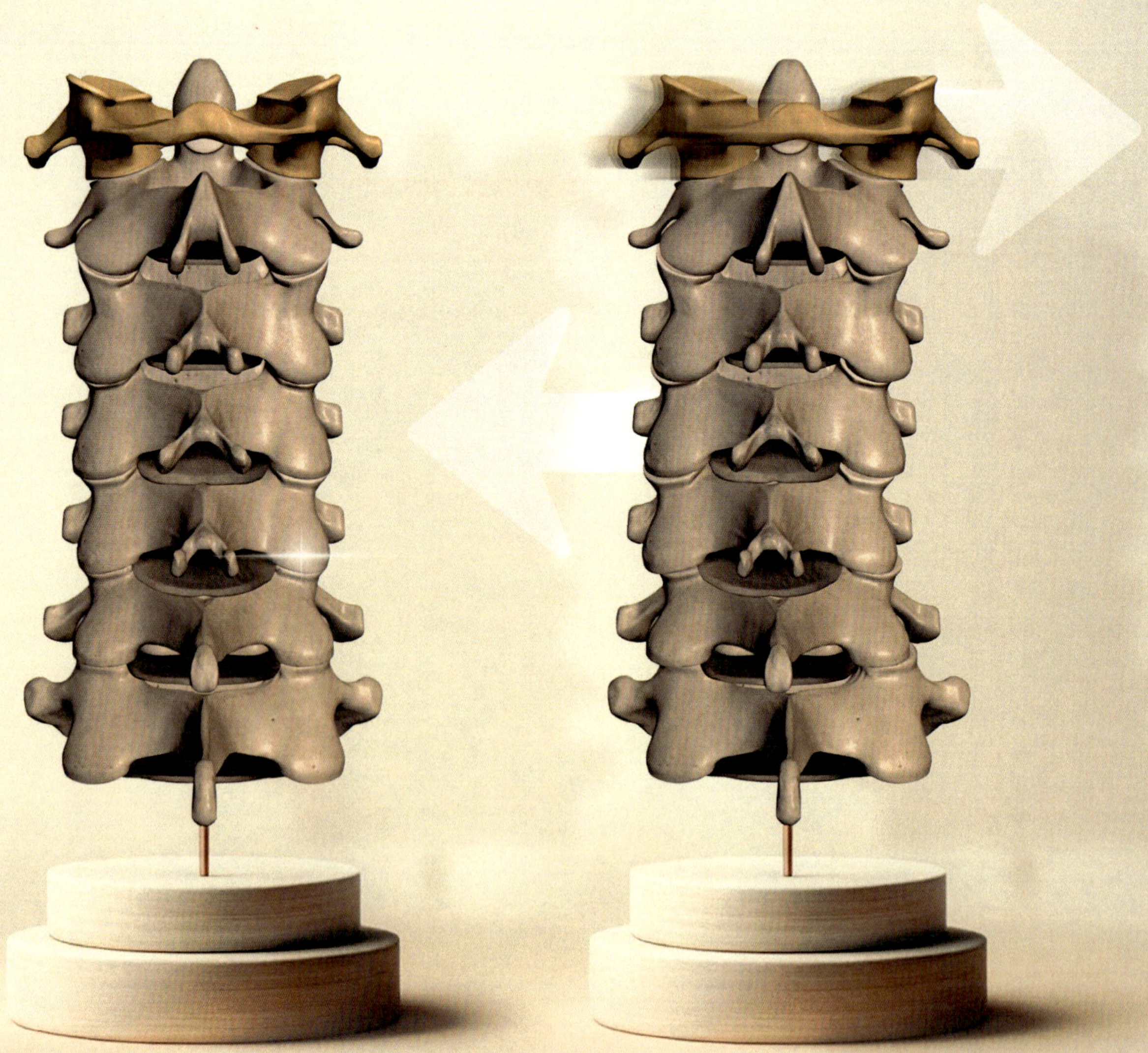

Compensation for Imbalance

Rightward atlas dislocation causes cervical scoliosis, tilting the head left to compensate. This often progresses to full spinal scoliosis, with the right shoulder dropping and the right side of the pelvis lifting. These adjustments aim to maintain balance but can lead to further complications and discomfort.

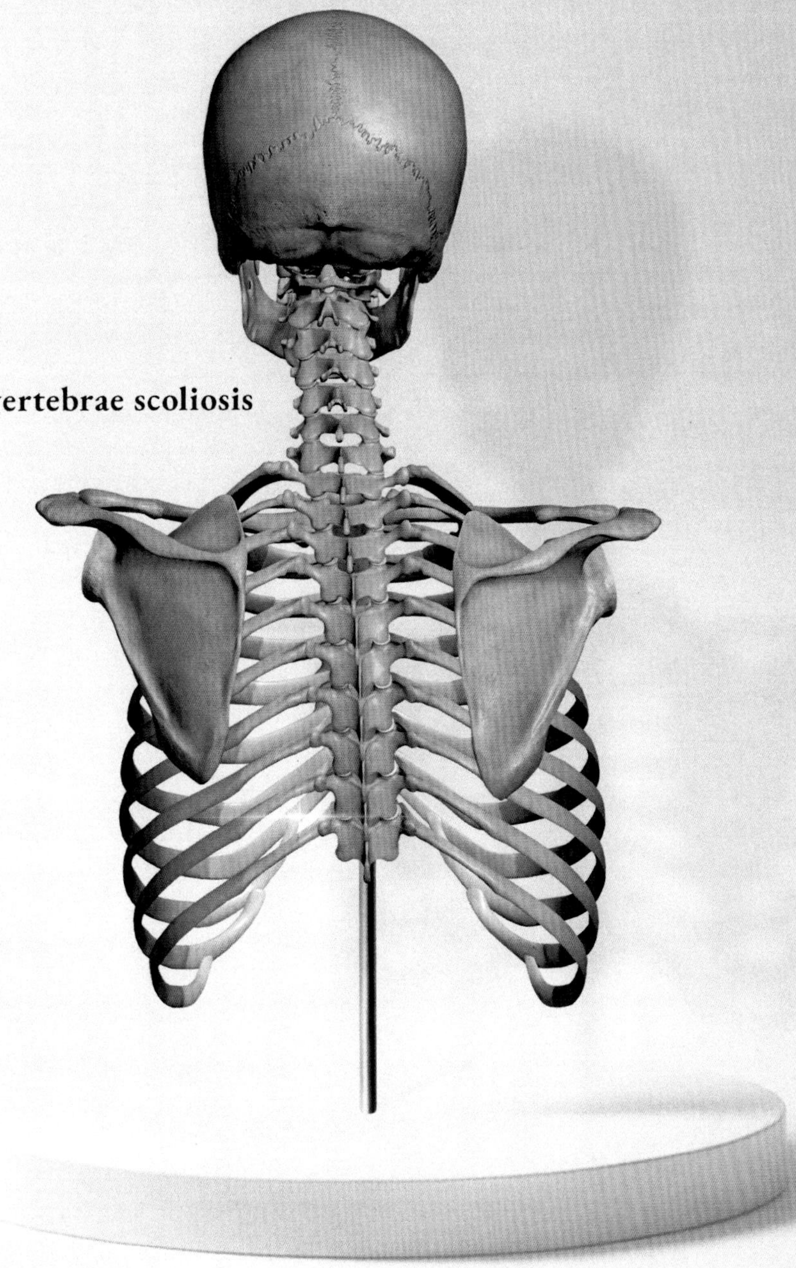

Compression of Cervical Spinal Nerves

Compression of cervical spinal nerves (C1-C8) can cause pain, tingling, numbness, or weakness in the neck, shoulders, arms, and hands, depending on the affected segment. For example, C5 compression affects the shoulders, while C7 impacts the arms and hands.

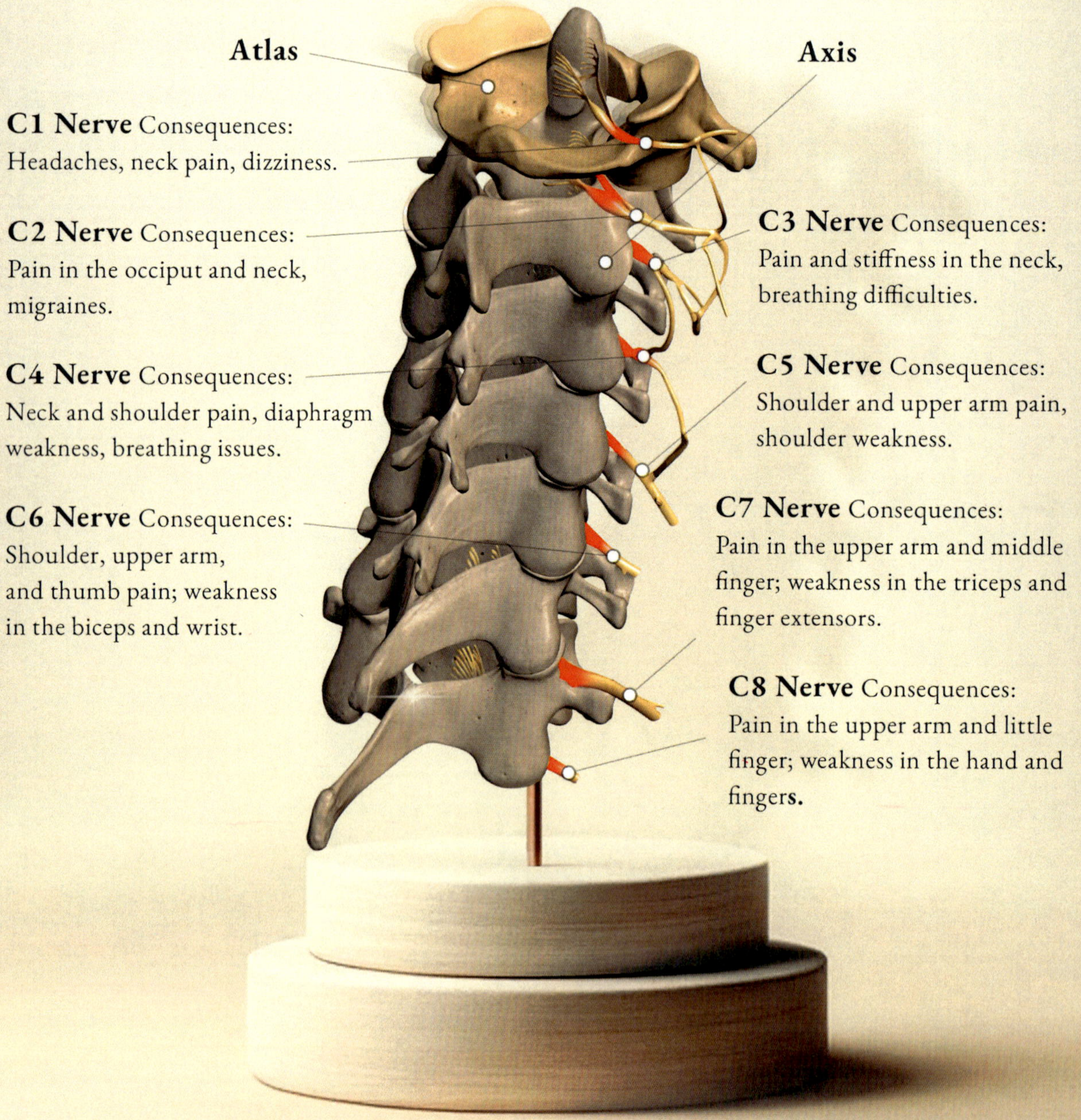

Vestibular System Disorders

Right lateral atlas subluxation and cervical vertebrae scoliosis can disrupt the vestibular system. Misalignment compresses nerves, including the vestibulocochlear nerve, leading to dizziness and balance issues. Displacement affects the vertebral arteries, restricting blood flow to the brain.The asymmetrical head and neck position creates muscle tension and imbalance, causing unsteadiness. Altered postural reflexes send incorrect signals to the vestibular system, leading to disorientation. Vagus nerve stimulation by cervical changes can trigger dizziness and nausea.

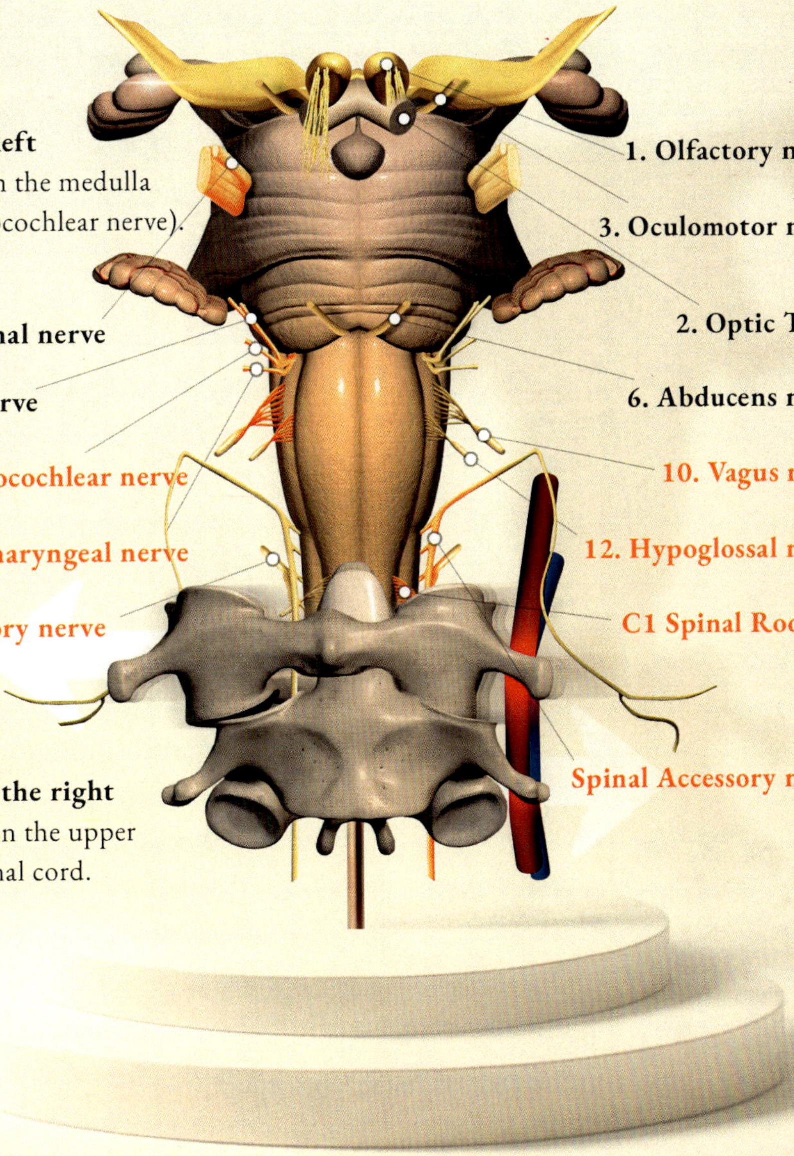

Levator Scapulae Strain in Right Atlas Shift

When the atlas vertebra is displaced to the right, the head tilts to the left to compensate for the imbalance. This compensation increases tension in the levator scapulae muscle on the right side. The levator scapulae, which connects the upper cervical vertebrae to the scapula, is responsible for elevating the scapula and supporting neck movements.

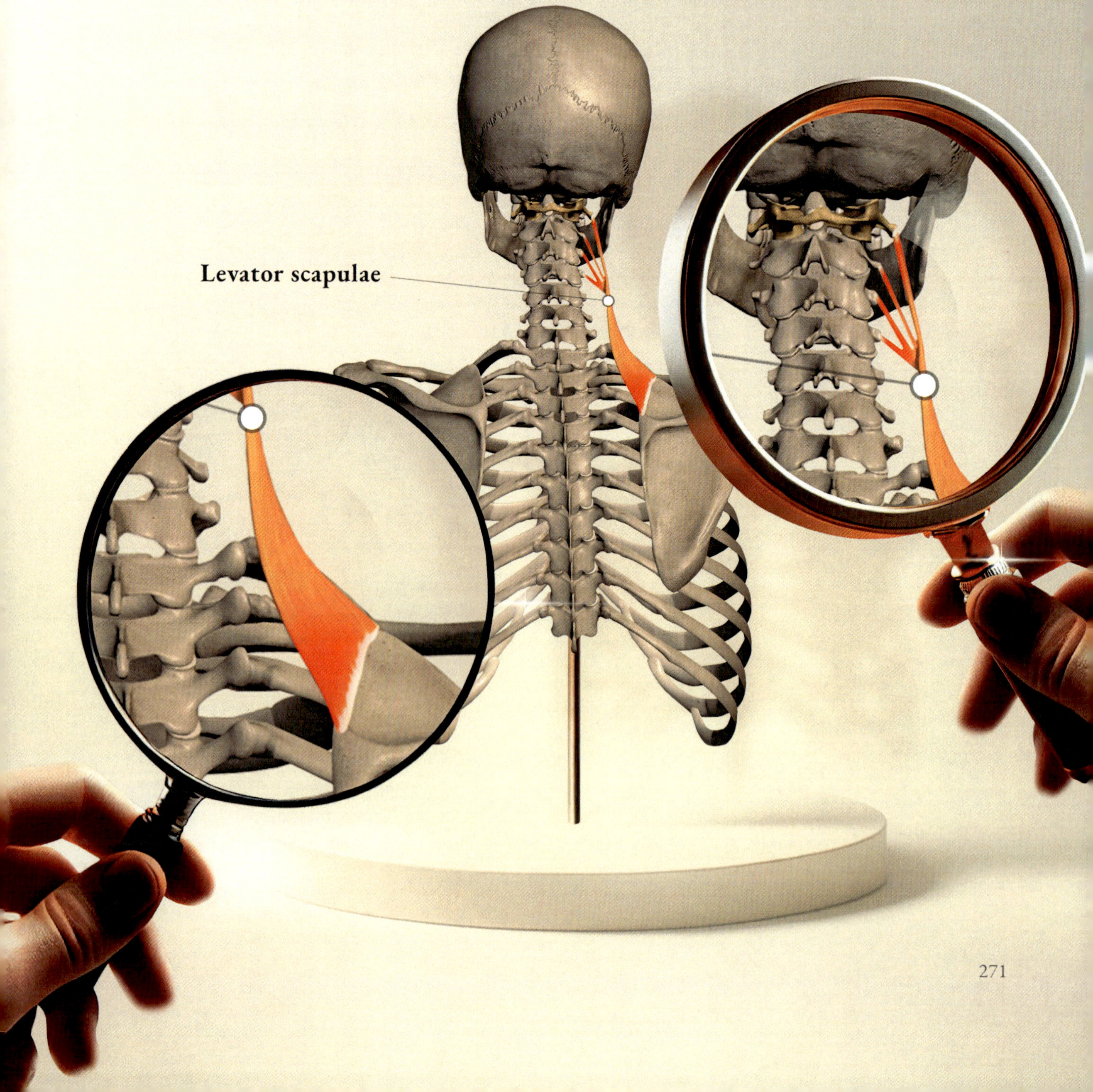

Pain in the Sternocleidomastoid Muscle

Right lateral subluxation of the atlas vertebra, combined with cervical vertebrae scoliosis, causes the head to tilt to the left to stabilize the imbalance. This can compress the spinal accessory nerve, leading to strain and inflammation in the sternocleidomastoid muscle. Correcting the atlas vertebra alignment is the only way to alleviate these symptoms.

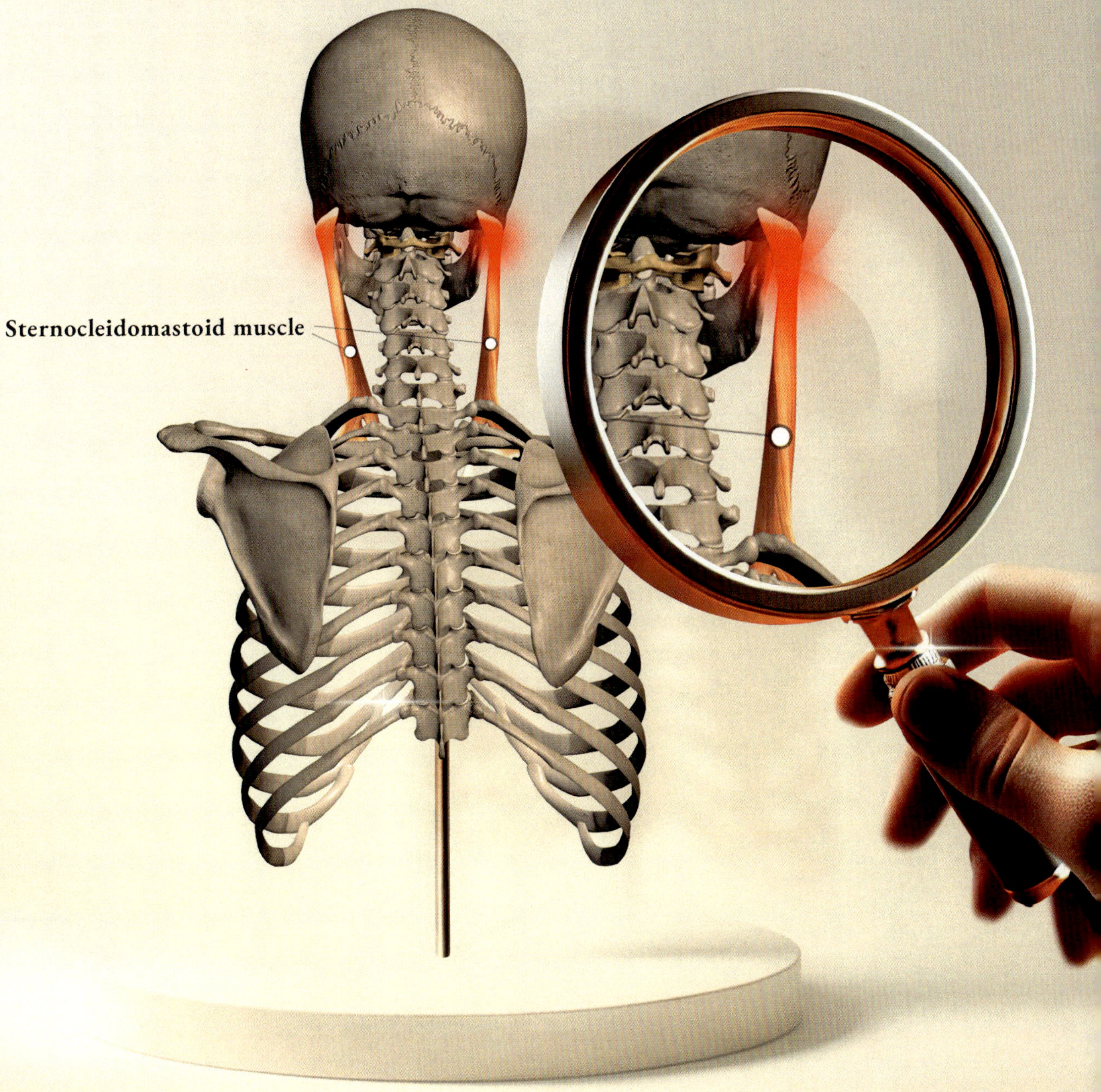

Pain in the Trapezius Muscles

When the atlas is displaced to the right and cervical vertebrae scoliosis is present, the head tilts to the left to maintain balance. This can put pressure on the spinal accessory nerve, leading to tension and inflammation in the trapezius muscle. Correcting the position of the atlas is necessary to alleviate these symptoms.

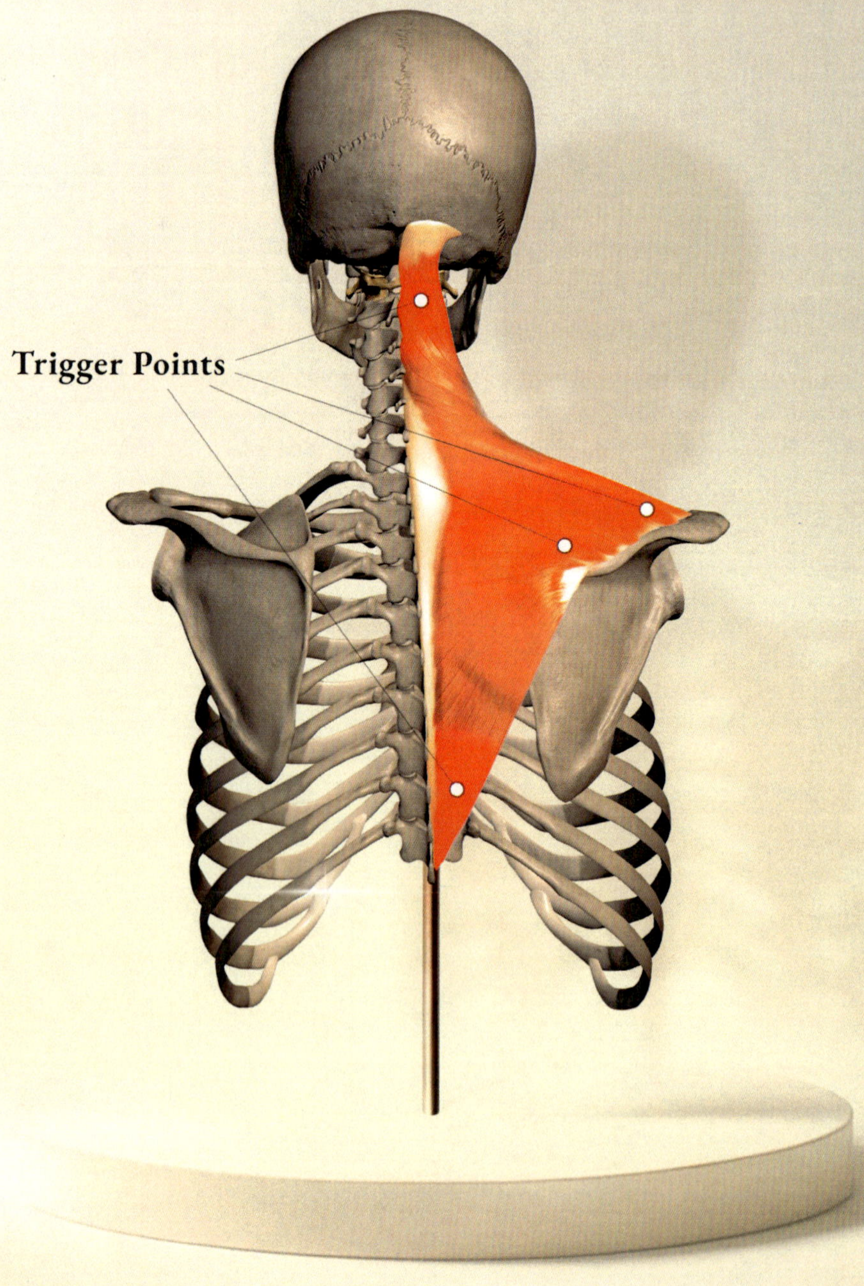

Right Shoulder Drooping

When the atlas is displaced to the right and cervical vertebrae scoliosis is present, the right shoulder drops downward and rotates the head by straining the sternocleidomastoid and trapezius muscles. Additionally, this shoulder drooping pulls the right side of the atlas downward, causing the atlas to lower on the right side relative to the axis.

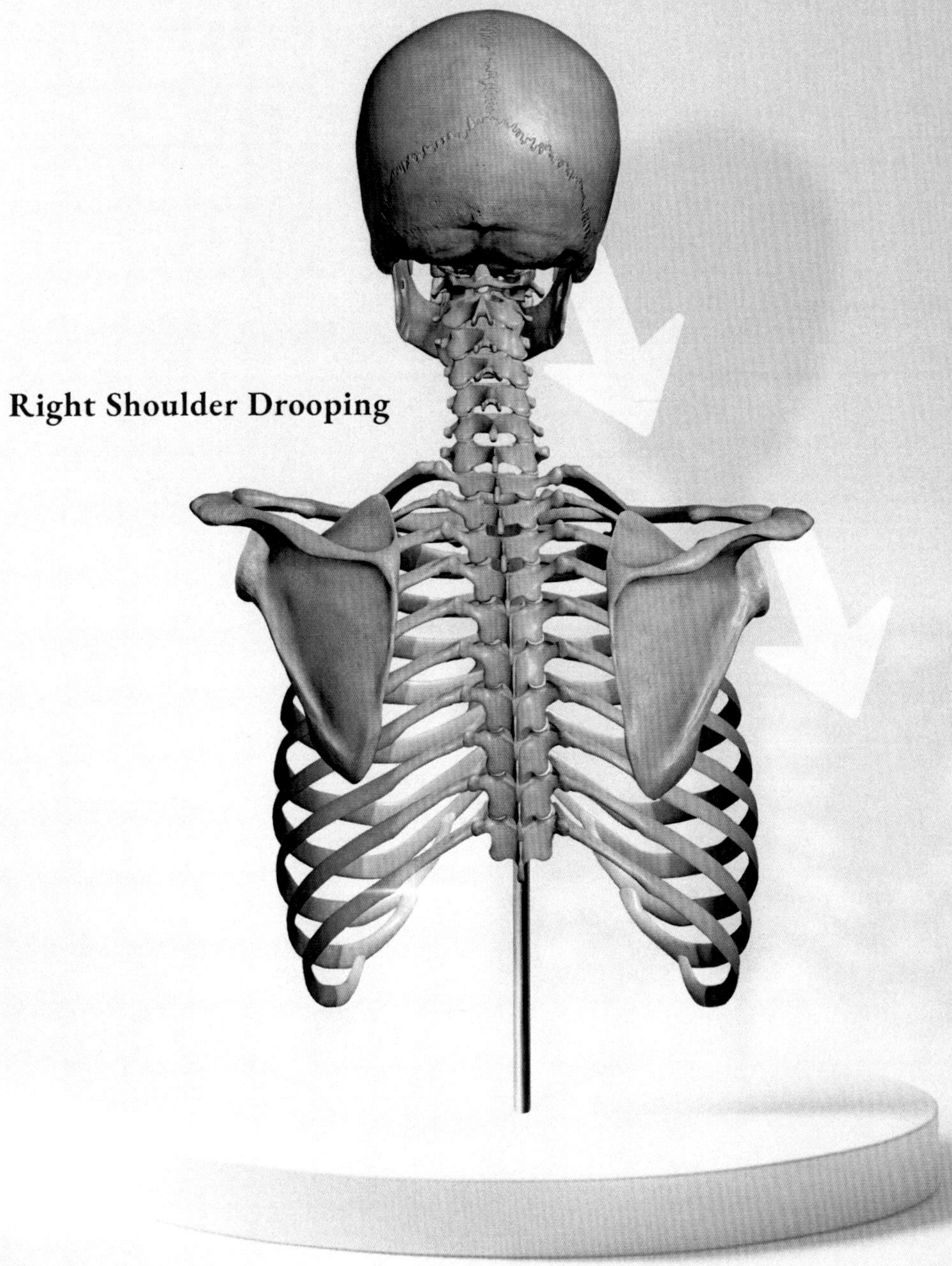

Exercise cannot straighten a curved spine

The cause of a curved spine is not weak and inactive muscles, but rather a misaligned atlas vertebra and poor head positioning, which, on average, weighs 5 kilograms. This weight disrupts the symmetrical activity of the neck and shoulder muscles. When the atlas vertebra is misaligned, it additionally compresses the nerves that innervate the muscles of the neck, shoulders, and back, leading to poor innervation and muscle weakness, causing them to adapt (by stretching or shortening) to the curvature of the skeleton. This weakness is not the cause, but rather a consequence of the spinal curvature and nerve compression.

Muscle weakness and inflammation occur as the body's response to disturbed balance. Muscles stretch and become inflamed as they attempt to correct the body's positional irregularities. However, these inflammations, which represent microtears in muscle structures, cannot be resolved through exercise.

The skeleton, composed of bones, is a stronger structure compared to muscles. Muscles follow the curvature of the spine; the spine cannot be straightened by strengthening the muscles. Therefore, correcting the misalignment of the atlas and ensuring proper innervation of the muscles are crucial for correcting body posture and resolving spinal problems that cause muscle weakness and inflammation.

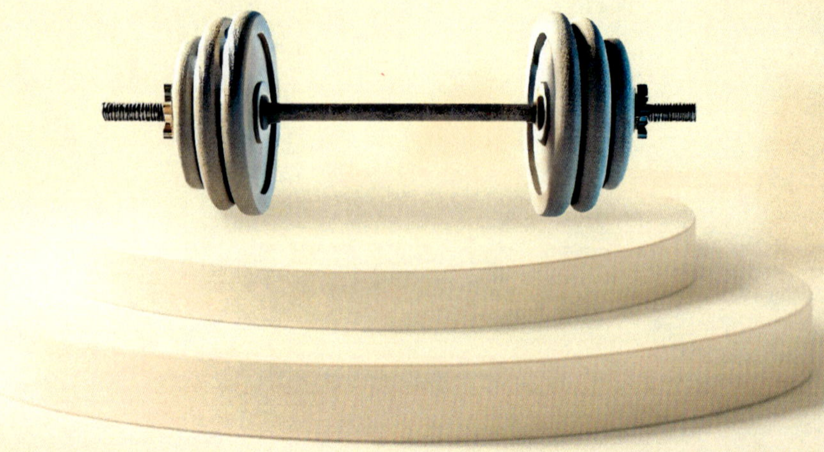

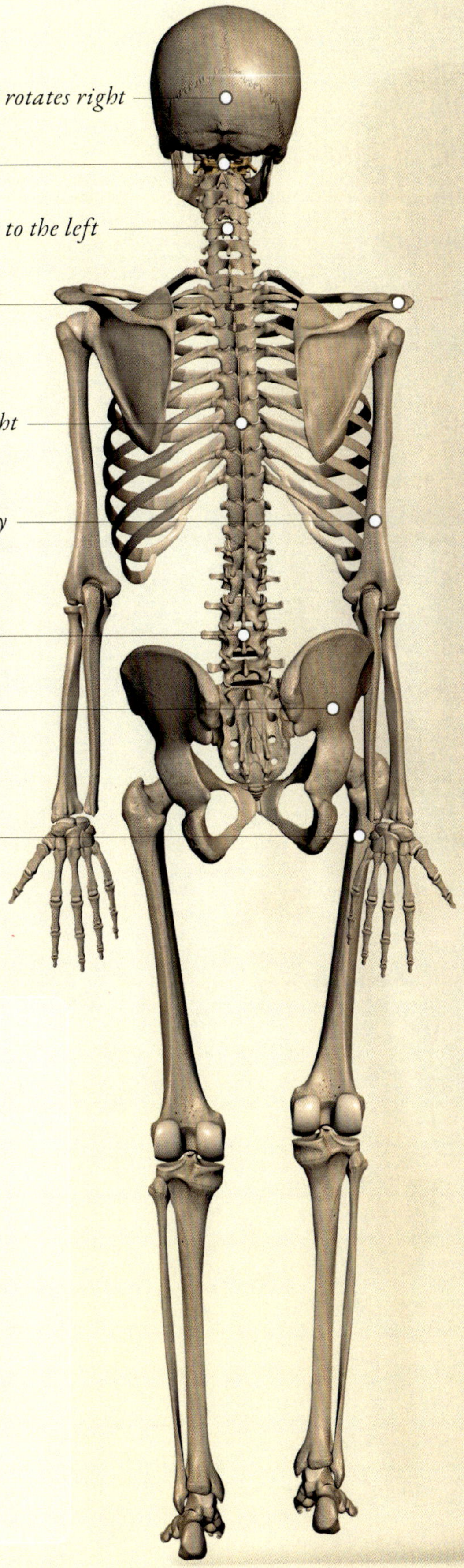

Body Posture

In cases of lateral subluxation, when the atlas shifts to the right, the head moves to the left, and its weight causes cervical scoliosis. This is compensated by right thoracic scoliosis and the dropping of the right shoulder in the thoracic spine, and left lumbar scoliosis, lifting the right side of the pelvis.

Chapter 6

Atlantoaxial Rotation

Atlantoaxial Rotation

Atlas rotation, which refers to the rotation of the first cervical vertebra, represents a complex disorder [Image 1]. When the atlas rotates, the entire dynamics of the neck can be disrupted, leading to various symptoms and issues.

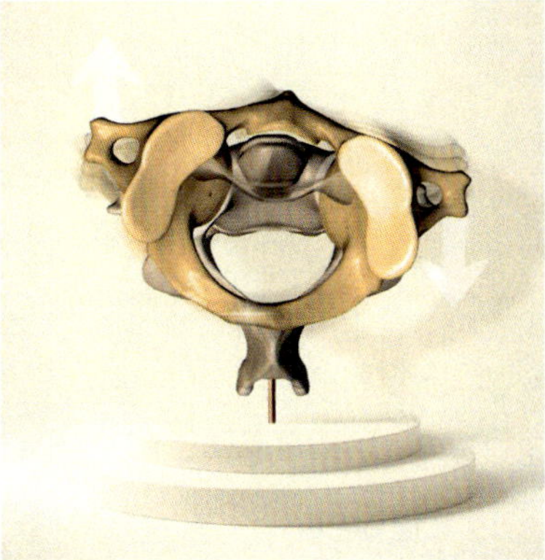

[Image 1] Atlantoaxial rotation

This disorder not only disturbs neck function but can also have broader consequences. It particularly affects the clear and precise communication between the head and body, as well as the functioning of blood, nerve, and lymphatic pathways [Image 2]. Additionally, atlas rotation can lead to neurological and other issues in the lumbar spine and lower limbs due to spinal twisting.

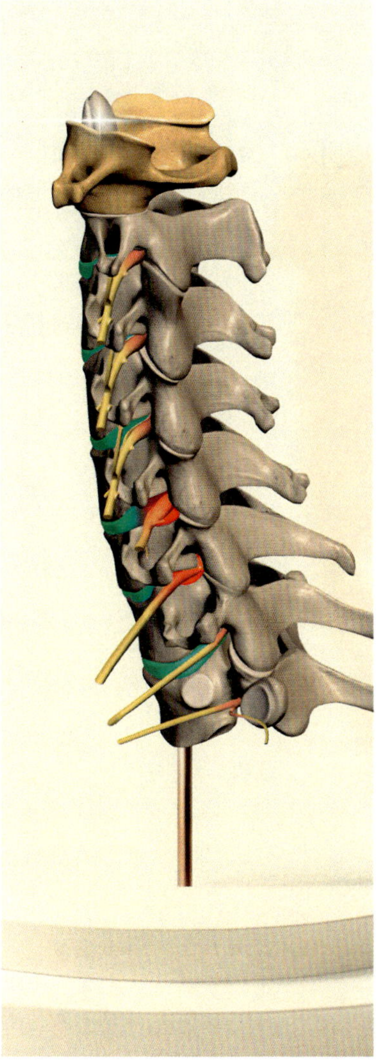

[Image 2] Nerve impact

Atlas rotation, which can be acute or chronic, can be caused by various factors, including trauma, poor posture, sleeping on the stomach, repetitive movements that strain the cervical spine, or irregularities in the spinal anatomy from childhood.

One of the key factors contributing to atlantoaxial instability is the rotation of the head during childbirth. During passage through the birth canal, a baby's head may experience rotational forces affecting the position of the first cervical vertebra. This rotation can be induced by physical exertion during childbirth and can result in the displacement of the atlas's normal position. Additionally, if the childbirth procedure involves rotating the baby's head for quicker and easier delivery of the shoulder, there is a possibility of rotating the baby's atlas vertebra, which affects the improper development of the child moving forward.

Poor posture is often a consequence of a misaligned atlas vertebra, and it can further accelerate the subluxation of the atlas towards the path of atlantoaxial dislocation, with atlantoaxial rotational subluxation being the most dramatic. When the atlas vertebra is already misaligned, the body tends to compensate by adopting improper postures and alignments [Image 1]. This maladaptive response to the misalignment exacerbates the condition, leading to a vicious cycle where poor posture perpetuates the misalignment of the atlas, and in turn, the misalignment worsens posture. This continuous cycle can result in increased strain on the surrounding muscles, ligaments, and nerves, contributing to a variety of symptoms and discomfort throughout the body, including neck pain, headaches, and decreased range of motion. Therefore, addressing both the underlying misalignment of the atlas and correcting poor posture are essential for restoring proper spinal alignment and overall musculoskeletal health.

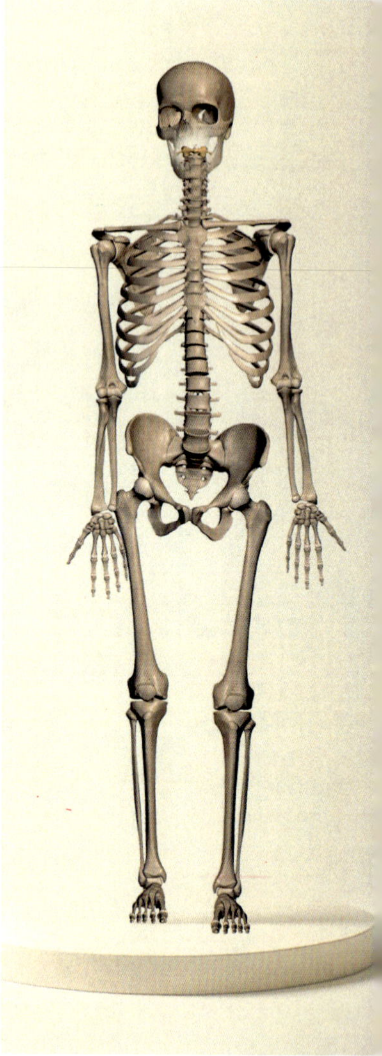
[Image 1] Posture of scoliosis

Sleeping on the stomach is one of the first life experiences we encounter as infants, often nestled against our mother's chest. The presence of care, the scent of maternal pheromones, the warmth, and the proximity of her voice create a sense of security that encourages us to develop the habit of sleeping on the stomach. For these reasons, sleeping in this position often feels pleasant and natural. However, sooner or later, this habit may result in the rotation of the atlas vertebra. The body position during stomach sleeping can exert irregular pressure on the cervical spine, which over time can lead to disturbances in the position of the first cervical vertebra. This rotation of the atlas can cause various issues with the cervical spine and nervous system, underscoring the importance of maintaining proper sleeping posture to preserve cervical spine health and prevent potential complications.

Repetitive movements that strain the cervical spine can significantly impact our health and posture. These movements, especially when performed improperly or with poor posture, can lead to various issues with the cervical spine. An intriguing dimension of this problem is the difference between right-handed and left-handed individuals. Right-handed individuals often favor the right side and right hand for everyday activities, while left-handed individuals rely more on the left side of their body. This asymmetry in muscle usage and movements can result in muscle imbalances in the neck and back, which leads to its further rotation in a specific direction. Being right-handed or left-handed can directly influence the rotation of the atlas. For example, right-handed individuals often have stronger muscles on the right side of their neck and back, while left-handed individuals have a stronger left side. This imbalance in muscle strength can affect the muscles around the atlas, leading to its rotation in a specific direction. It's essential for both arms and sides of the body to be equally developed and strong to avoid postural irregularities and atlas rotation. Exercises that strengthen muscles on both sides of the body, along with stretching and massage techniques, can help maintain muscle balance and cervical spine health. Additionally, awareness of how we perform movements and hold our bodies can be crucial in preventing issues with the cervical spine and atlas rotation.

However, traumas such as impacts to the front of the chest or sudden twisting of the head, blows to the lower jaw, or even slaps can exert force transmitted through the cervical spine and lead to rotation of the atlas. These events are often sudden and unexpected, especially in sports-related incidents and traffic accidents. We will delve further into these common causes in the following chapter.

Restricted neck movement and pain are among the main symptoms of atlas rotation. Individuals with a rotated atlas often experience tension, stiffness, or pain in the neck, especially when attempting to rotate the head or tilt the neck. Additionally, atlas rotation can irritate nerves and blood vessels in the surrounding tissues, leading to symptoms such as tingling, numbness, or a sensation of 'pins and needles' in the arms, shoulders, or even the head.

In addition to local symptoms in the cervical spine, atlas rotation can have further consequences on overall spinal health and overall body health. An improper atlas position can cause imbalance in the muscles of the neck and shoulders, leading to additional issues such as back pain, headaches, or even postural disturbances.

Treating atlas rotation typically requires a multidisciplinary approach. However, in practice, atlas adjustment has proven to be the most effective choice, tailored to the needs of each individual. This may involve therapy customized to each patient, including therapeutic exercises to strengthen the muscles of the neck and back, techniques for correcting body posture, and manual therapy such as muscle massage to expedite the correction process.

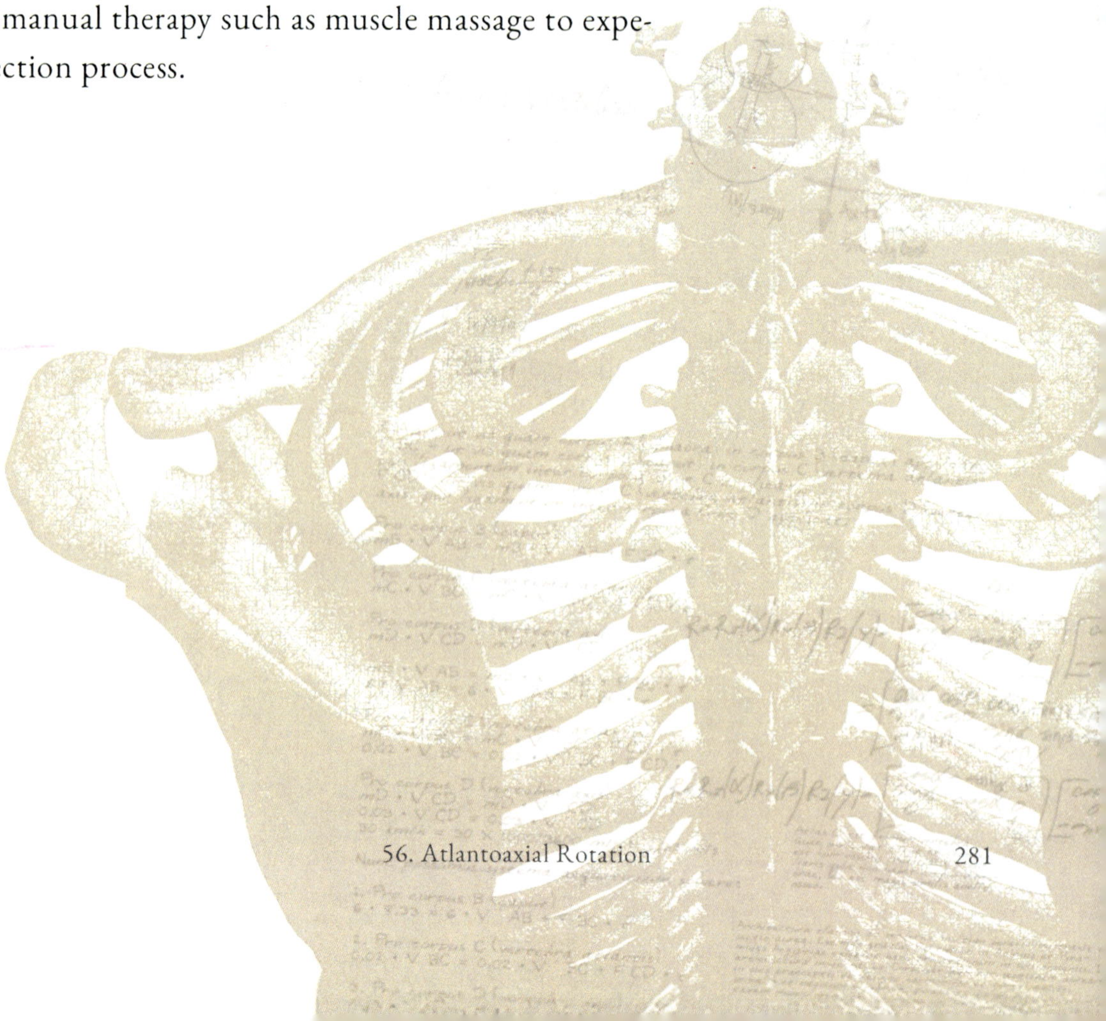

Impact of Rotational Atlas Subluxation

Rotational subluxation of the atlas, although it may have various causes, is often linked to our lifestyle and physical activities. In today's world, filled with dynamic events and rapid changes, a restless life has become the norm. We often expose ourselves to unnecessary physical activities without consciously considering the consequences they may have on our bodies. The modern way of life often drives us to be part of traffic, whether as drivers, passengers, or pedestrians. This exposure to the risks of traffic accidents cannot be ignored, as even minor incidents can have serious consequences for our health.

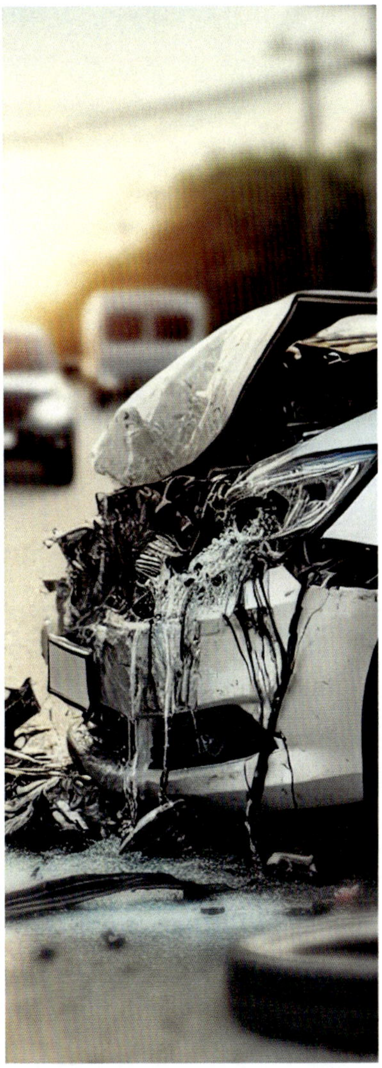

[Image 1] Traffic accidents

One significant observation I have noticed in my work is that most patients facing atlas rotation and other atlas subluxations have been direct participants in traffic accidents [Image 1]. Many of them are active individuals who have enjoyed physical activities for entertainment or recreational sports [Image 2]. This suggests that even everyday, seemingly harmless activities such as cycling, running, or jumping can cause atlas rotation following a fall. This is an important realization that reminds us to carefully choose our physical activities and pay attention to our bodies' signals. Because, although we may not face extreme risks, routine activities can have long-term consequences on our health, including atlas rotation.

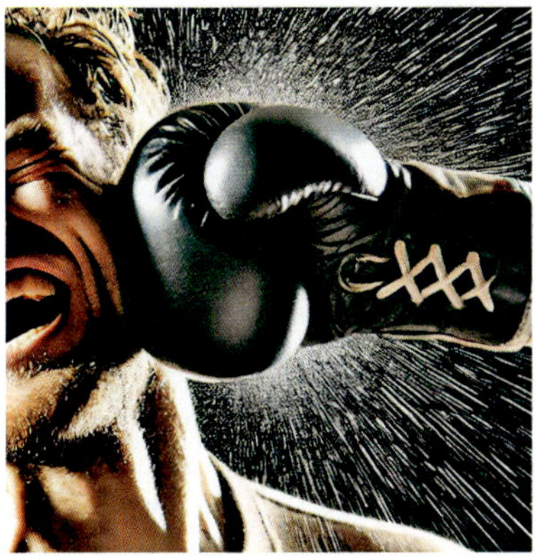

[Image 2] Restless life

Rotational subluxation of the atlas, especially when occurring uncontrollably, carries with it the consequence of twisting the spinal column. This rotation can cause not only an imbalance in the cervical spine but also twisting of the entire spinal column. As a result, the entire spine can be twisted, leading to a range of issues.

The consequences of spinal column twisting can be serious. Firstly, this disorder can cause pain and discomfort, especially in the cervical spine. Additionally, twisting of the spinal column can cause restricted movement and reduced mobility, making daily activities more challenging. Furthermore, this problem can affect body alignment, causing an irregular stance. In severe cases, twisting of the spinal column can lead to complications such as nerve compression or blood vessel damage, further worsening the condition and necessitating proper treatment and rehabilitation.

The rotation of the atlas vertebra not only affects the cervical spine but can have far-reaching consequences on the alignment of the entire spinal column, including the pelvis. When the atlas rotates, it can trigger a chain reaction throughout the spine, leading to pelvic rotation. This pelvic rotation places additional pressure on motor nerves, such as the femoral, fibular, and sciatic nerves, which pass through the lower back and pelvis.

As the atlas rotates, the pelvis shifts in the opposite direction of the shoulders, further disturbing the body's balance and creating uneven strain on the nerves. This asymmetry in body posture can cause nerve compression, leading to pain, tingling, and weakness in the legs and lower back. For instance, pressure on the sciatic nerve can result in sciatica, causing severe pain and discomfort along the back of the leg. Similarly, compression of the femoral and fibular nerves can impair mobility and leg function, making activities like walking or bending the knee difficult.

These issues complicate everyday activities and require prompt recognition and treatment. Correcting atlas rotation can help restore the body's balance, reducing pressure on the pelvis and motor nerves. Aligning the atlas, shoulders, and pelvis frees nerve pathways, reducing pain, improving mobility, and enhancing the spine and lower extremities' condition.

Mechanics of Rotational Atlas Subluxation

Let's recall the calculation we performed analyzing the mechanical forces acting on the atlas after a strike to the left side of the head. The result showed that, due to inertia and the force of impact, the atlas tends to move in the opposite direction of the strike, toward the left side of the body, the side from which the strike is directed. This happens due to the distribution and balance of forces on the spine after the impact, leading to a shift of the atlas to the left.

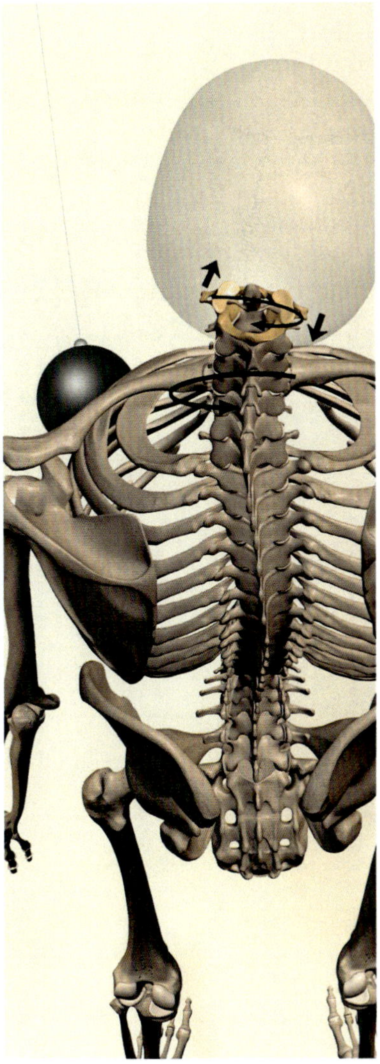

[Image 1] Vector forces and torque

We could consider an equation for the rotation of the atlas after an impact to the right shoulder or chest area of the chest. According to the principle of conservation of momentum, we can derive an equation describing the rotation of the atlas in response to an external force. However, it is important to note that this equation would be more complex than the simple linear analysis we applied for the displacement of the atlas. Rotation of the atlas concerning its normal position in a particular plane (e.g., the sagittal plane) may result from a combination of mechanical forces and factors such as inertia, body shape, point of force application, and others. This analysis would require a more detailed biomechanical study and modeling, including the use of the moment of inertia and other rotational parameters.

In the analysis of the rotation of the atlas after an impact to the right shoulder or the right area of the chest, we can utilize some basic principles of mechanics. Let us assume the body is at rest before the impact, with no initial rotational velocity [Image 1].

The equation describing the rotation of the atlas can be expressed through the moment of force (torque) acting on the vertebra. If we denote this moment as M, and the moment of inertia of the atlas (in the sagittal plane) as I, then we can use the basic equation of mechanics:

$$M = I \cdot \alpha$$

where α represents the angular acceleration of the atlas. This acceleration depends on the force F acting on the atlas, the moment of inertia I, and the body's structural characteristics. In this case, a strike to the right shoulder or chest area induces a moment of force M, causing the atlas to rotate.

Such calculations require a detailed understanding of the anatomy and biomechanics of the spinal column, as well as specific parameters of the impact, including its magnitude, angle of impact, point of force application, and other factors.

However, due to the complexity of the equation compared to the linear analysis we applied for the displacement of the atlas, it is possible to describe the general form of an equation that would model the rotation of the atlas after an impact, considering some of the aforementioned parameters. One possible description of such an equation is:

Atlas rotation = f (Impact magnitude, Angle of impact, Point of force application, Atlas properties, Surrounding structures)

In this equation, f represents a function that models the rotation of the atlas based on various impact parameters and anatomical characteristics of the atlas and surrounding structures.

The parameters included in this equation can be specified as follows:

Impact magnitude: Expressed in appropriate units of measurement, such as N (newtons) or kg*m/s^2 (kilograms times meters per second squared).

Angle of impact: The angle at which the impact acts on the body, expressed in degrees.

Point of force application: The location on the body where the impact acts, expressed in suitable coordinates.

Atlas properties: Anatomical characteristics of the atlas that influence its response to impact, such as shape, size, strength, elasticity, and other physical attributes.

Surrounding structures: The presence and characteristics of surrounding structures, such as ligaments, muscles, and other parts of the spine, which may affect the rotation of the atlas.

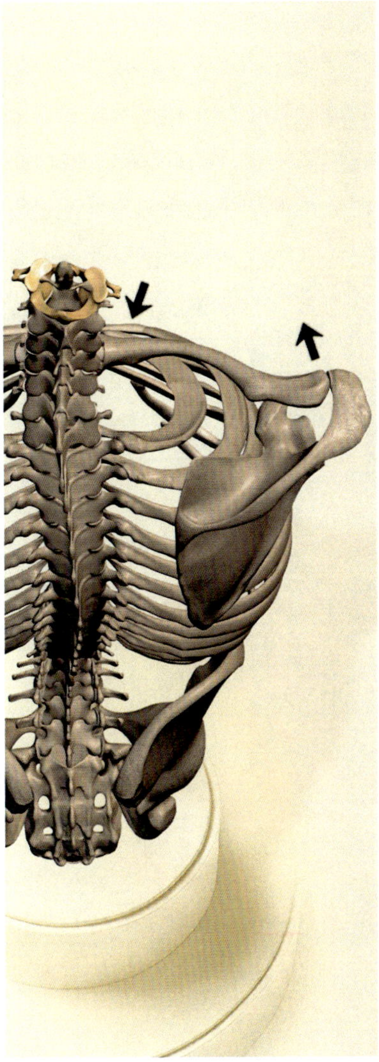

[Image 1] Swing

Practice has revealed that the most common rotations of the atlas are diagnosed through imaging or palpation relative to the horizontal plane of the shoulders. When it comes to the rotation of the atlas, particular attention should be paid to the position of the lateral processes of the atlas, which are considered key indicators of rotation. Typically, when the rotation of the atlas is directed towards the right side, the lateral process of the atlas rotates backward, resulting in the forward movement of the right shoulder, while the left shoulder moves backward [Image 1]. On the other hand, when the rotation of the atlas is to the left side, the lateral process of the atlas rotates forward, causing the left shoulder to move forward and the right shoulder to move backward.

This phenomenon is particularly pronounced in rotational dislocations, where changes in body position are visually more apparent than in rotational subluxations. In cases of rotational dislocations, symptoms are often more pronounced and obvious, making diagnosis easier through the observation of body posture. However, in rotational subluxations, where changes are less pronounced, diagnosis requires skills and experience.

This change in shoulder and body position indicates the complexity of atlas rotation and its impact on overall body posture. Understanding these characteristics enables healthcare professionals to accurately identify atlas rotation and make a proper diagnosis.

The consequences of atlas rotation are varied and complex, potentially having a long-lasting impact on overall body posture and spinal biomechanics. Besides causing changes in shoulder position, atlas rotation can directly affect the position of the pelvic bone, further complicating body posture and movements.

When the atlas is rotated backward along its right side, opposite to the rotation of the right shoulder, it triggers a chain reaction in the body. This disturbance in the position of the atlas leads to the torsion of the entire spinal column, including the pelvis. As a result, the right side of the pelvis rotates backward, aligning with the rotation of the atlas.

This process is particularly significant because the pelvis plays a crucial role in body stability and balance. Pelvic rotation can lead to muscle imbalances in the lower back and hips, affecting gait and movements. Additionally, this change in pelvic position can cause discomfort and pain in the lower back and hips, making everyday activities more difficult and affecting quality of life.

Rotational subluxations of the atlas present a complex problem with potentially serious consequences for spinal health and the nervous system. One of the key complications of this condition involves problematic blood flow and pressure on the nerve structures passing through the atlas apertures.

When a rotational subluxation of the atlas occurs, the processes of this vertebra can shift and compress the arteries passing through these apertures. This can disrupt normal blood flow to the brain, especially to the cerebellum, causing oxygen and nutrient deficiencies in this vital region. Insufficient blood flow to the brain can cause a range of symptoms, including dizziness, loss of balance, and fainting, further complicating everyday activities and quality of life.

In addition to issues with blood flow and nerve function, rotational subluxations of the atlas can also compress nerve pathways in surrounding tissues. This can lead to the compression of motor nerves that innervate the limbs, resulting in mobility and functionality issues in the extremities. Herniated discs in the lumbar spine can also result from uneven weight distribution caused by atlas rotation, further exacerbating the situation and leading to pain and discomfort.

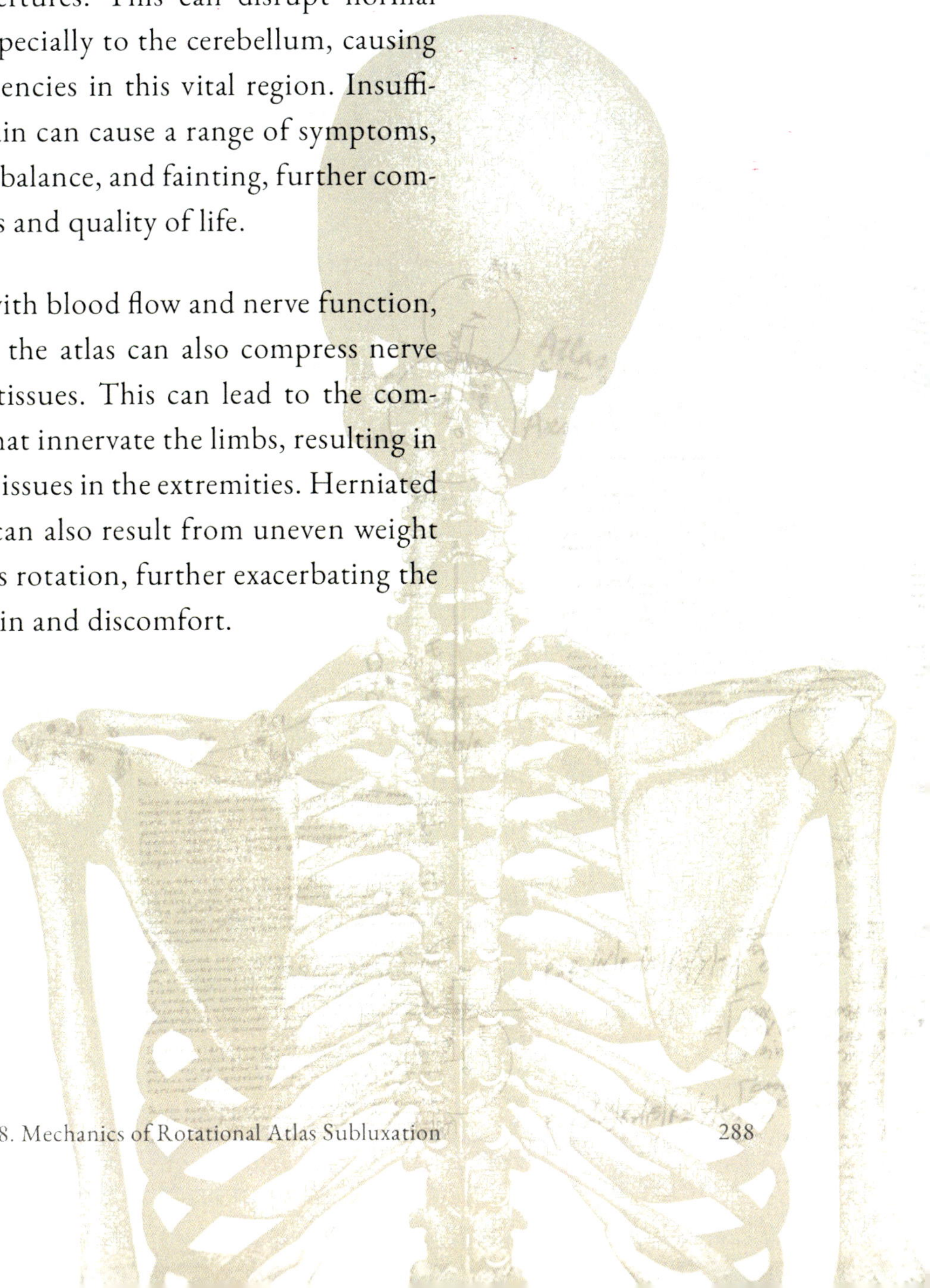

Treating Rotational Atlas Subluxations

Considering the impact of traumatic injuries and intensive physical activities on the occurrence of atlas rotational subluxations is crucial for understanding the complexity of this condition and its potential consequences for spinal health and the nervous system. In this analysis, we will focus on several key aspects directly related to atlas rotational subluxations that can lead to serious complications.

It is important to consider how traumatic injuries like impacts, falls, or traffic accidents can cause atlas rotation. The intense force exerted on the cervical spine during these events can result in shifts and rotations of the atlas, causing subluxations and disrupting the normal functioning of this part of the spinal column. This rotation can be gradual or sudden, but in both cases, it can lead to serious problems.

In cases of sudden trauma, such as traffic accidents or falls, a rapid and severe impact can directly displace the atlas from its normal position, causing immediate rotation and misalignment. On the other hand, repetitive strain or minor injuries over time can gradually weaken the ligaments and structures supporting the atlas, eventually leading to gradual rotation. This gradual onset of rotation may not be immediately noticeable but can worsen over time, causing chronic pain and dysfunction.

Moreover, the specific mechanics involved in transmitting these traumatic forces to the cervical spine play a crucial role in determining the direction and degree of atlas rotation. Factors such as the angle and direction of impact, the position of the head and neck at the time of trauma, and the overall biomechanics of the cervical spine all influence how the atlas will respond to external forces.

Additionally, individual anatomical variations and pre-existing conditions can influence the susceptibility to atlas rotation. For example, a person with a congenital abnormality or underlying weaknesses in the ligaments supporting the atlas may be more prone to rotational subluxations following trauma.

Another important aspect is the compression of the arteries that supply blood to the cerebellum. Atlas rotation can impede normal blood flow through the atlas foramina, resulting in oxygen and nutrient deficiencies in this vital brain region. Insufficient blood supply to the cerebellum can lead to various neurological symptoms, including dizziness, loss of balance, and fainting, significantly impacting the patient's daily activities and quality of life.

When the arteries are compressed due to atlas rotation, there is a reduced blood flow through them, disrupting the brain's normal oxygen and nutrient supply. The cerebellum plays a crucial role in coordinating movements and maintaining balance, so inadequate blood circulation to this part of the brain can cause various neurological symptoms. Dizziness is a common symptom when there is a lack of blood flow to the cerebellum, which may manifest as a feeling of lightheadedness or instability when walking or changing body position. Additionally, loss of balance and fainting are possible consequences of inadequate blood supply to this vital brain region. These symptoms can significantly limit the patient's daily activities and negatively impact their quality of life; thus, it is essential to recognize and appropriately treat artery compression as a potential cause of these neurological symptoms in patients with atlas rotational subluxations.

Compression of the vagus nerve is another critical factor

to consider. This nerve is responsible for regulating vital functions in the body, including heart activity and breathing. Compression of the vagus nerve can lead to disturbances in heart and lung function, which can result in serious health problems and complications.

The vagus nerve plays a crucial role in maintaining the balance of the autonomic nervous system, controlling heart rate and rhythm, as well as respiratory function. Compression of this nerve can result in dysfunction in its regulation, leading to heart arrhythmias, bradycardia, or tachycardia, as well as breathing dysfunction. These changes in heart and lung function can pose a serious threat to the patient's health, especially in cases where compression of the vagus nerve is pronounced and prolonged.

Heart rhythm disturbances can lead to various complications, including syncope (fainting), hypertension or hypotension, as well as life-threatening cardiac arrhythmias. Additionally, respiratory dysfunction can cause hypoxia (oxygen deficiency) and hypercapnia (elevated carbon dioxide levels) in the blood, which can further lead to organ and tissue damage due to inadequate oxygenation. Therefore, it is crucial to adequately diagnose and treat vagus nerve compression as a potential cause of health problems in patients with atlas rotational subluxations.

Furthermore, atlas rotation can cause uneven weight distribution across other vertebrae in the lumbar spine, leading to compression of the motor nerves of the lower extremities. This can result in mobility and functionality issues in the legs, further complicating daily activities and negatively impacting the patient's quality of life.

When pressure on motor nerves increases due to uneven spinal loading, damage and compression of these nerves can occur, further disrupting the normal flow of information between the brain and the muscles of the lower extremities. This can result in various neurological symptoms, including weakness, tingling, pain, and loss of sensation in the legs.

Issues with mobility and functionality in the legs can significantly hinder the patient's daily activities, such as walking, standing, climbing stairs, or performing tasks that require motor skills of the lower extremities. Additionally, limited leg mobility can seriously impact the patient's quality of life, restricting their ability to live independently and causing emotional and psychological discomfort. Therefore, it is important to recognize and adequately treat this complication of atlas rotational subluxations to improve functionality and the quality of life for patients.

Overall, considering these factors helps us better understand the complexity of atlas rotational subluxations and underscores the importance of accurate diagnosis and treatment to prevent potential complications and preserve patient health.

"Health is not merely the absence of disease, but the presence of complete physical, mental, and social well-being."

(Hippocrates)

Preventing Rotational Atlas Subluxations

Preventing rotational subluxations of the atlas is vital for maintaining spinal health and overall well-being. There are numerous preventive measures individuals can take to reduce the risk of this condition and keep their cervical spine in optimal condition.

First and foremost, it's important to lead a calm life without unnecessary exposure to trauma and risks. This includes avoiding activities that could lead to serious neck injuries, such as extreme sports or unsafe driving. Maintaining a cautious and mindful attitude towards daily activities can significantly reduce the chances of developing rotational subluxations of the atlas.

Additionally, respecting physical and ethical laws plays a crucial role in preventing this condition. Driving safely, obeying traffic rules, and wearing a seatbelt while driving can reduce the risk of traffic accidents and potential neck injuries. Furthermore, avoiding violent situations and conflicts can help preserve the physical integrity of the neck.

It's also important to recognize responsibility for one's own health and the health of others. Regular check-ups with a physician, especially with an orthopedist or physiotherapist, can help in early detection of any cervical spine problems and prevent the development of rotational subluxations of the atlas. It's also important to follow experts' recommendations on maintaining proper posture, performing neck and back strengthening exercises, and lifting heavy loads correctly.

One of the key preventive strategies is maintaining proper weight and physical fitness. Regular exercise, such as stretching, aerobic exercise, and strength training, can strengthen the muscles around the neck and spine, reducing the risk of injuries and atlas subluxations. Additionally, avoiding prolonged sitting or standing in unnatural positions can help maintain spinal health.

Moreover, it's important to be aware of proper lifting techniques and avoid excessive use of mobile devices, such as cell phones or tablets, which can cause strain on the neck and spine.

In summary, preventing rotational subluxations of the atlas requires careful living, adherence to safety measures, taking responsibility for one's health and the health of others, regular medical check-ups, maintaining proper weight and physical fitness, as well as awareness of proper posture and lifting heavy objects. Implementing these preventive measures can significantly reduce the risk of rotational subluxations of the atlas and maintain spinal health.

In this book, we will explore the method of atlas adjustment that has already been applied to over 3000 patients of different genders, ages, and occupations. This method is not just treatment but an approach leading to healing from symptoms and pains, focusing on eliminating the root cause of the problem that has disrupted the proper functionality of the body.

The core of this method is focused on the atlas, the first cervical vertebra, often a key factor in many neurological and musculoskeletal issues. Through careful and precise adjustment of the atlas, this method works to reestablish the optimal position of the vertebra and proper flow of nerve impulses, enabling the body to self-heal and restore its natural balance.

What's fascinating about this method is that the relief experienced by patients and the processes of health improvement are seen as a true renaissance in the art of healing. Patients not only free themselves from pain and discomfort but also experience deeper changes in their physical and emotional well-being. It's not just symptom relief but a journey towards holistic health and revitalization of the body and mind.

Through in-depth research, this book reveals the depth and complexity of this method, as well as its accessibility and applicability in various situations. Its goal is not only to inform readers about the principles behind this method but also to inspire them to explore new paths to health and well-being.

Rotational subluxations of the atlas affect physical and psychological health by impacting the central nervous system and hormone-producing glands. When misaligned, it can press on nerves and blood vessels, leading to hormonal imbalances.

Hormones regulate vital functions such as mood, motivation, and willpower. When atlas subluxation disrupts hormonal balance, it can impair the function of glands like the pituitary, thyroid, and adrenal glands, causing symptoms such as fatigue, loss of motivation, and anxiety.

Correcting atlas misalignment restores physical balance and stabilizes the hormonal system, improving mental clarity, energy, and emotional well-being. Realigning the atlas helps the body regain its natural balance, allowing hormones to function properly and restoring strength and motivation. We should take care of our health and adopt a preventive approach to avoid countless hours of unpleasant symptoms and pain, even though these problems are largely solvable.

Atlantoaxial Rotation

Atlantoaxial rotation most commonly involves the backward rotation of the right side of the atlas vertebra. This subluxation results in symptoms like the rotation of the chest and hips. It causes the spinal column to twist, with the shoulders rotating opposite to the atlas and the pelvis rotating in the same direction as the atlas.

Atlas is rotated with the right side backward

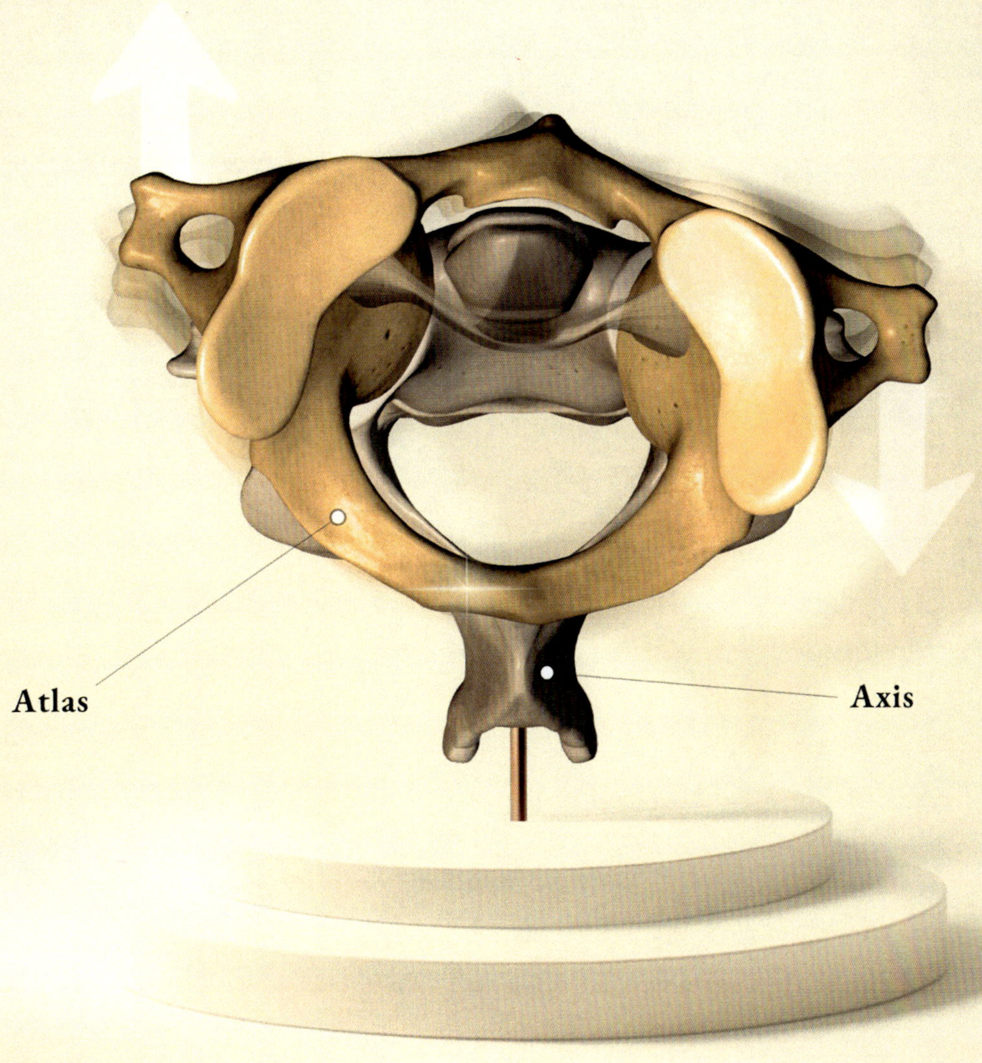

Head and Atlas Rotation: Angle of Rotation

The rotation of the head and atlas (C1) is essential for understanding neck and head movements. When the head is turned so that the nose aligns with the shoulder, the total rotation is about 90 degrees. However, the atlas itself only rotates up to 45 degrees relative to the axis (C2). The remaining rotation comes from the other cervical vertebrae. Thus, while the nose is aligned with the shoulder, the atlas provides up to 45 degrees of rotation, with the rest resulting from the movement of the other cervical vertebrae.

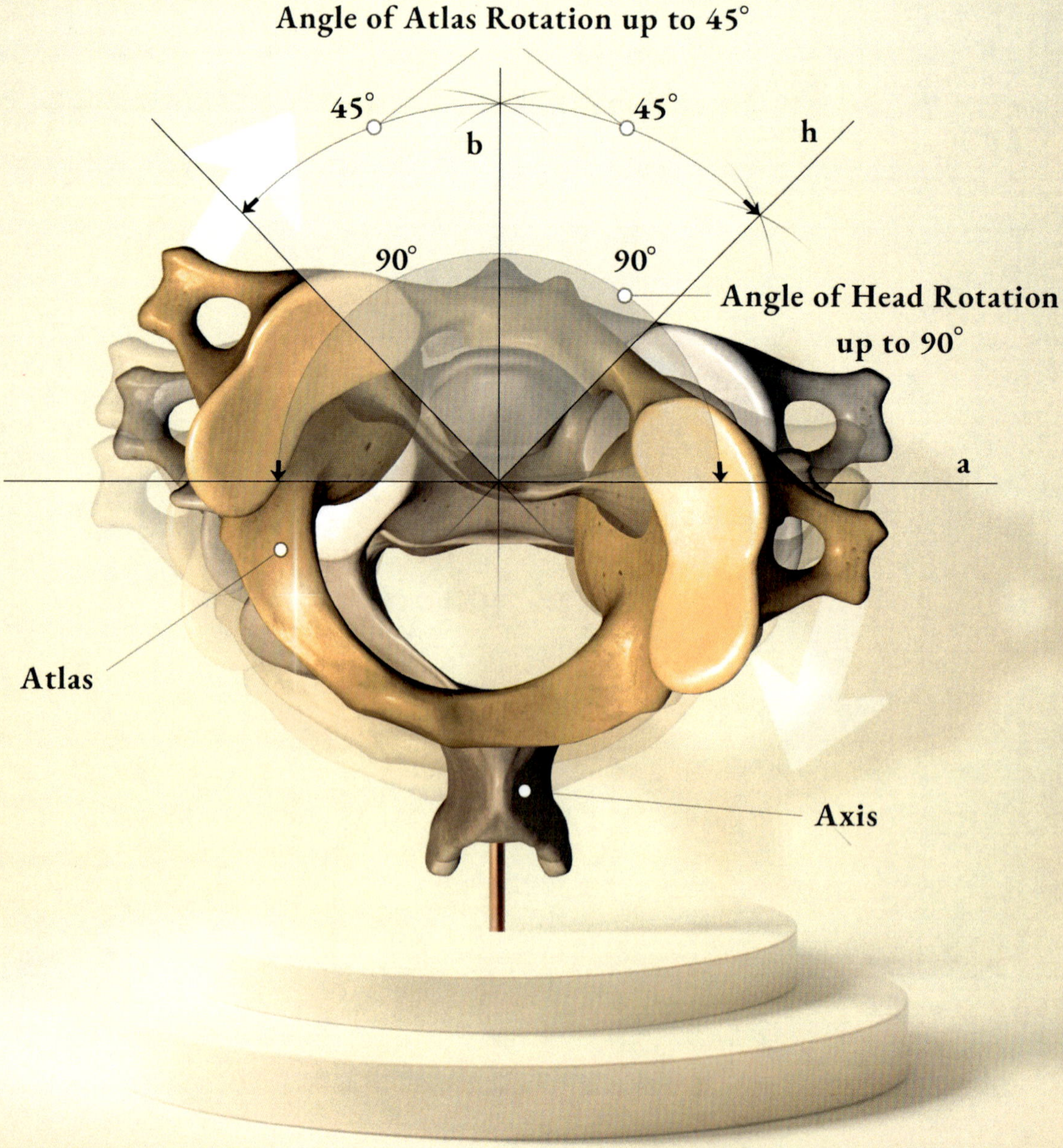

Atlas Rotation and Subluxation

Given that atlas rotation is a natural state and function, an anomaly that appears with rotational subluxation is a slight rotation of the atlas and head relative to the axis vertebra if there is inflammation (shortening or stretching) of the neck muscles due to other present atlas subluxations.If there is a slight rotation of the atlas and head (the head slightly rotates to the side), it occurs as a result of lateral subluxation (most commonly to the right) and the dropping of the right side of the atlas (inflammation of the neck and shoulder muscles). Therefore, the slight rotation of the atlas in alignment with the axis is a consequence of posterior subluxation and inclinational subluxation of the atlas.

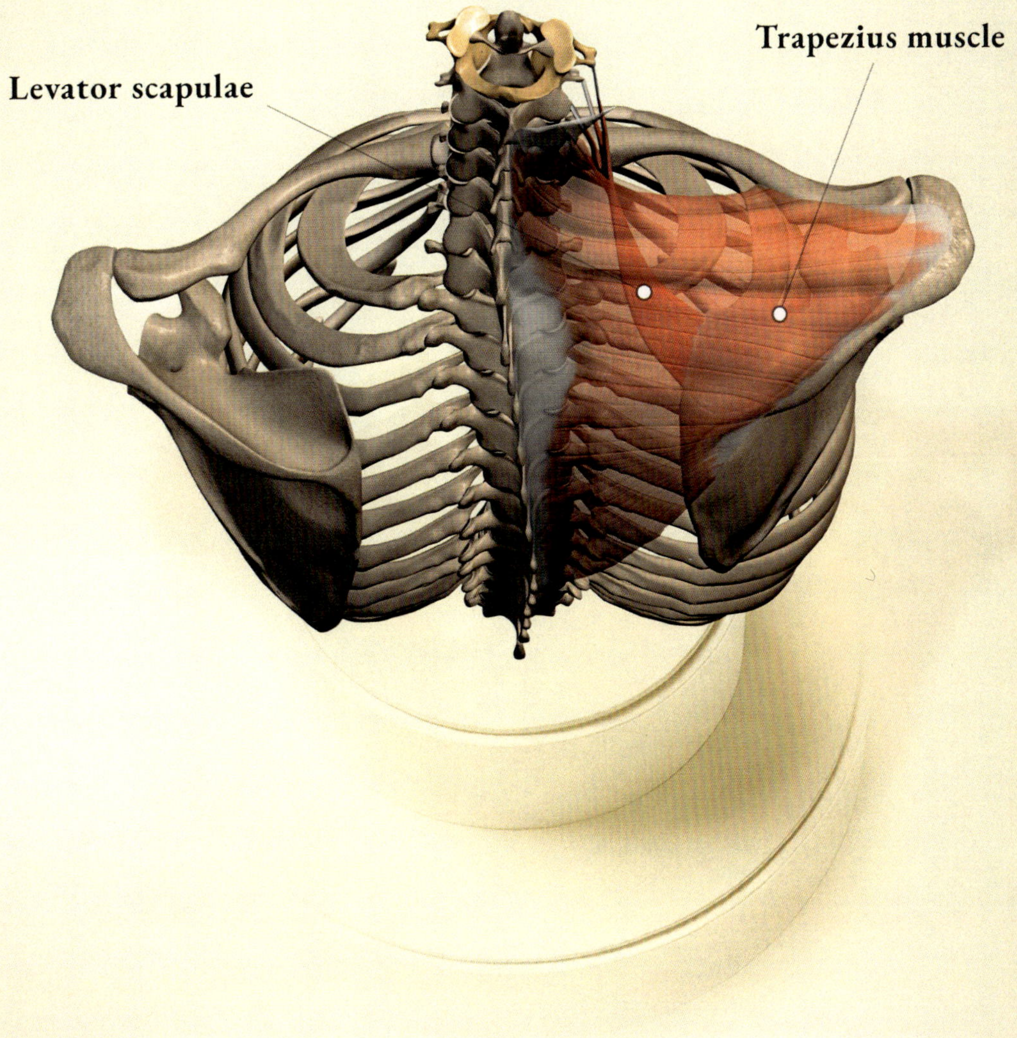

Spinal Twisting Due to Atlas Rotation

Spinal twisting occurs due to the rotation of the atlas (C1) caused by muscle tension. Tense or inflamed neck muscles pull the atlas, leading to its rotation and triggering a chain reaction along the spine. Upper cervical vertebrae (C2-C7) adapt, causing slight rotations. This rotation transfers down, twisting the thoracic and lumbar vertebrae, leading to muscle tension, pain, stiffness, and reduced mobility. The right shoulder moves forward, and the right side of the pelvis moves backward. The shoulders rotate opposite to the atlas rotation, while the pelvis follows its rotation. Rotation of the atlas backward on the right side always involves lateral displacement (usually to the right) and tilting to the right.

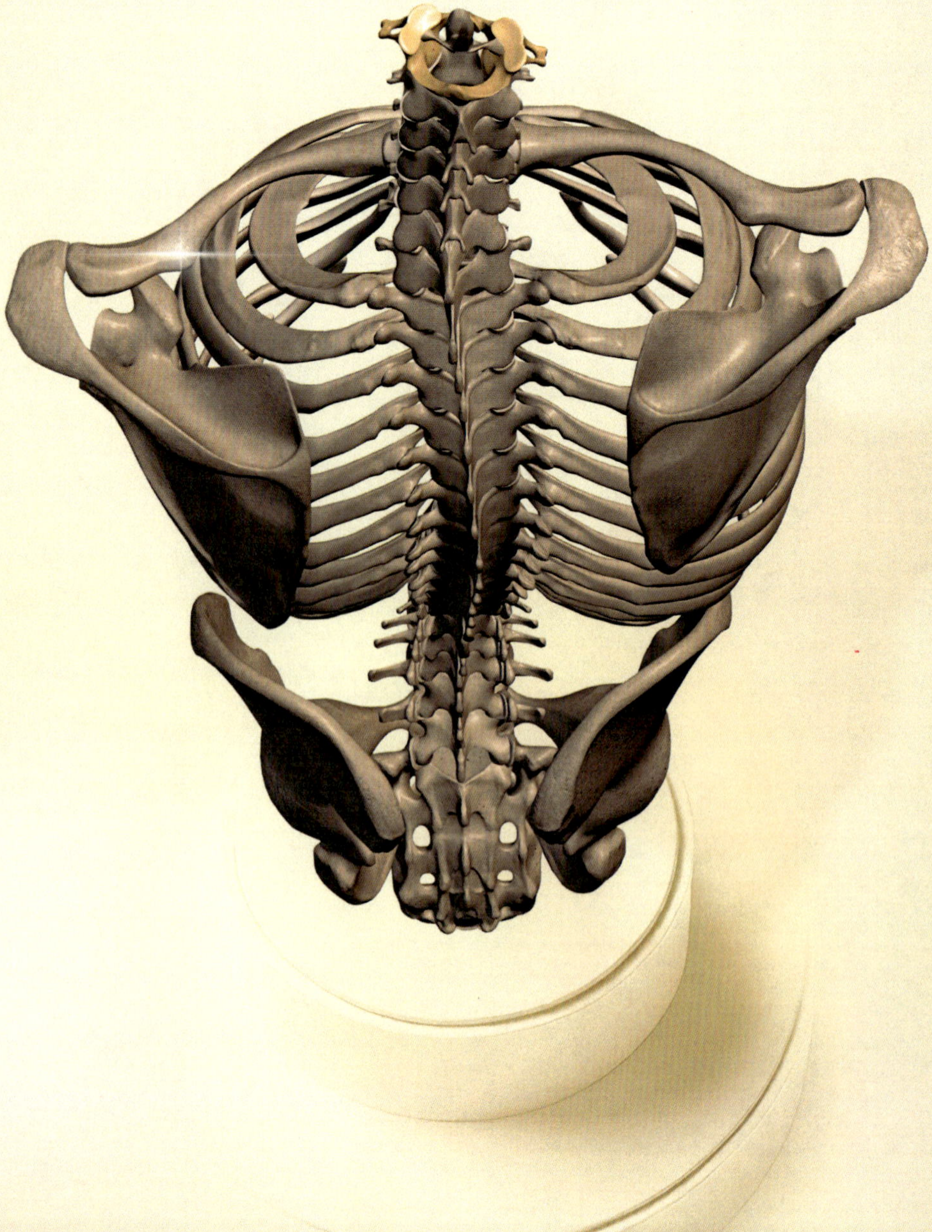

Multifidus Muscle Response

Multifidus muscles become overactive to compensate for postural changes caused by atlas displacement, leading to tension, fatigue, and pain. Overload reduces their ability to stabilize the spine, increasing the risk of injury. Additionally, disrupted proprioception affects postural control and movement.

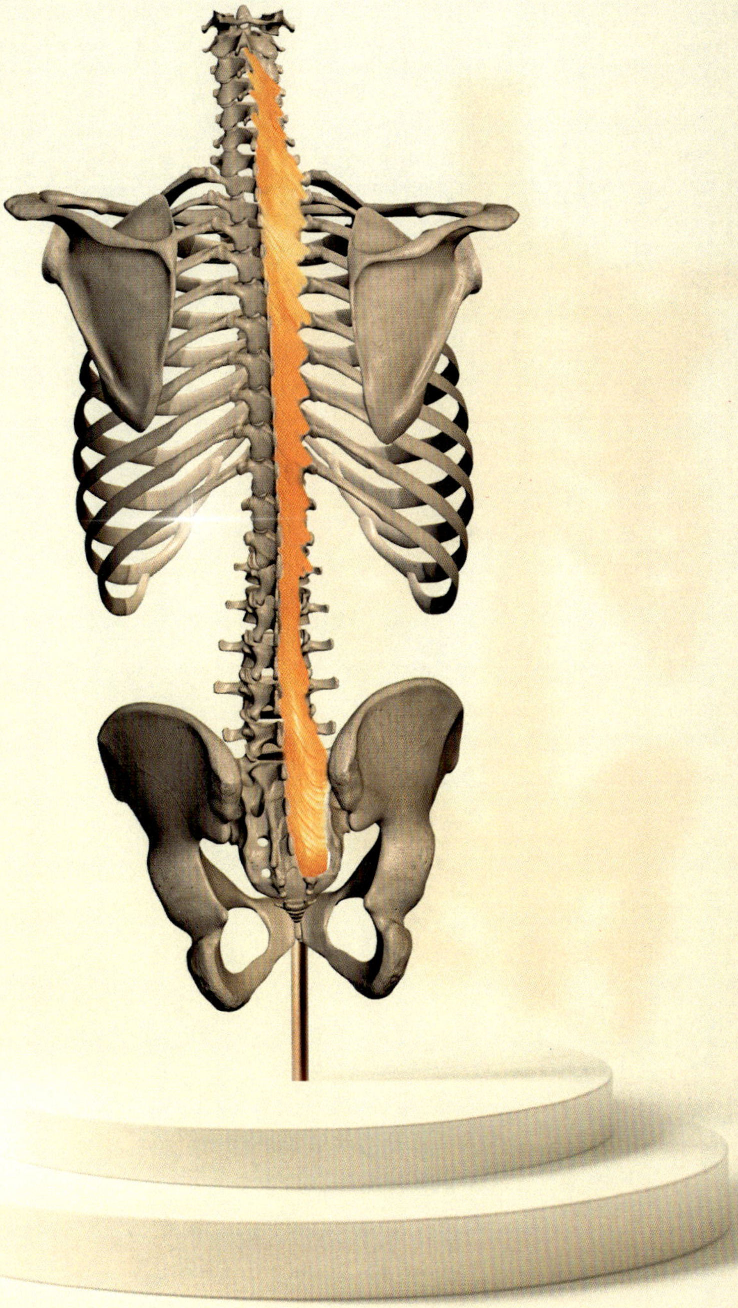

Spinalis Thoracis Muscle Response

The spinalis thoracis muscle may become overactive on one side to compensate for atlas displacement, leading to imbalance and tension. Constant stress from improper spine mechanics causes fatigue and pain, potentially resulting in spasms and reduced flexibility. Overload reduces the muscle's ability to stabilize the thoracic spine, increasing injury risk.

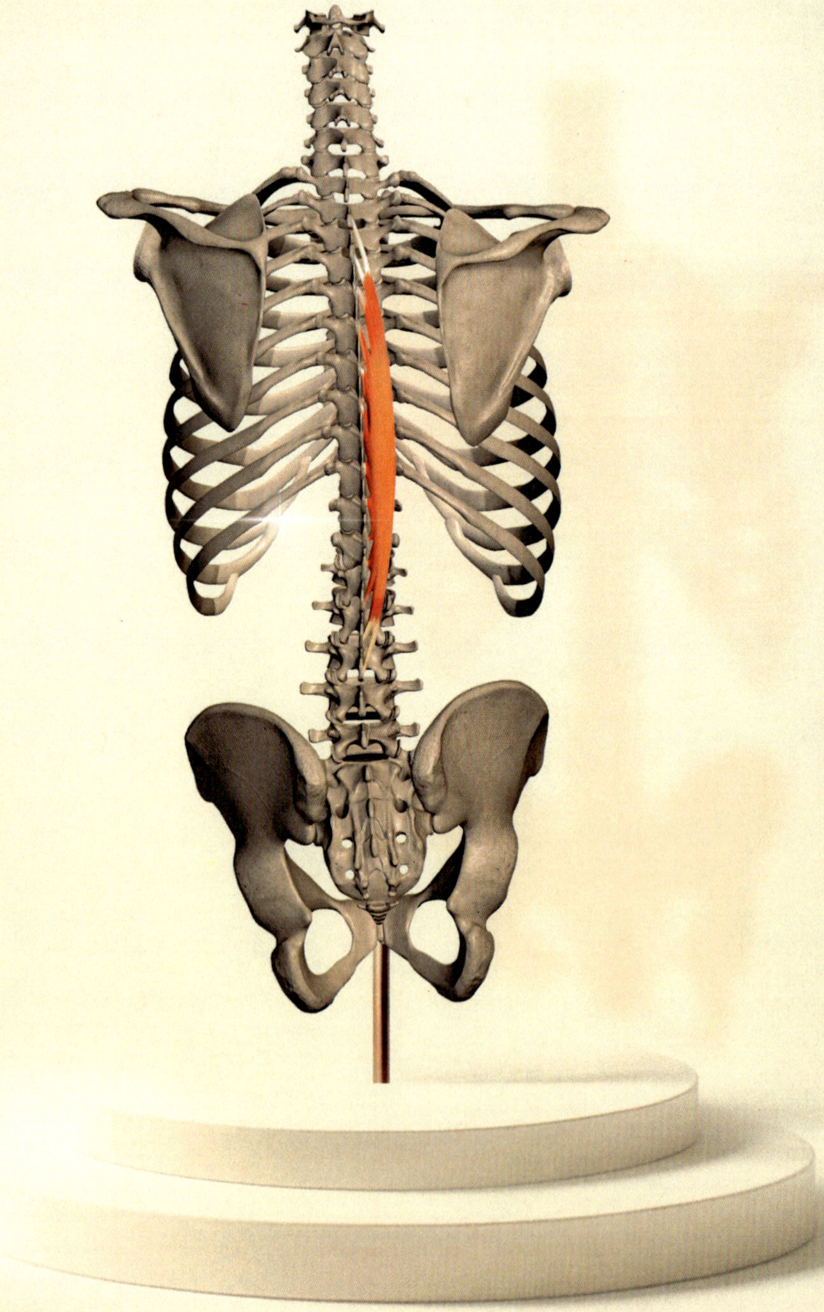

Splenius Cervicis Muscle Response

The splenius cervicis muscle may become overactive on one side to compensate for changes caused by atlas displacement. When it is overloaded or asymmetrically activated, its ability to stabilize the neck is compromised. Tension in this muscle can contribute to tension headaches and neck pain by pulling on structures in the neck and skull, creating pressure.

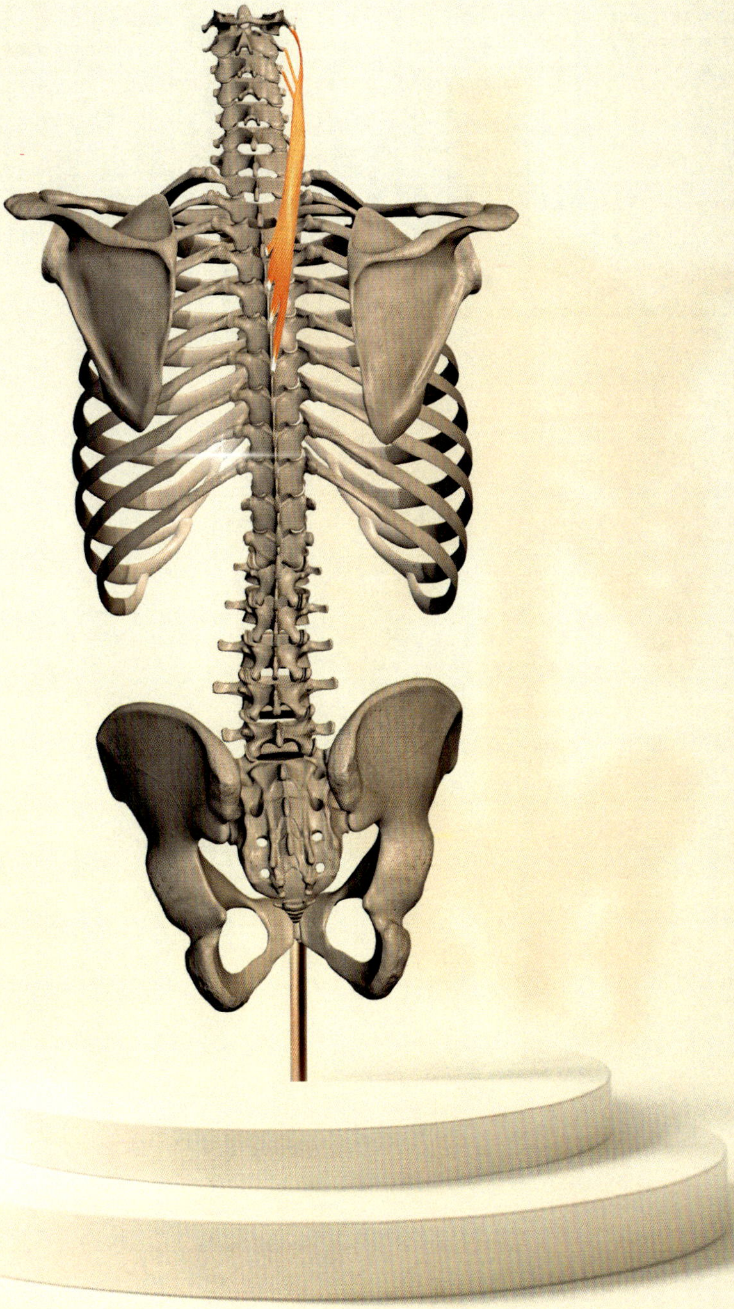

Splenius Capitis Muscle Response

Tension in the splenius capitis muscle can cause occipital headaches, neck and shoulder pain, and limited mobility. It can also lead to tingling and numbness in the neck, shoulders, and arms. Secondary tension in the trapezius muscle can increase discomfort. Chronic tension may alter posture, straining neck and upper back muscles.

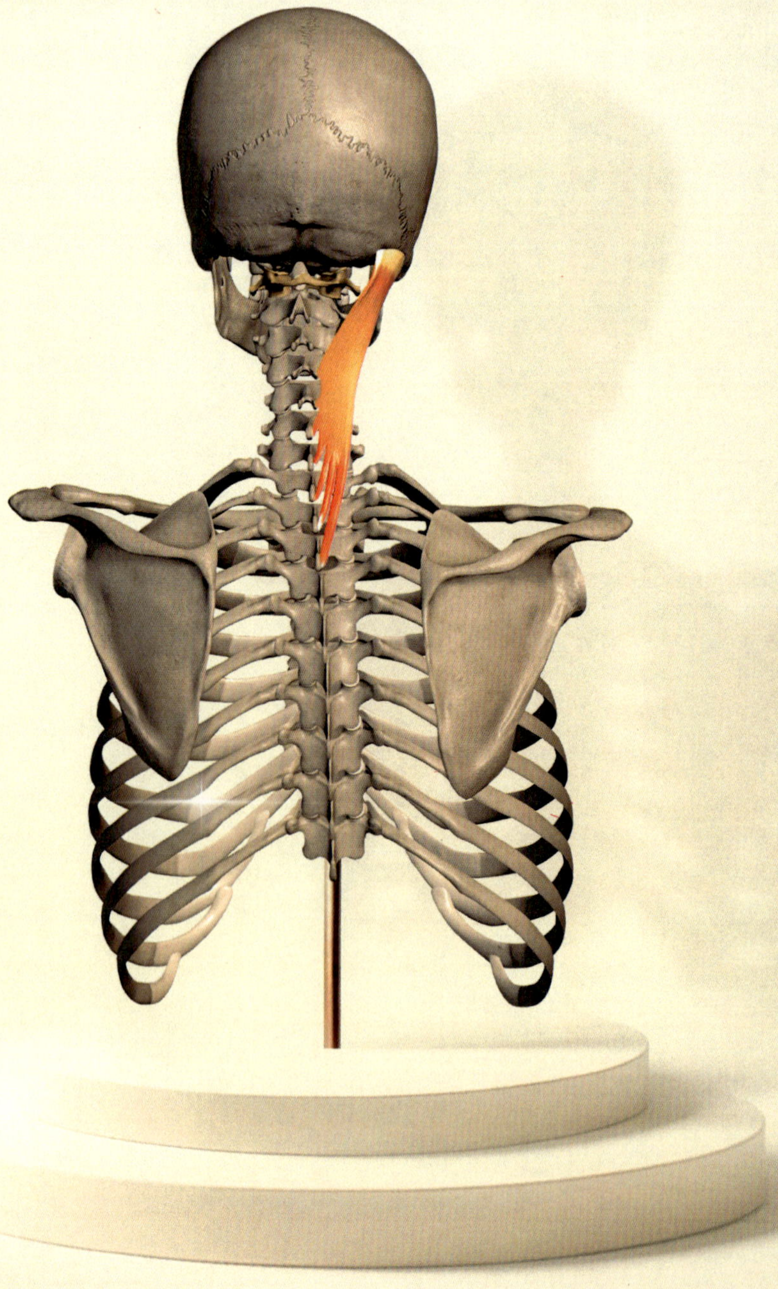

Impact of Semispinalis Capitis Muscle Tension

Tension in the semispinalis capitis muscle can lead to tension headaches, particularly in the occipital region where the Greater Occipital and Third Occipital nerves are located. Increased tension can cause restricted and painful movements of the head and neck, and tingling in the arms due to compression of the brachial plexus nerves.

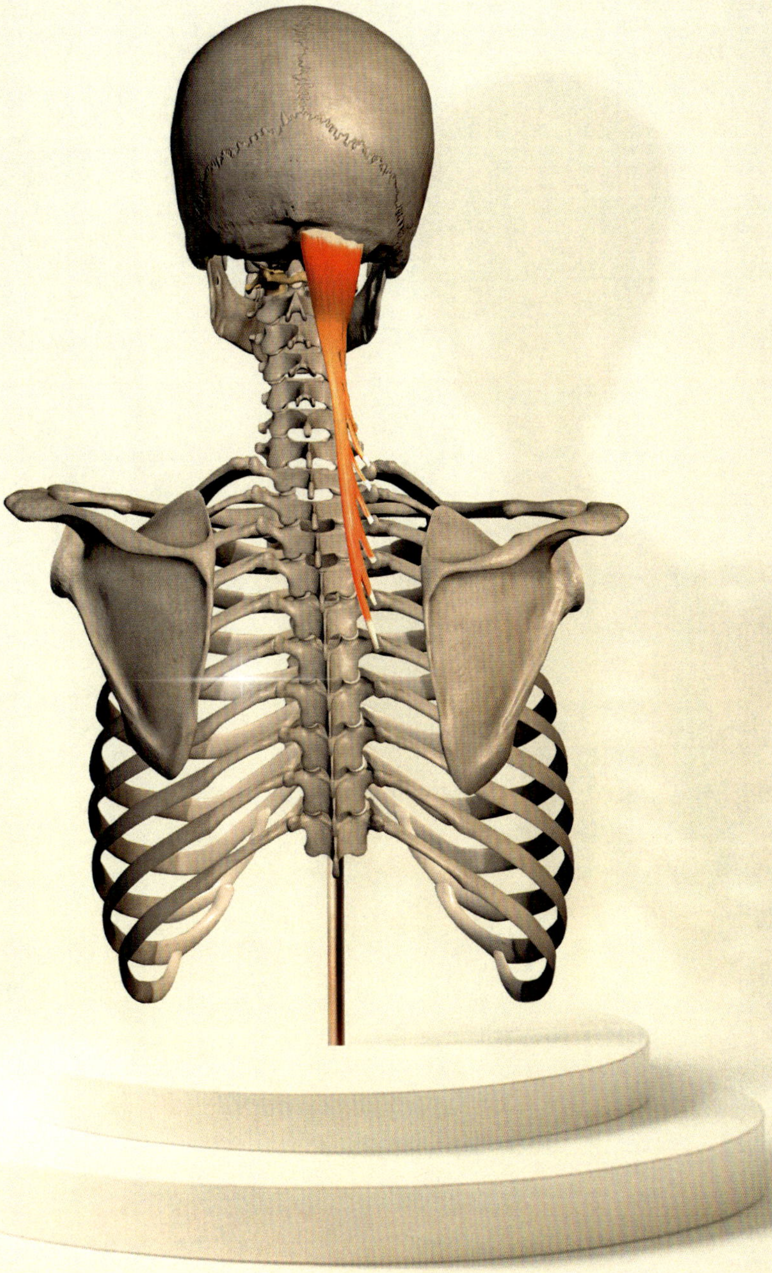

Cervical Disc Herniation

Cervical disc herniation, particularly in the C5-C6 and C6-C7 discs, can be caused by rotation and displacement of the atlas (the first cervical vertebra) to the right. These biomechanical imbalances lead to improper load distribution and vertebral twisting, increasing pressure on the discs, leading to their degeneration and herniation.

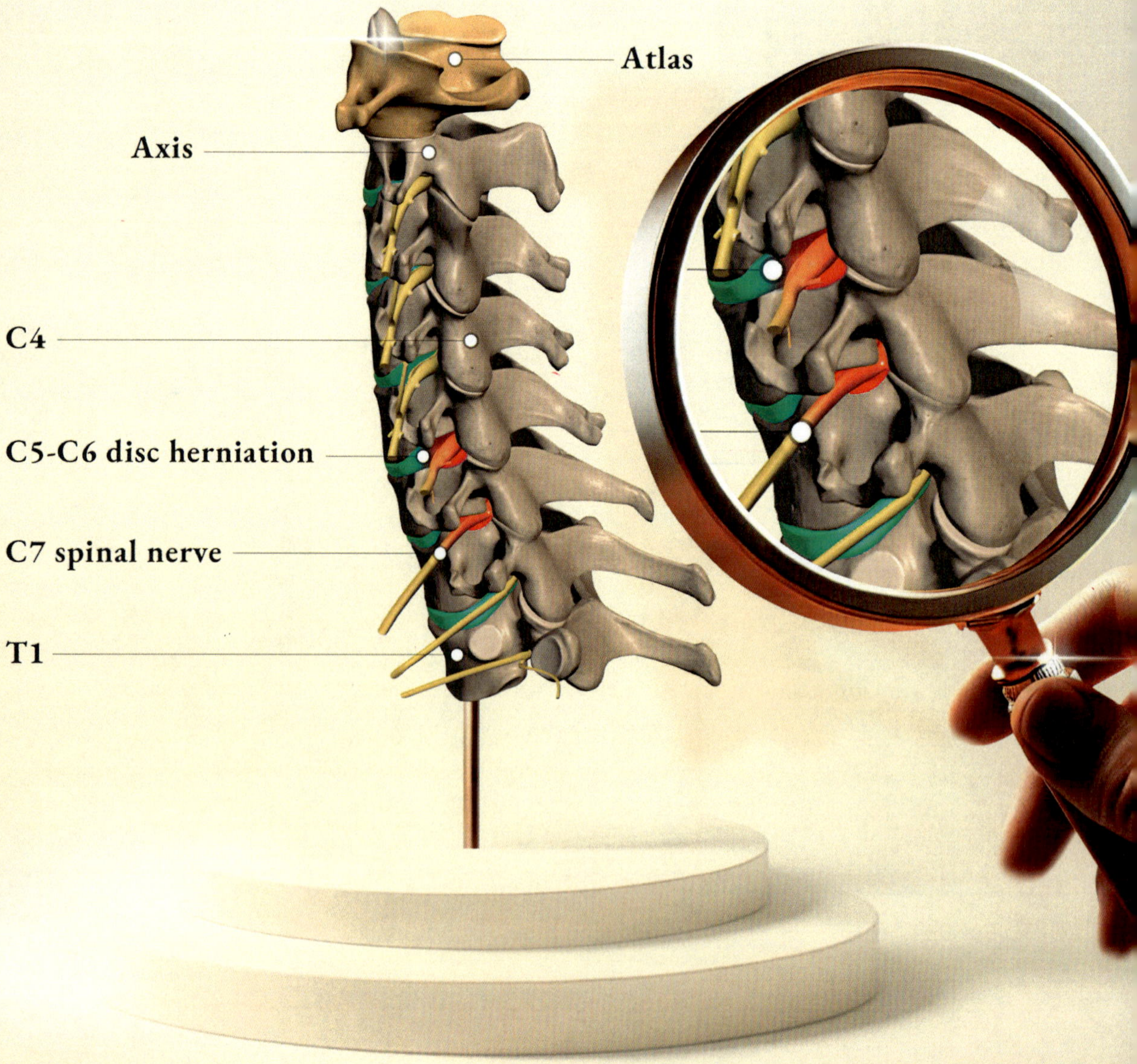

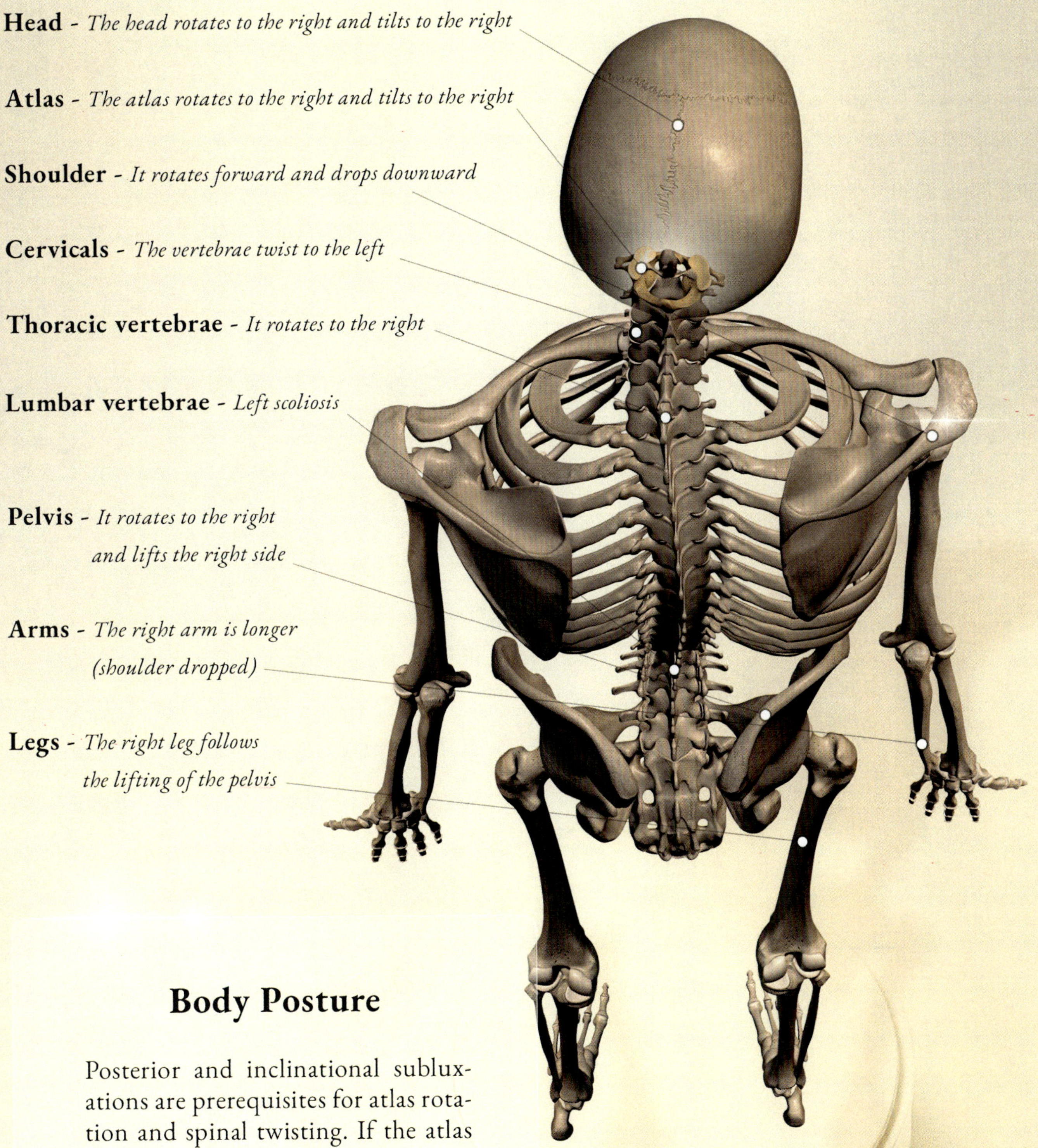

Body Posture

Posterior and inclinational subluxations are prerequisites for atlas rotation and spinal twisting. If the atlas rotates to the right, the cervical vertebrae rotate to the left, the thoracic vertebrae to the right, and the lumbar vertebrae typically rotate to the left to maintain balance and alignment of the spinal column.

Rotation, Shifting, and Elevation of the Pelvis

When the atlas vertebra rotates, most commonly involving a rightward rotation and a downward displacement on the right side, cervical vertebral scoliosis consequently affects all the vertebrae in the spinal column. In such cases, the rotation of the pelvis follows the rotation of the atlas vertebra, while the shoulders are rotated in the opposite direction of the atlas and the pelvis. Besides the rotation, which is generally backward, lumbar vertebral scoliosis shifts the pelvis to the right and elevates it, resulting in the right hip being higher than the left hip. The hip pulls the right leg, and during measurement, a shortened right leg may be diagnosed, although it is not genetically shorter but pulled up due to the elevated pelvis.

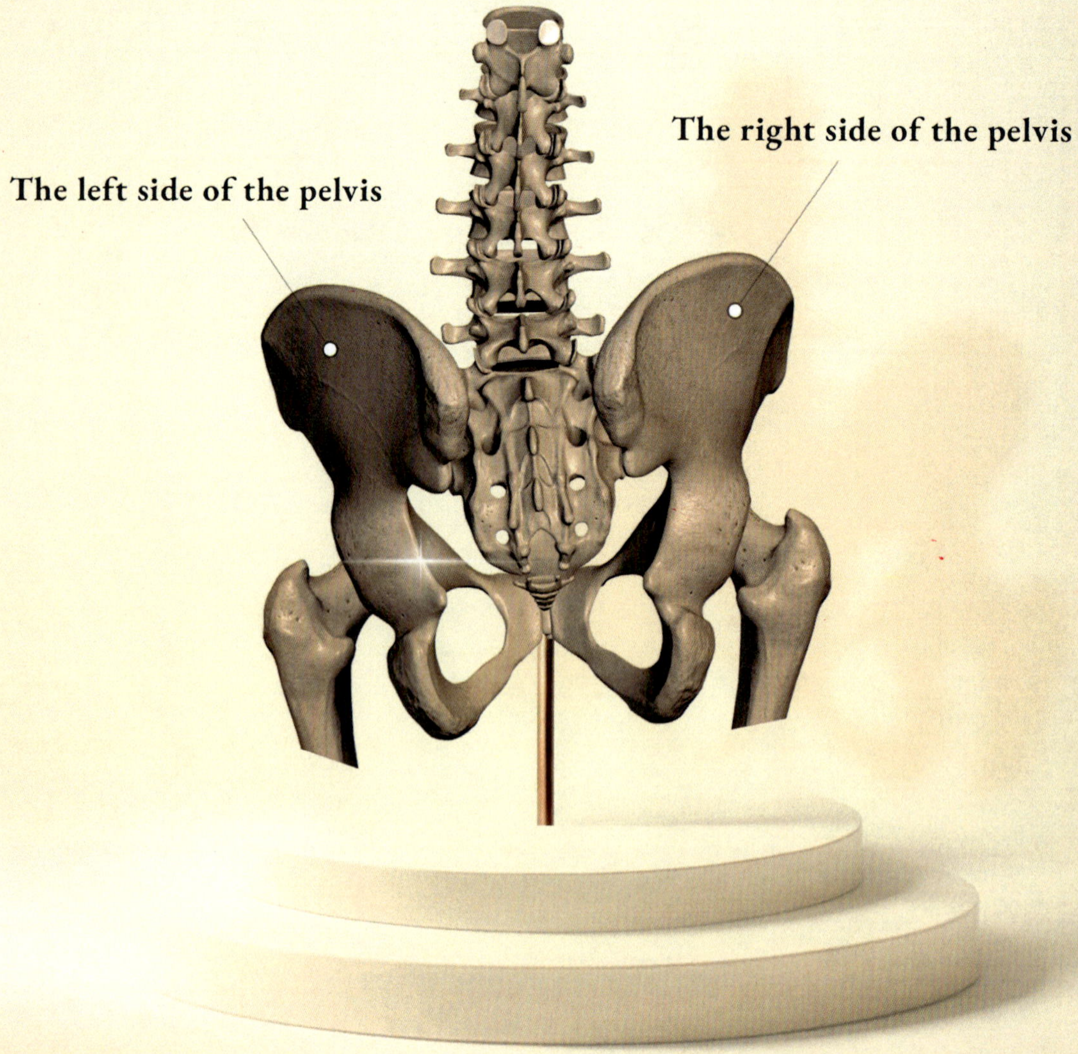

Impact of Pelvic Elevation on Gluteus Muscles

Since the right hip is elevated, the right gluteus muscle is shortened and tightened. This can lead to increased tension and potential discomfort or pain in this muscle. Conversely, since the right hip is elevated, the left gluteus muscle is stretched. This side may be prone to weakness or reduced tone due to prolonged elongation. Such an imbalance in the length, tightness, and stretching of the gluteus muscles affects all the remaining muscles in the lumbar region of the spine and the femoral muscles of the legs. Therefore, the pain that occurs in the back muscles and the femoral muscles of the legs is a consequence of the disturbed balance in the gluteus muscles, not the cause of the pain and stiffness.

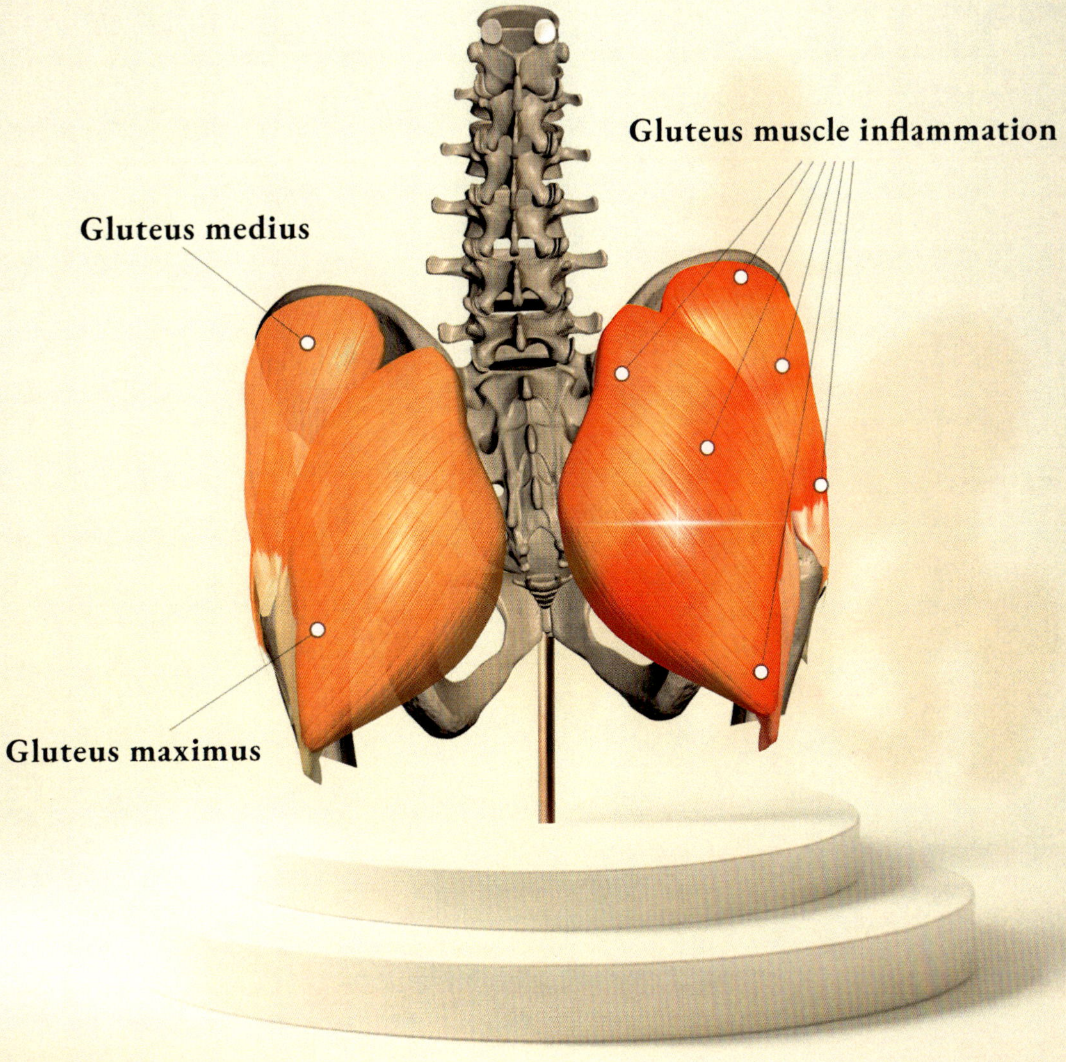

Lumbar Disc Herniation

Lumbar disc herniation in the L4, L5, and S1 discs can result from scoliosis and spinal twisting. The rotation of the pelvis and disruption of body alignment contribute to uneven pressure on the lumbar discs. Over time, this imbalance leads to degeneration and herniation, causing pain, nerve compression, and reduced mobility. Atlas adjustment resolves this issue.

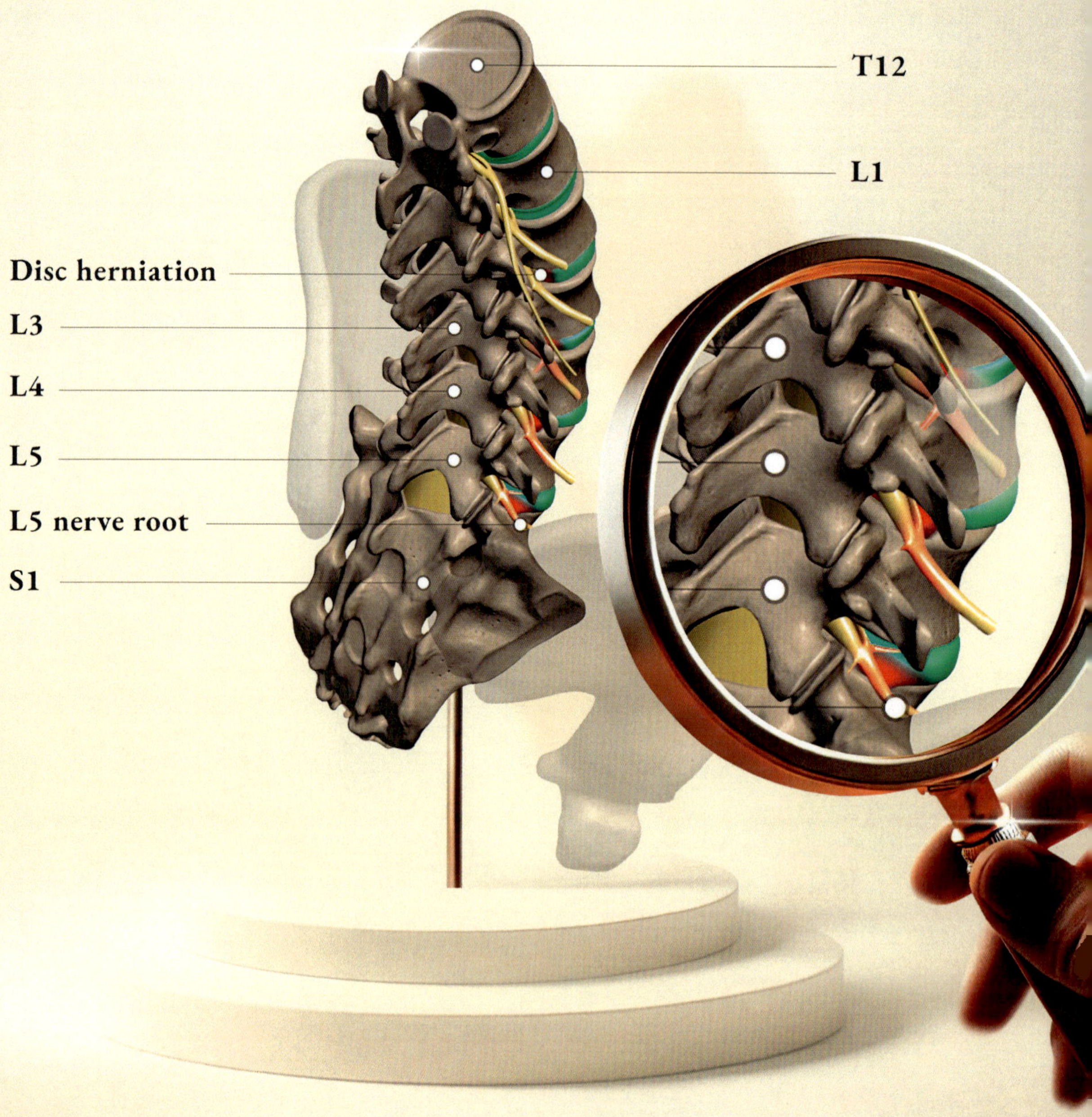

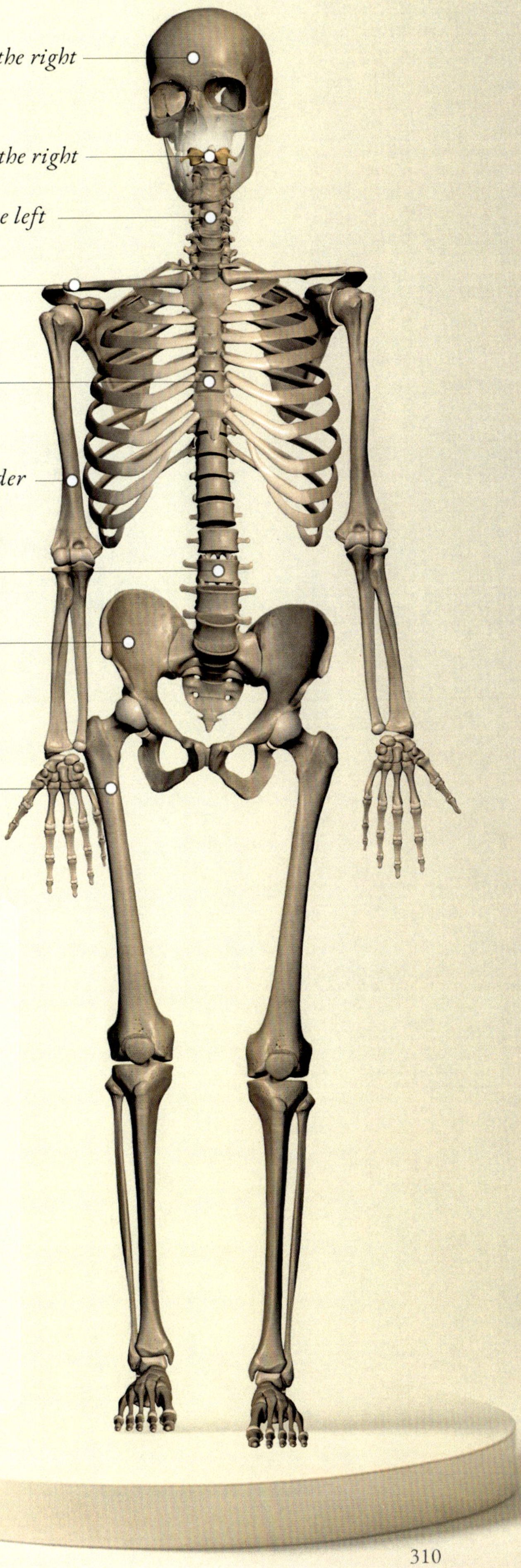

Body Posture

Rotation of the atlas to the right and its downward displacement on the right side, causing spinal scoliosis, result in the head being rotated to the right, the right shoulder lowered and rotated forward, and the right hip elevated, shifted to the right, and rotated backward. Elevation of the hip pulls the leg up and shortens it.

Chapter 7

Atlas Inclinational Subluxation and Anterolisthesis

Atlas Inclinational Subluxation and Anterolisthesis

Physical trauma in childhood and youth can have profound and long-lasting consequences on the health of the spinal column, including the potential occurrence of atlas inclination subluxation. Atlas inclination subluxation represents a condition in which the first cervical vertebra, known as the atlas, is tilted out of its normal position. This condition can result from various factors, and understanding the causes and mechanisms contributing to its development is crucial for prevention and appropriate treatment.

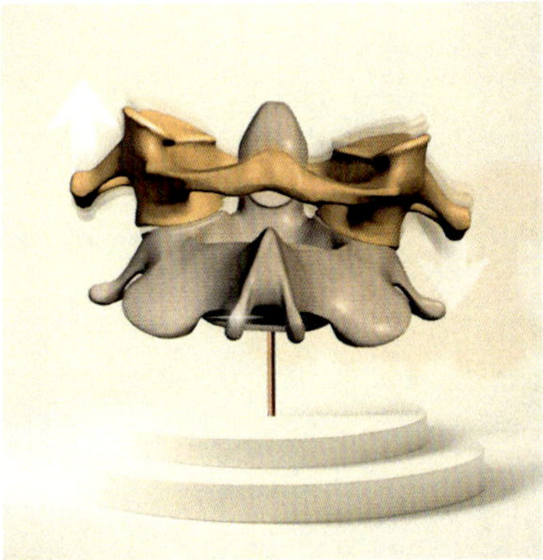

[Image 1] Horizontal tilt

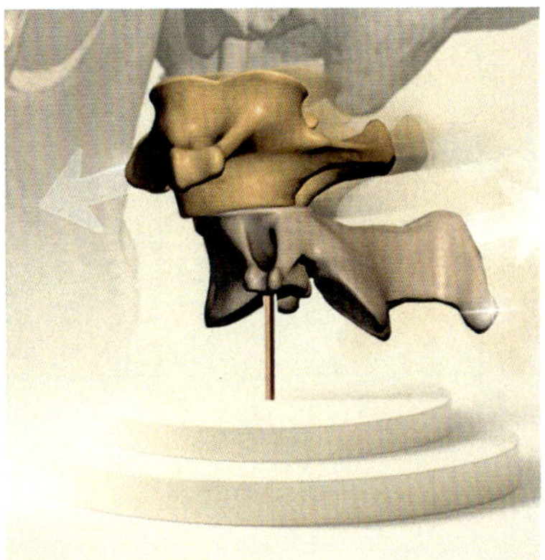

[Image 2] Vertical tilt

Typically, atlas inclination subluxation does not occur suddenly but gradually develops over time, often beginning as a slight tilt of the atlas that progressively worsens if not identified and addressed promptly. When diagnosing this condition, the most common observations include the tilt to the right side of the atlas on the horizontal axis and the forward tilt on the vertical axis of the atlas vertebra [Image 1][Image 2].

There are various factors that can contribute to the development of atlas inclination subluxation over time. One key factor is poor head posture, which can result from prolonged sitting in an incorrect position or excessive use of mobile devices. These incorrect postures can cause gradual strain on the cervical spine, which over time can lead to atlas inclination subluxation.

Additionally, genetic predisposition plays a role in an individual's susceptibility to this type of subluxation. People with natural ligamentous laxity or weaker neck muscle structure may be at greater risk. Lack of muscle activity and strength in the neck muscles responsible for head stabilization can also contribute to this problem.

It is important to emphasize that prevention of this condition begins in early childhood. Encouraging proper body posture, maintaining an active lifestyle, and regular exercise can help preserve spinal health and prevent the development of atlas inclination subluxation. Additionally, awareness of correct posture during daily activities, as well as regular medical check-ups, especially for individuals prone to genetic factors or who have been exposed to childhood traumas, are crucial.

Overall, understanding the factors contributing to the development of atlas inclination subluxation and taking appropriate preventive measures can help preserve spinal health and reduce the risk of this condition. This underscores the importance of continuous attention to spinal health and proper posture in all stages of life.

Anterolisthesis of the atlas refers to the forward displacement of the first cervical vertebra in relation to the second cervical vertebra, the axis. This condition occurs as a result of atlas inclination subluxation, where the atlas is tilted relative to its normal position. The inclination of the atlas creates pressure and stress on the cervical spine, which can lead to gradual forward displacement of the first vertebra.

When atlas inclination subluxation occurs, the first cervical vertebra is subjected to unnatural stress and displacement, which can gradually cause anterolisthesis. This displacement can further compromise the stability of the cervical spine and affect the function and comfort of the patient.

Managing atlas anterolisthesis typically involves treating the underlying cause, which in this case involves treating atlas inclination subluxation.

Causes and Effects

Atlas inclination subluxation can result from various factors, and one of the key contributors to this condition is the weight of the head. The head is one of the heaviest parts of the body relative to its size, and its weight can vary among individuals depending on genetics, body structure, and other factors.

The average weight of an adult human head is around 4.5 to 5.5 kilograms. However, it's important to note that this weight can vary among individuals. For example, some people may have larger heads that are heavier than average, while others may have smaller heads that are lighter. These variations can result from genetics, bone structure, tissue density, and other factors.

During the embryonic development phase, the neural crest is the primary structure that forms and provides the foundation for the development of various tissues and organs in the body, including the skull and brain. The process of head formation begins when neural crest cells transform into mesenchymal cells, which are precursors to many different cell types, including those that will differentiate into bones, cartilage, and connective tissue.

In this process, mesenchymal cells differentiate into cartilage cells that gradually form the bones of the skull. One of the key factors in this process is the interaction between cells and various biochemical signals that regulate growth and development. One of these signals can be salt, specifically sodium chloride, which plays a role in regulating osmotic pressure inside cells and contributes to tissue formation and growth.

When there is a disruption in this process, oversized head development can occur as a genetic factor. Genetic mutations or variations can affect various factors that regulate growth and development, including the process of head formation. For example, genetic changes that affect salt receptors or enzymes involved in salt metabolism can disrupt the regulation of osmotic pressure inside cells and disrupt the growth and development of skull tissues.

As a result, individuals with genetic factors contributing to oversized head development may develop a larger head compared to the average. This enlargement can be the result of increased skull bone growth or an irregular head shape. These genetic factors can be hereditary or may occur as new mutations during embryo development.

Overall, the process of head formation through salt in the embryonic development phase of neural crest cells plays a crucial role in skull and brain formation. However, disruptions in this process, such as genetic factors leading to oversized head development, can have a significant impact on skull and brain development during the embryonic phase.

The weight of the head can have a significant impact on the body, especially on the cervical spine. When the head is improperly positioned or when it bears a load greater than what the cervical spine can adequately support, it can lead to gradual strain on the cervical vertebrae and ligaments. This strain can cause atlas inclination, primarily due to disproportionate loading on this vertebra.

Additionally, constant wearing of heavy loads on the head, such as motorcycle helmets, can further increase pressure on the cervical spine and contribute to the development of atlas inclination subluxation. Unnatural body positions during sleep or prolonged sitting can also cause imbalance and overloading of the cervical spine, which can contribute to this problem.

Overall, understanding the weight of the head as a factor that can contribute to atlas inclination subluxation highlights the importance of maintaining proper posture, avoiding excessive strain on the cervical spine, and caring for spinal health. This emphasizes the importance of awareness of proper body ergonomics in daily activities to preserve the balance and functionality of the cervical spine.

Stretchable ligaments have greater elasticity and flexibility compared to normally non-stretchable ligaments. This difference arises from the structure and composition of the ligaments. Normally non-stretchable ligaments are typically dense, strong fibrous tissues that provide stability and restrict movements between bones, while stretchable ligaments are usually composed of multiple elastic fibers that give them the ability to stretch and return to their original shape.

The causes of ligament stretchiness can be genetic in nature, as well as factors such as a lack of connective tissue, hormonal changes (such as pregnancy), physical inactivity, or excessive activity. Genetic mutations can affect the structure and composition of ligaments, making them more susceptible to stretching. A lack of certain components of connective tissue, such as collagen or elastin, can also contribute to increased ligament stretchiness.

Ligament stretchiness can affect the muscle-bone connection in several ways. When ligaments are overly stretched, they can become looser and less effective in maintaining joint stability. This can lead to joint laxity and increased mobility, but at the expense of stability. This can result in joint dislocation, as ligaments cannot adequately restrict joint movements.

When it comes to the mechanism of head movement in relation to the atlas and axis, ligament stretchiness can have a significant impact. The atlas and axis are the first and second cervical vertebrae, and their connection forms the main joint for rotating the head. If the ligaments between these vertebrae are overly stretched, it can lead to joint laxity and increased mobility, making it difficult to maintain head stability during movement. This can result in irregular or excessive head movements, which can cause pain and discomfort, as well as increase the risk of injury.

Weak neck muscles can have a significant impact on the position of the head and overall body posture. When neck muscles are not strong enough to support the weight of the head, they may droop forward, which encourages atlas inclination subluxation, a condition in which the first cervical vertebra is tilted out of its normal position.

This tilted position of the atlas can compress nerves in the neck, resulting in pain and discomfort. Additionally, atlas inclination subluxation can contribute to the development of thoracic kyphosis, which is a forward curvature of the spine, chest deformity, and forward rotation of the shoulders. Inflammatory processes in the T2 vertebra can manifest as a hump, further complicating the body's posture.

This condition can also affect lumbar lordosis, which is an inward curvature of the spine in the lumbar region. As we age, atlas inclination subluxation can pull us towards a cane, making it even more challenging to maintain proper posture and body movement.

The reasons for weak neck muscles can vary, including a lack of exercise or improper exercise technique, excessive use of mobile devices that strain the neck muscles, poor body posture, as well as more serious issues such as injuries or neurological conditions.

The best way to maintain neck muscle strength is through regular exercises targeting these muscles, including stretching, strengthening, and neck stabilization exercises. Exercises such as lifting the head from a lying position, stretching the neck in different directions, and neck rotation can help strengthen neck muscles and maintain their functionality. It is also important to pay attention to body posture during daily activities and avoid prolonged sitting or standing in improper positions. Regular check-ups with a physiotherapist or trainer can also be beneficial for maintaining and improving neck muscle strength.

Atlas inclination subluxation occurs concurrently with atlas anterolisthesis, which is a situation where the first cervical vertebra, atlas, slides forward in relation to the second cervical vertebra, axis. This combination can cause various neurological and musculoskeletal problems, as the displaced atlas can exert pressure on surrounding structures and nerves in the cervical spine.

This condition can result from various factors, and one of the main causes is the weight of the head on the cervical spine. Head weight can be a significant factor contributing to atlas anterolisthesis, especially if the head is larger or heavier than average. As the head continuously exerts pressure on the cervical spine, particularly on the first vertebra, it can cause gradual shifting of the atlas forward. This displacement can be even more pronounced if there is a lack of muscular strength in the neck region that should support and stabilize the atlas.

When atlas anterolisthesis occurs, pressure on surrounding structures, such as nerves and blood vessels in the cervical spine, can occur. This can result in various symptoms, including neck pain, headaches, dizziness, and a feeling of weakness or numbness in the arms. Additionally, atlas anterolisthesis can affect the stability of the cervical spine and make normal functioning of this part of the body more challenging.

Atlas anterolisthesis further exacerbates this situation, making it more complex and demanding to treat. Therefore, it is important to recognize the relationship between atlas inclination subluxation and atlas anterolisthesis.

"What? know ye not that your body is the temple of the Holy Ghost which is in you, which ye have of God, and ye are not your own?"

(1 Corinthians 6:19)

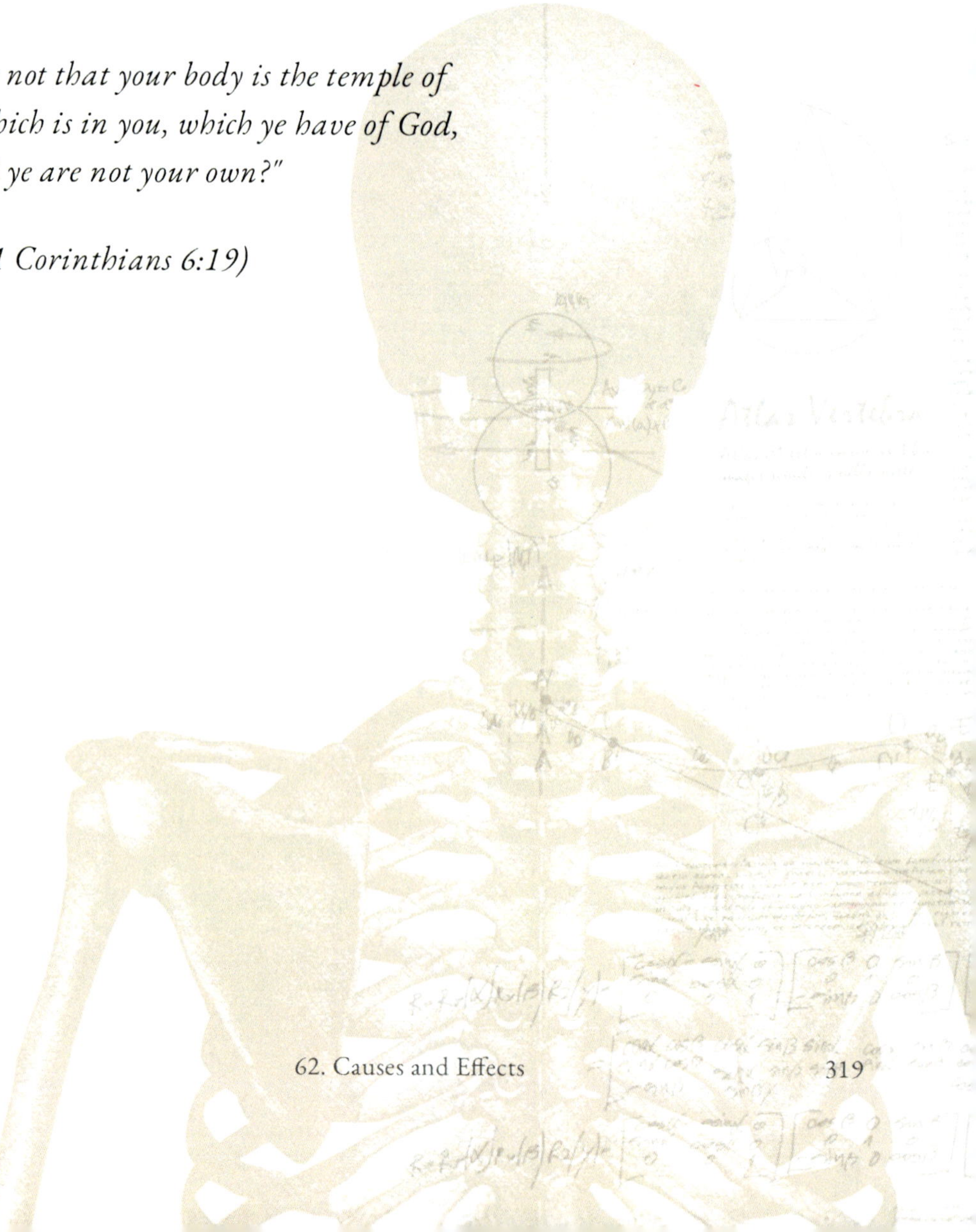

Posture and Health Impacts

Atlas inclination subluxation and atlas anterolisthesis are conditions that reflect the shifted position of the atlas, the first cervical vertebra [Image 1]. These disorders directly affect body posture, causing thoracic kyphosis and lumbar hypelordosis. Visually, this body posture creates an appearance that is far from optimal, often described as stooped or in the shape of a question mark, especially when viewed from the side.

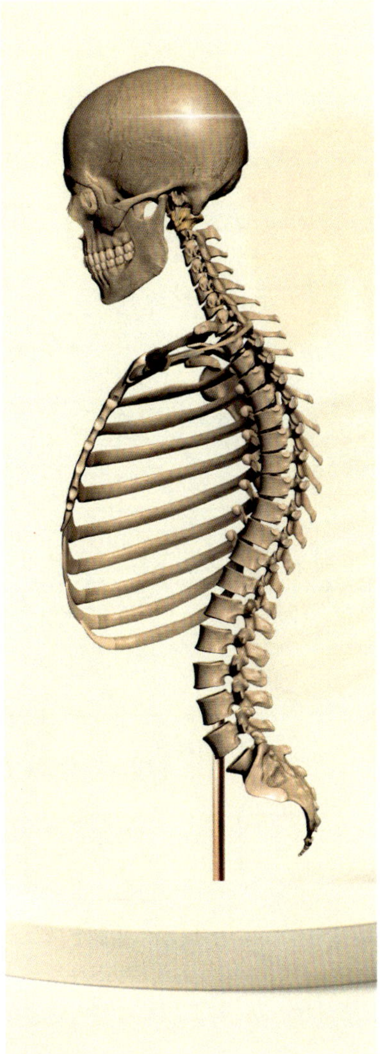

[Image 1] Unbalanced appearance

When the head is tilted forward, the entire body posture appears unbalanced. The head moves forward, deviating from the vertical axis of the spine, while the shoulders are shifted forward due to kyphosis in the thoracic spine, further deforming the shape of the chest. The pelvic bone tilts forward, creating a sense of instability and leaning the body forward. This posture also affects the arches of the feet, which follow the deformation of the spine and can lead to a diagnosis of pes planus, or "flat feet," further compromising the stability and aesthetics of the body posture.

Overall, these visual signs of atlas inclination subluxation and atlas anterolisthesis clearly indicate that disorders in the position of the atlas are not only a medical but also an aesthetic problem. This imbalanced posture not only disrupts the function of the spine and causes discomfort but also looks aesthetically unpleasant. Therefore, it is important to recognize and adequately treat these disorders to restore the optimal position of the atlas and achieve a harmonious body posture.

Analyzing the image of the atlas region using a 3D scanner provides deeper insight into the connection between the position of the atlas and the curvature of the body posture. It is clear that the atlas is shifted and tilted forward in relation to the axis vertebra, which significantly affects the overall body posture. This change in the position of the atlas is seen as a key factor in creating irregular postural dynamics.

The progression of the atlas towards the lower jawbone, with a tendency for further sliding, further complicates the situation. This shift also brings the processes of the atlas closer to the mastoid bone, further affecting the overall structure of the neck and head. Analysis shows that these changes in the position of the atlas are directly related to improper body posture, which can have a wide range of negative consequences for the health and functionality of the spine.

Using a 3D scanner, these specific vertebral positions can be identified and analyzed in detail, providing significant information essential for treatment and rehabilitation planning.

It is worth noting that a person's height can have a significant impact on spinal health and the frequency of certain conditions such as atlas inclination subluxation and atlas anterolisthesis. These conditions are more pronounced in tall individuals compared to those of average or shorter stature.

One of the key factors in this phenomenon is the greater curvature of the spine in taller individuals. Greater body mass and longer limbs can affect postural changes and increase pressure on the spine, resulting in a tilted or shifted position of the atlas. These spinal problems may be the result of not only increased weight pressing on the spine but also genetic factors that affect the structure and shape of the spine.

Taller individuals may also have a greater curvature of the spine due to attempts to compensate for their height or irregularities in posture. Improper posture can further strain the spine and cause changes in the position of the atlas and other vertebrae.

It is important to note that taller individuals often face greater health challenges than those of average or shorter stature, especially concerning spinal health. In addition to atlas inclination subluxation and atlas anterolisthesis, other issues such as back pain, joint damage, and degenerative changes in the spine may occur.

"Fear thou not; for I am with thee: be not dismayed; for I am thy God: I will strengthen thee; yea, I will help thee; yea, I will uphold thee with the right hand of my righteousness."

(Isaiah 41:10)

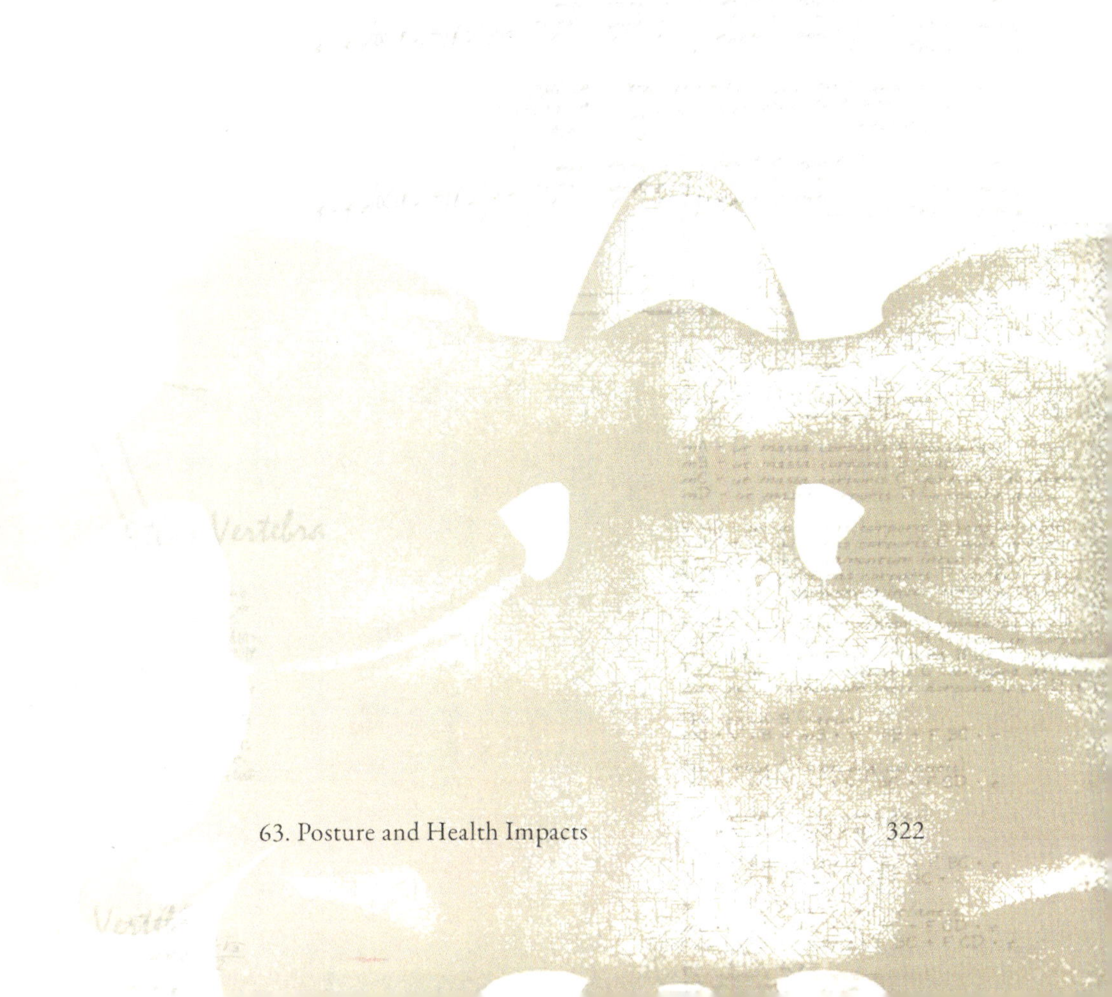

Inclinational Subluxation and Anterolisthesis

These are the most commonly diagnosed conditions where the atlas vertebra is lowered on its right side and tilted forward relative to the axis. This position transfers the weight of the head to the other cervical vertebrae and the entire spine, causing spinal scoliosis, straightened cervical lordosis, thoracic kyphosis, and straightened lumbar lordosis.

The atlas is lowered on the right side and tilts forward.

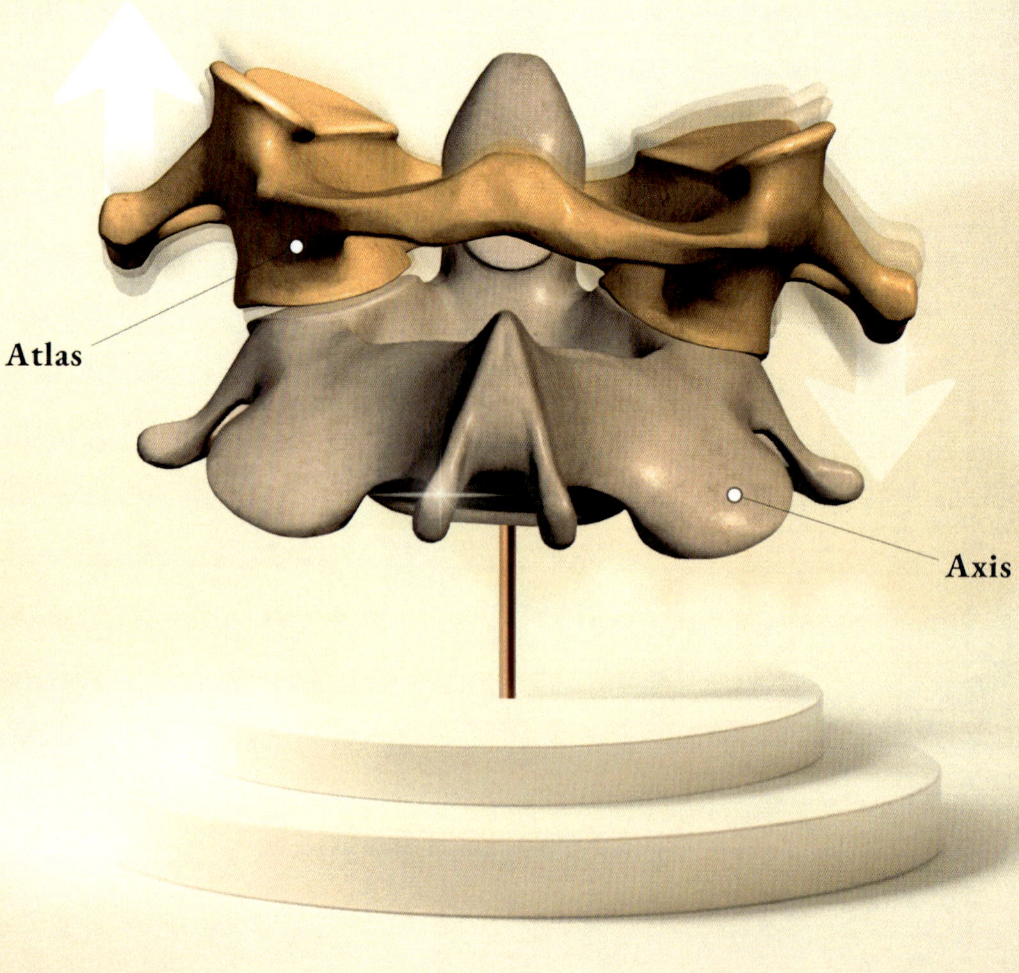

Frontal View

These conditions of the displaced atlas vertebra are best observed when viewing the patient frontally, face to face. A visibly lowered right shoulder and the appearance of a longer right arm compared to the left arm and shoulder are noticeable. The head is slightly rotated to the right, with the left ear visible and the right ear positioned behind the head. Additionally, the head appears visibly shifted to the left compared to the vertical axis of the straight spinal column.

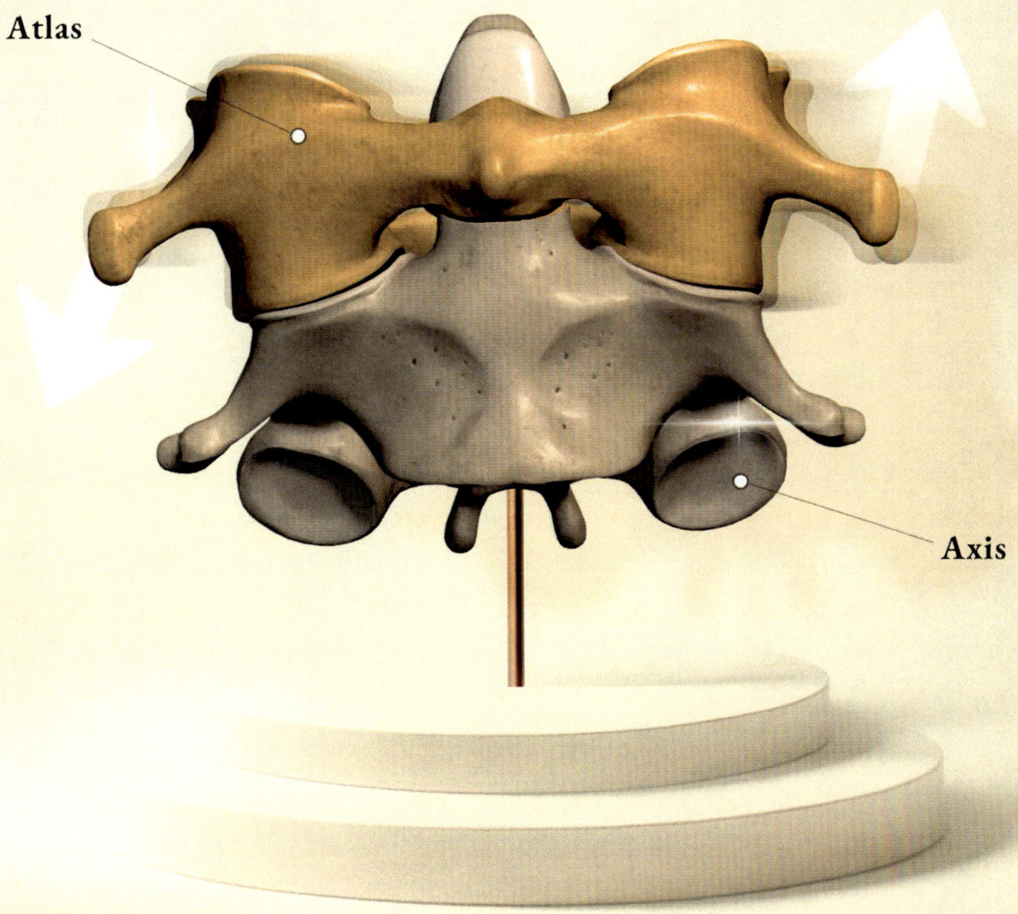

Head Position in Inclination Subluxation

Forward tilting of the atlas can cause the head to tilt slightly forward, leading to an unnatural position and neck muscle strain. This can result in pain in the neck, back of the head, and even the front of the head, potentially causing headaches. Inclination subluxation can straighten the natural cervical lordosis, placing additional strain on other cervical vertebrae. The atlas shift can also contribute to scoliosis in the cervical, thoracic (hyperkyphosis), and lumbar (hyperlordosis) regions due to improper weight distribution. Neck muscles, particularly the trapezius and sternocleidomastoid, can become tense and painful. Prolonged tension can lead to muscle weakness and fatigue, worsening head and neck stability. Compensatory movements by the neck muscles to maintain balance can cause asymmetry and additional strain.

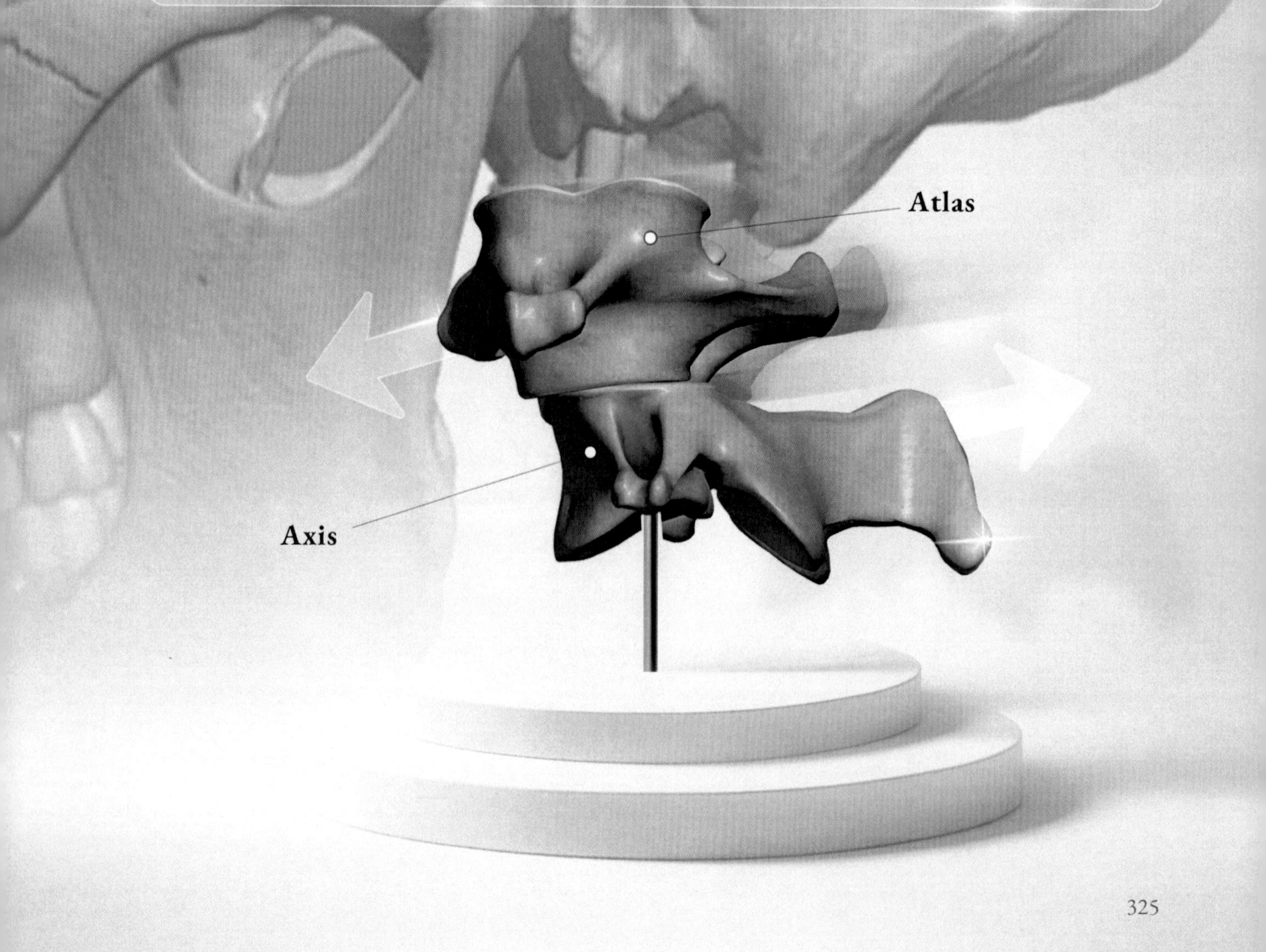

Ligament Stretching

In cases of Inclination Subluxation combined with Anterolisthesis Subluxation, the ligaments of the atlas vertebra stretch over time. This stretching mainly affects the ligaments on the side opposite to the subluxation. The transverse, alar, and accessory atlanto-axial ligaments stretch on the left side when viewed from the back. Meanwhile, the apical and transverse ligaments follow the weight of the head and further stretch the atlas forward relative to the axis and the dens.This imbalance can worsen the forward tilting of the atlas, increasing instability and misalignment of the cervical spine. As the ligaments stretch, their ability to stabilize the atlas decreases, leading to additional stress on surrounding structures and potential neurological symptoms.

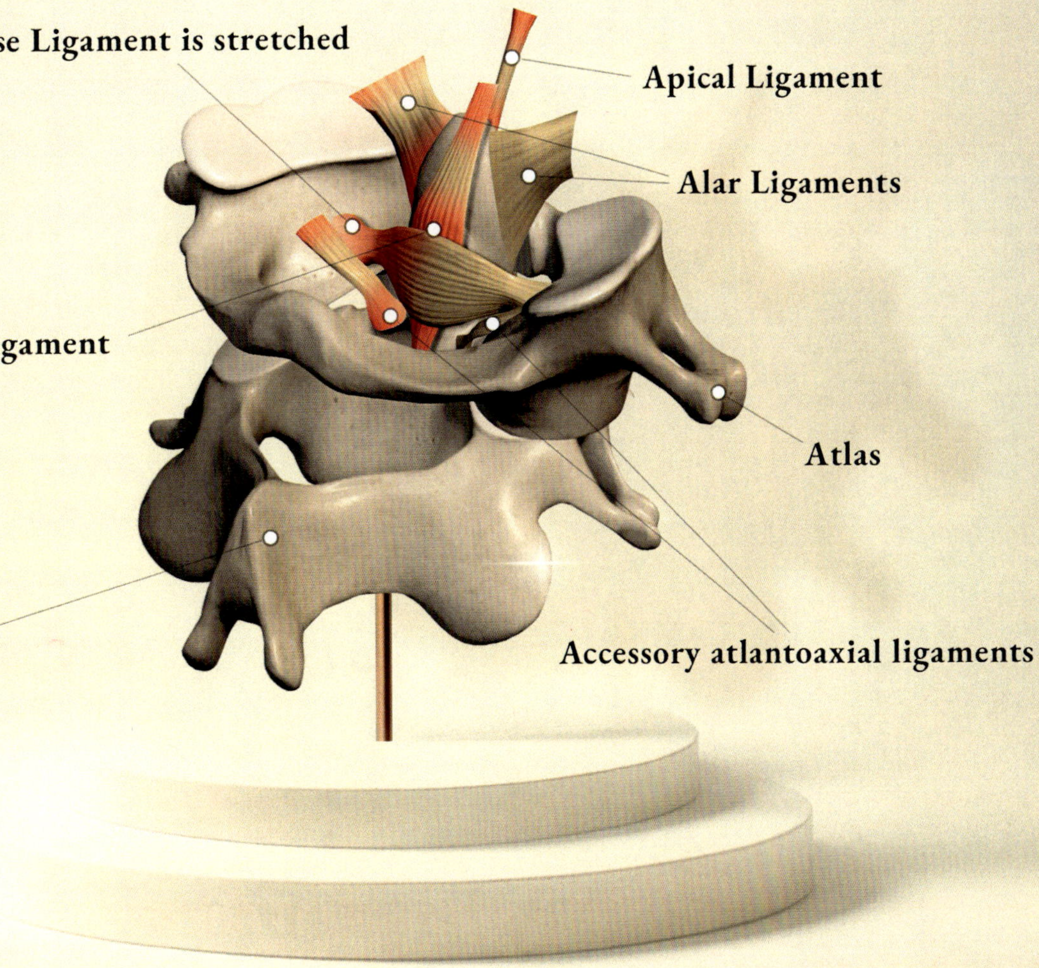

Straightened Cervical Lordosis

Forward tilting and displacement of the atlas vertebra gradually straightens cervical lordosis, creating thoracic hyperkyphosis and lumbar hyperlordosis. Acute neck pain transitions into chronic conditions, including neck and shoulder pain, a feeling of heaviness in the shoulders, pain in the upper arms, and lumbar pain. The only solution is to address the root cause by repositioning the atlas vertebra to its correct anatomical position.

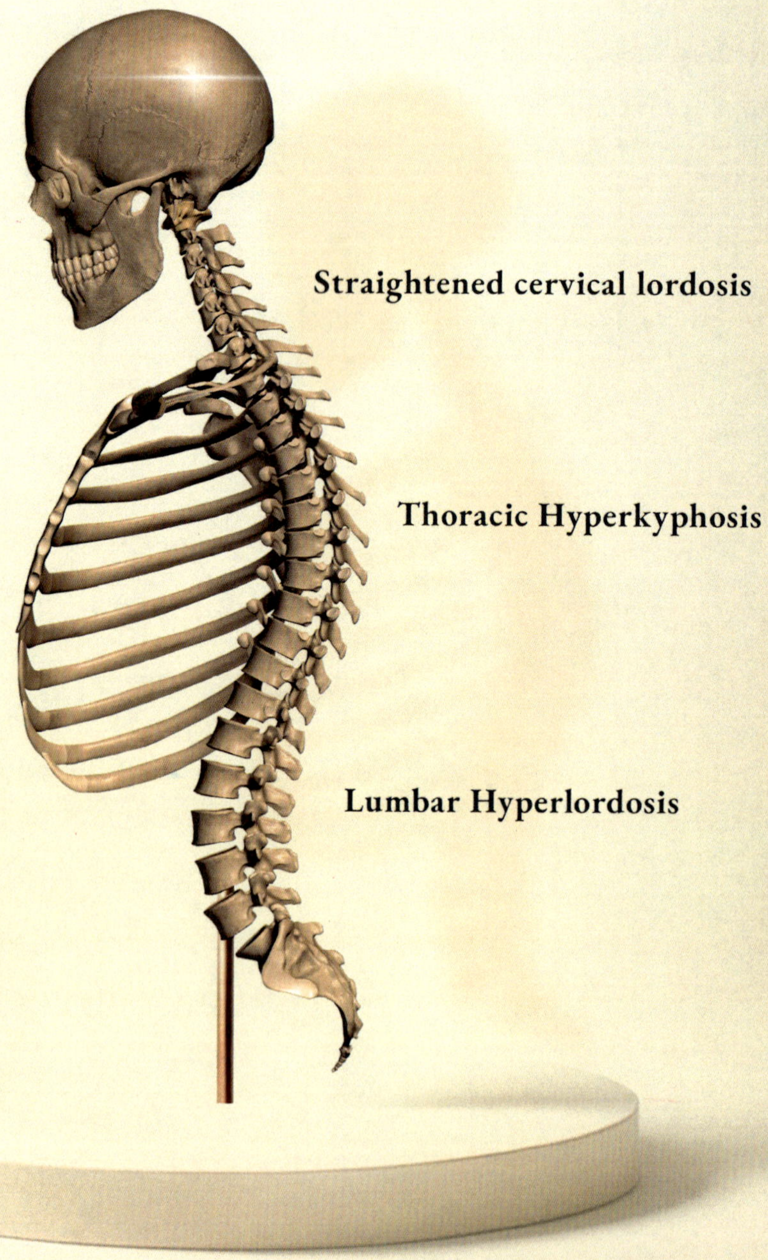

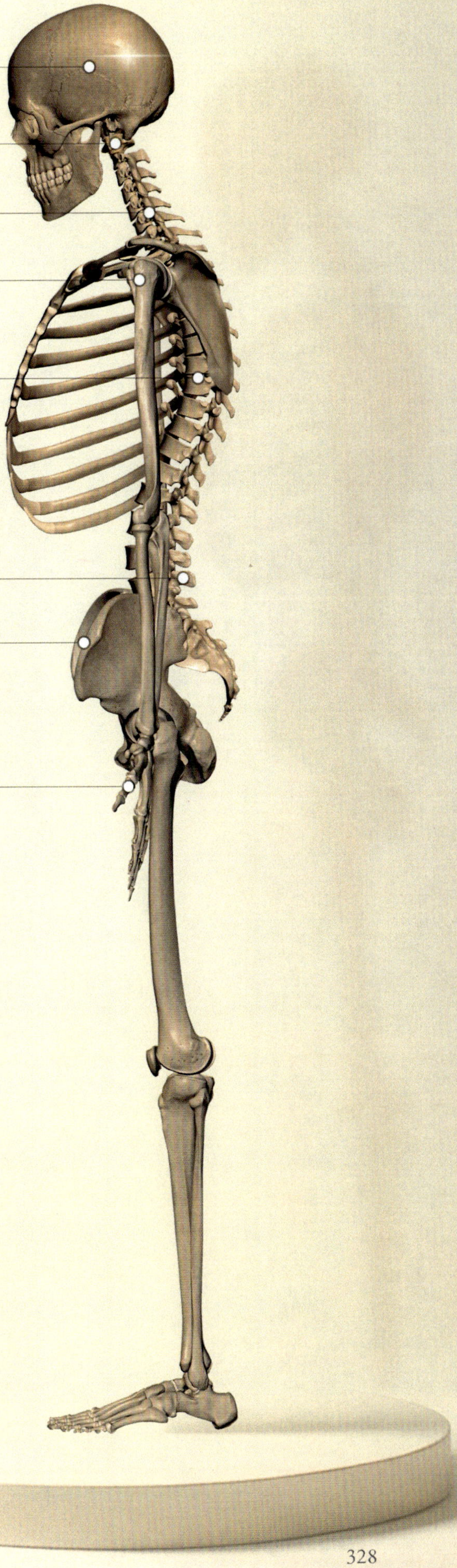

Body Posture

Inclination Subluxation and Anterolisthesis are common in individuals who have experienced head or chest trauma or long-term atlas displacement, particularly in older adults. In all these cases, regardless of the degree of trauma or age, practice has shown successful results after atlas vertebra repositioning.

Chapter 8

Complex Combined Atlas Subluxation

Complex Combined Atlas Subluxation

Complex combined subluxation of the atlas is a common diagnosis in my medical practice. This complex dislocation of the atlas usually involves at least three, and sometimes four, combined dislocations, often accompanied by a minor or major degree of anterolisthesis of the atlas. In most patients, this diagnosis involves a forward tilt, anterior displacement, rightward deviation, and rotation to the right side with anterolisthesis of the atlas with a tendency to slide to the right side.

These variations in the position of the atlas can cause various symptoms and complications, including pain, discomfort, and limited mobility, often represented by similar symptoms that patients report. Patients often face challenges in maintaining proper posture and may experience headaches, migraines, back pain, shoulder burden, tingling in the left leg, knee pain, poor digestion, and nausea. Additionally, symptoms such as heart arrhythmias, high blood pressure, and shallow breathing may also occur.

It is not uncommon for symptoms of a disruption in the center for coordination and orientation to be a very unpleasant consequence of complex combined subluxation of the atlas, especially in women. This condition can cause serious balance disturbances and difficulty maintaining proper body posture. In women, these symptoms can be particularly pronounced and uncomfortable, affecting daily activities and quality of life. Besides physical discomfort, these symptoms can also cause emotional stress and anxiety.

The diagnosis of complex combined subluxation of the atlas should require careful analysis and detailed examination, often using various medical images and imaging techniques. However, experienced atlas therapists can often accurately diagnose the position of the atlas through palpation. In treating this condition, the "Harmony Balance" method stands out for its ability to reset all present variations in the position of the atlas and return the atlas vertebra to the correct anatomical position. This method differs from other approaches that deal only with individual variations, offering a holistic approach to treating complex subluxations of the atlas.

The diagnosis of complex combined subluxation of the atlas is of paramount importance in the context of spinal disorders, as it can provide crucial information about the position of the atlas and its impact on the overall body posture. This diagnosis allows medical personnel to identify specific variations in the position of the atlas, including tilt, displacement, rotation, and sliding of the atlas vertebra, which can be vital for proper treatment planning and rehabilitation.

In addition to causing pain, discomfort, and limited mobility, complex combined subluxation of the atlas can lead to various spinal disorders, including kyphosis, lordosis, and scoliosis. These disorders can further affect the function of the nervous system, muscles, and joints, leading to various neurological symptoms.

In essence, the proper diagnosis of complex combined subluxation of the atlas plays a crucial role in managing spinal disorders, enabling precise targeting of the problem and providing adequate treatment to improve the quality of life of patients.

Combined Atlas Subluxation

The primary cause of the development of complex combined subluxation of the atlas is a lack of prevention, due to the complexity of the mechanism of the head, atlas, and axis, with all their structures. When trauma occurs, attention is rarely paid to the possibility of atlas dislocation. Pain from body trauma or injuries elsewhere distracts attention from monitoring the position of the atlas vertebra, which should be one of the first measures of control after physical trauma, especially in cases of traffic accidents, sports injuries, or dramatic falls that typically involve jarring of the head. Complex combined subluxations of the atlas following trauma, unless extremely severe, do not cause pain that indicates the need to check the atlas's position. Complex combined subluxations of the atlas develop slowly, insidiously, and over many years. Sometimes it may even take a decade for them to evolve into conditions we recognize as scoliosis, kyphosis, and lordosis of the spine.

The complexity of the mechanism of the head, atlas, and axis, along with all their structures and their interconnection and synergy, is the reason these elements influence each other, moving together if shifted from their correct anatomical positions, just as setting the atlas vertebra into its correct anatomical position can restore them to the right anatomical position. The connection of ligaments is a key bridge in their connectivity.

Minimal dislocation of the atlas vertebra during physical trauma such as accidents, falls, or sports incidents that can evolve over time into greater dislocation, causing various symptoms and diseases. Although the severity of this dislocation may not be apparent at first glance, the long-term effects can be significant. Over time, the lack of adequate control and proper treatment can lead to the progressive worsening of the atlas's condition, which further affects the overall posture of the body and the function of the spine.

The fundamental cause of complex combined subluxation of the atlas lies in its indistinguishability, a result of the complexity of the mechanism of the head, atlas, and axis, with all their structures. When trauma occurs, few pay attention to the possibility of atlas dislocation. The pain and discomfort felt after trauma often distract from controlling the position of the atlas vertebra, which should be one of the first measures after a physical injury, especially in traffic accidents, sports incidents, or dramatic falls that can result in the head being jerked.

Complex combined subluxations of the atlas often do not cause pain that would indicate the need for their control after trauma, unless the cases are extremely serious. They develop slowly and insidiously over a long period, often years or even decades, before manifesting as conditions such as scoliosis, kyphosis, and lordosis of the spine.

The complexity of the mechanism of the head, atlas, and axis, along with all their structures, and their mutual connection and synergy, play a crucial role in the impact of these elements on each other. When one element moves out of its correct anatomical position, the other elements often move along with it. However, the same ligament connection that enables this connectivity can also serve as a key pathway for returning these elements to their correct anatomical position, particularly when it comes to adjusting the atlas vertebra.

Neurological Impact of Atlas Subluxation

Atlas subluxation can affect the nervous system due to the proximity of the atlas to the brainstem and the first cervical nerves. This can lead to various neurological symptoms such as headaches, dizziness, and even changes in sensory functions such as vision and hearing. Damage to nerve tissue can also cause secondary neurological issues like neuropathic pain.

1. Migraine

Migraine is a neurological condition that manifests as an intense, throbbing headache, often localized on one side of the head. This type of headache can last from several hours to several days and can significantly disrupt daily activities. In addition to severe pain, migraines are often accompanied by other symptoms such as nausea, vomiting, and increased sensitivity to light and sound. These symptoms make migraine much more than just a common headache, creating a complex condition that requires careful management and understanding.

One possible cause of migraines is the compression of the greater occipital nerve, which is located at the back of the head. This nerve is responsible for transmitting sensations from the back of the scalp to the cerebral cortex. When the greater occipital nerve is compressed, it can lead to excessive stimulation of nerve pathways associated with pain, resulting in a migraine.

Compression of the greater occipital nerve can be caused by the abnormal positioning of the atlas, the first cervical vertebra in the spinal column. Two specific positional disorders of the atlas that can lead to this compression are inclinational subluxation and anterolisthesis of the atlas. Inclinational subluxation of the atlas occurs when the atlas tilts forward or backward, which can lead to pressure on surrounding nerve structures. Anterolisthesis of the atlas refers to a condition where the atlas slides forward relative to the axis vertebra below it, creating additional pressure on nerve channels.

2. Parkinson's Disease

Parkinson's disease is a neurodegenerative disorder characterized by the progressive loss of nerve cells in the brain, especially those that produce the neurotransmitter dopamine. This results in numerous symptoms, including tremor, slowed movements, muscle stiffness, and balance problems. The medulla oblongata, part of the brainstem, contains the reticular formation, which plays an important role in regulating movement, including tremor. Additionally, the medulla oblongata contains neurons responsible for controlling muscle tone, which may play a role in regulating muscle stiffness. These neurons form part of the reticular formation, which extends through the brainstem and plays a key role in regulating various functions, including muscle tone.

In the medulla oblongata, there are neurons responsible for regulating the speed and coordination of movements. This region may be associated with the control of movement speed and could be considered part of the system that controls the body's motor functions. Neurons in the medulla oblongata that play a crucial role in maintaining balance belong to the vestibular system, which is located in the inner ear and sends information about the position of the head and body to the brain to maintain balance. These signals are processed in parts of the brain connected to the medulla oblongata, allowing the central nervous system to coordinate the muscle movements needed to maintain stability and balance.

In cases of inclined subluxation of the atlas, rotational subluxation of the atlas, and anterior displacement of the atlas, there can be compression of these medulla oblongata neurons that mimic the loss of nerve cells in the brain, especially those that produce the neurotransmitter dopamine, and produce symptoms of Parkinson's disease. Adjusting the atlas vertebra has, over time, reduced and eventually completely eliminated all listed symptoms.

3. Alzheimer's Disease

Alzheimer's disease is a neurodegenerative disorder that leads to the gradual progressive loss of cognitive functions. A factor that can contribute to the development of neurodegenerative diseases like Alzheimer's is a disorder in the cervical spine.

For example, research has shown that an improper position of the neck, such as inclinational subluxation of the atlas, can affect blood flow to the brain and disrupt the circulation of cerebrospinal fluid. This can affect the nutrition and function of the brain, which may contribute to the development or progression of neurodegenerative diseases like Alzheimer's disease.

Additionally, some researchers have suggested that abnormalities in the cervical spine can affect the autonomic nervous system and cause chronic stress, which may be a risk factor for the development of Alzheimer's disease.

Musculoskeletal Disorders

Improper positioning of the atlas can lead to muscle imbalances in the neck and shoulders, resulting in additional stress and tension in these areas. These altered biomechanics can affect overall body posture, potentially causing conditions like scoliosis, kyphosis, and lordosis. Postural disorders can lead to chronic pain in the back and other areas of the body.

Osteoarthritis

Osteoarthritis is a progressive joint disease characterized by the gradual deterioration of cartilage, leading to pain, stiffness, and limited mobility. Two key factors that can significantly exacerbate the condition of osteoarthritis are poor circulation and a lack of cartilage regeneration. Understanding how these factors are connected to the function of the medulla oblongata, which plays a crucial role in regulating blood circulation, can further explain how systemic issues affect localized conditions like osteoarthritis.

The medulla oblongata, located in the brainstem, plays a vital role in regulating vital functions, including blood circulation and blood pressure. Poor circulation can lead to reduced blood flow to various parts of the body, including the joints. Cartilage, which does not have its own blood supply, relies on the diffusion of nutrients from synovial fluid, which is vital for its maintenance and regeneration. When circulation is compromised, the amount of nutrients and oxygen reaching the synovial fluid decreases, slowing down or disrupting the cartilage regeneration process.

Cartilage is a smooth, elastic tissue that allows joints to move smoothly. With aging or due to injury, cartilage can become damaged, and without adequate regeneration, this damage becomes progressive, leading to osteoarthritis.

Factors such as poor diet, lack of physical activity, and poor circulation contribute to a reduction in the body's ability to renew cartilaginous tissue. When cartilage regeneration is insufficient to compensate for its wear, joints become increasingly exposed to bone-on-bone friction, causing pain and inflammation.

Given that the medulla oblongata regulates autonomic functions such as circulation, problems in this area of the brain can directly affect overall circulation and indirectly impact joint health. For instance, dysfunction in the medulla oblongata can lead to reduced efficiency of the circulatory system, further limiting the transport of essential nutrients and oxygen needed for the maintenance and repair of cartilage tissue.

The atlas's misalignment may exert pressure on the medulla oblongata, potentially disrupting its normal function. Since the medulla oblongata plays a pivotal role in controlling blood flow and blood pressure, any interference with its activity can lead to compromised blood circulation. Poor circulation can affect the entire body, but especially the extremities and areas that require consistent blood flow for proper function and health, such as joints.

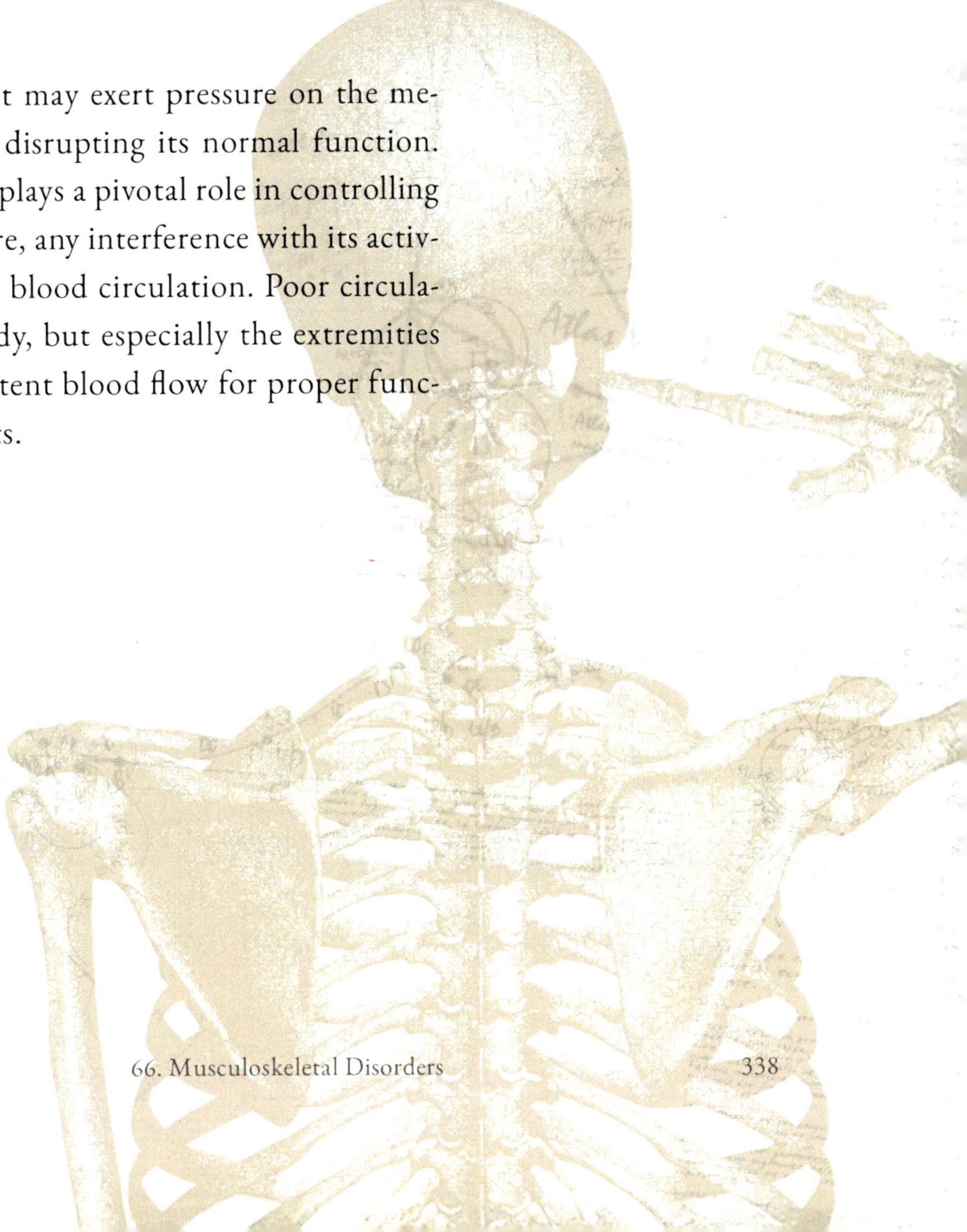

Scoliosis

Scoliosis is a musculoskeletal disorder characterized by an abnormal lateral curvature of the spinal column [Image 1]. Although it can have various associated causes, one of the lesser-known but fundamentally significant factors that contribute to both the development and worsening of scoliosis is the misalignment of the atlas vertebra.

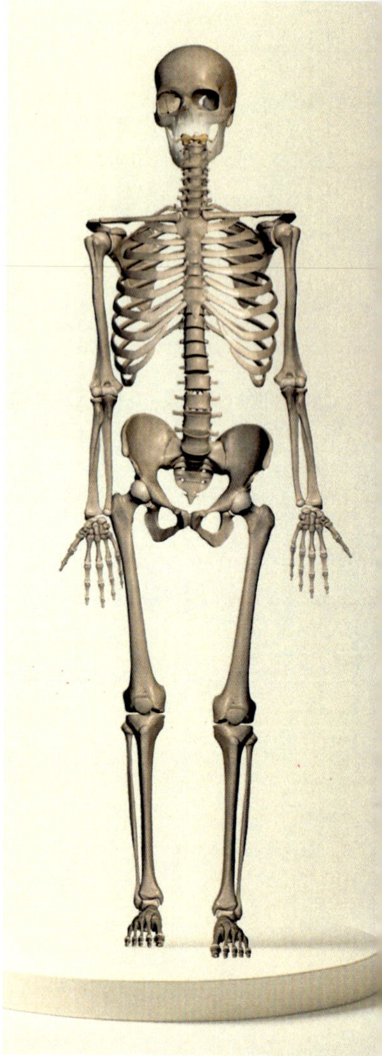
[Image 1] Scoliosis

When the atlas is displaced from its normal position, it can cause a chain reaction of problems along the entire spine [Image 2]. An improper position of the atlas can disrupt the normal balance and symmetry of the spinal column, potentially leading to the development of scoliosis. This disorder can affect the muscles, ligaments, and even the nervous system that controls posture.

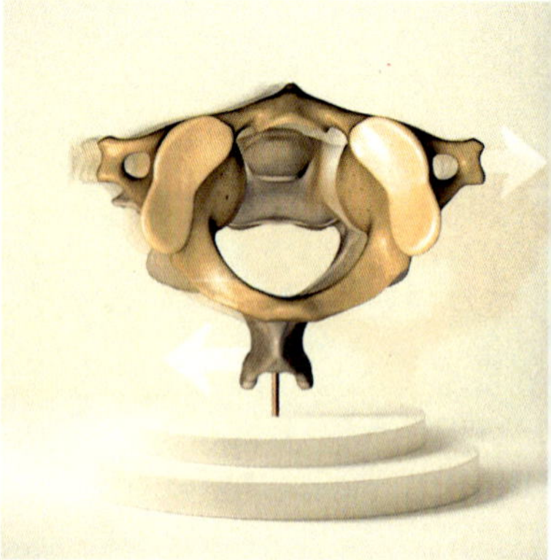
[Image 2] Cause of scoliosis

When the atlas is misaligned, it can affect how the spinal column distributes weight and bears loads. The atlas is crucial for the proper alignment of the neck and head, and its displacement can lead to an asymmetrical head position. This can provoke compensatory changes in body posture, where the lower parts of the spine adopt improper positions to compensate for the imbalance. Such biomechanical changes can lead to a permanent curvature of the spine, known as scoliosis.

Symptoms of scoliosis caused by a misaligned atlas can include not only visible curvature of the spine but also neck pain, headaches, fatigue, and even balance issues.

Scoliosis of the Cervical Vertebrae

Stiffness in the arm and cramps in the hand can result from pinching or compression of a nerve in the cervical spine (neck spine). The nerves that innervate the arm and hand exit the spinal cord between the C2 and C7 vertebrae.

Here is how problems with these nerves can cause symptoms in the arm and hand [Image 2]:

C3 - C4: Nerve compression at this level may result in pain and stiffness in the neck and shoulders.

C4 - C5: At this level, compression of the nerve might lead to pain and weakness in the shoulder.

C5 - C6 (C6 nerve root): Here, the compression may cause pain, tingling, stiffness, and weakness in the biceps and the outer part of the forearm. It can also result in symptoms in the thumb and index finger.

C6 - C7 (C7 nerve root): Compression occurring at this point could result in pain, tingling, stiffness, and weakness in the triceps, middle finger, and part of the forearm.

C7 - T1 (C8 nerve root): At this level, the nerve compression can cause symptoms in the little finger, ring finger, and part of the hand. It might also lead to weakness in gripping the hand.

If there is stiffness in the arm and cramps in the hand, the nerve roots C6, C7, or C8 are most likely affected. Pinching these nerves can cause pain, stiffness, tingling, and weakness in various parts of the arm and hand.

Although the cervical spine (neck spine) has seven vertebrae (C1-C7), there are eight cervical nerve roots (C1-C8) [Image 1]. This is due to the way the nerves exit the spinal cord.

Cervical Nerve Roots C1-C7: These nerves exit above the corresponding vertebra. For example, the C1 nerve root exits above the first cervical vertebra (C1), the C2 nerve root exits

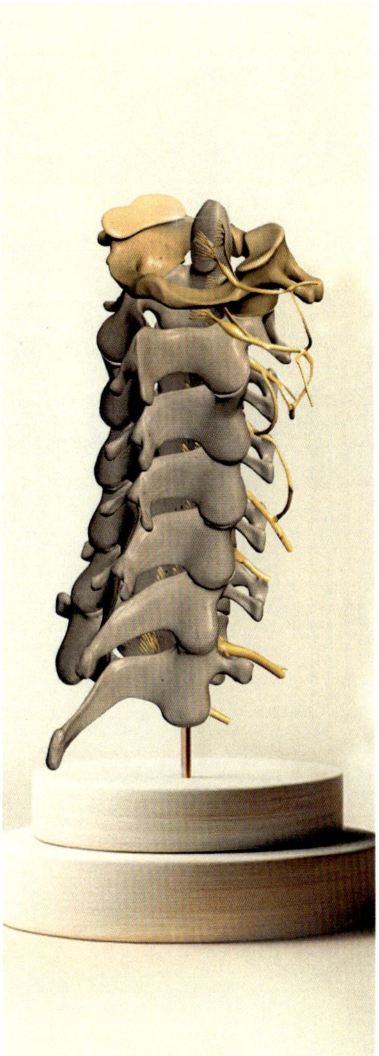

[Image 1] Cervical nerve roots

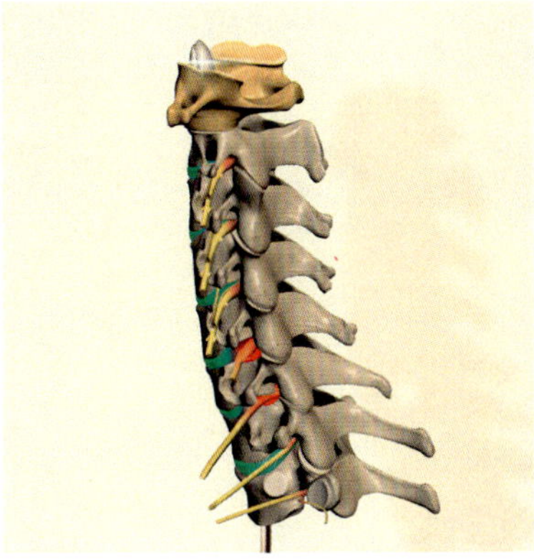

[Image 2] Cervical nerve compression

above the second cervical vertebra (C2), and so on.

Cervical Nerve Root C8: The C8 nerve root exits between the seventh cervical vertebra (C7) and the first thoracic vertebra (T1) [Image 1]. This means that the C8 nerve is the last cervical nerve, even though there is no eighth cervical vertebra. Therefore, pinching the C8 nerve root can occur between the C7 and T1 vertebrae, causing symptoms in the arm and hand, including pain, tingling, and weakness in the little finger, ring finger, and part of the hand.

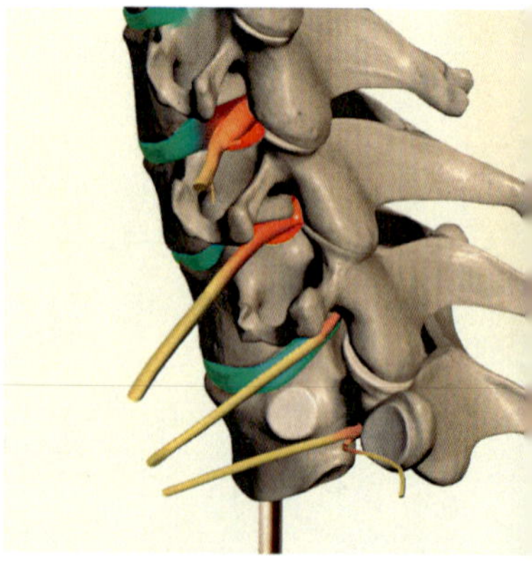

[Image 1] Arm nerves

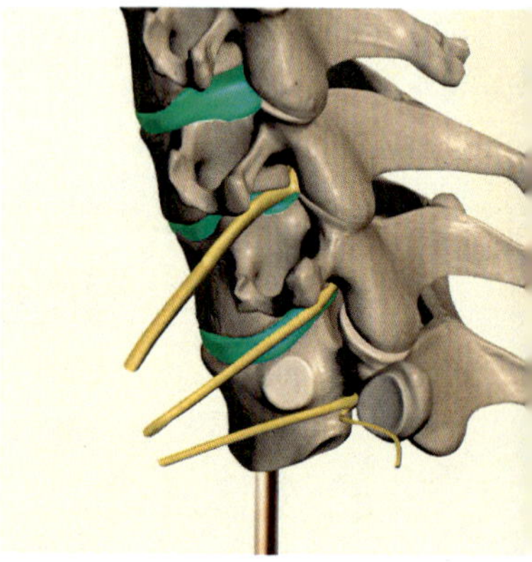

[Image 2] Brachial plexus roots

Nerves Exiting from the C6, C7, C8 Nerve Roots

The C6, C7, and C8 nerve roots contribute to the formation of the brachial plexus, which innervates the arm [Image 2].

C6 Nerve Root: The C6 nerve root exits between the fifth and sixth cervical vertebrae (C5-C6). The sensory innervation includes parts of the outer side of the forearm, thumb, and index finger, while the motor innervation includes the biceps brachii (elbow flexion), brachialis, brachioradialis, and partly the wrist extensors.

C7 Nerve Root: The C7 nerve root exits between the sixth and seventh cervical vertebrae (C6-C7). The sensory innervation includes the middle finger and the center of the forearm, while the motor innervation includes the triceps brachii (elbow extension), wrist extensors, and finger extensors.

C8 Nerve Root: The C8 nerve root exits between the seventh cervical vertebra (C7) and the first thoracic vertebra (T1). The sensory innervation includes parts of the little finger, ring finger, and the inner side of the hand and forearm, while the motor innervation includes the finger flexor muscles, including the flexor digitorum profundus, flexor digitorum superficialis, and hand muscles such as the lumbricals.

The C6, C7, and C8 nerve roots contribute to the formation of specific nerves that innervate different parts of the arm. These nerves are part of the brachial plexus.

C6 Nerve Root:

Nerve: *Musculocutaneous nerve*

Innervates: Biceps brachii, brachialis, and coracobrachialis muscles.

Nerve: *Radial nerve*

Innervates: Partly innervates wrist and finger extensors.

C7 Nerve Root:

Nerve: *Radial nerve*

Innervates: Triceps brachii, wrist and finger extensors.

Nerve: *Median nerve*

Innervates: Wrist and finger flexors, as well as thumb muscles.

C8 Nerve Root:

Nerve: *Ulnar nerve*

Innervates: Flexor digitorum profundus, flexor carpi ulnaris, and intrinsic hand muscles.

Nerve: *Median nerve*

Innervates: Finger flexors, as well as thumb muscles.

All these nerves are spinal nerves that originate from the cervical nerve roots (C6, C7, C8) and are part of the brachial plexus. The brachial plexus is a network of nerves that originates from the cervical and thoracic nerve roots (from C5 to T1) and innervates the shoulder, arm, and hand.

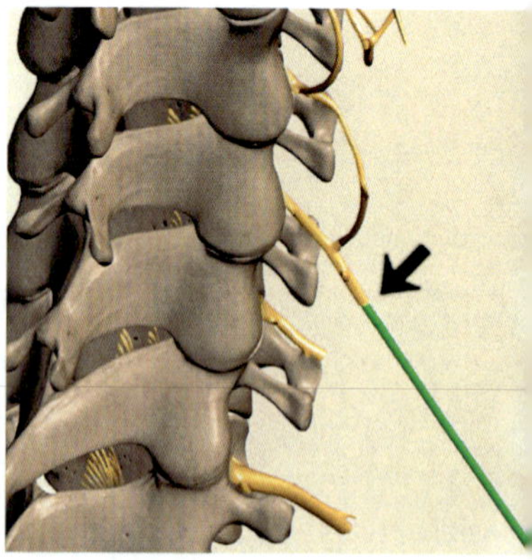

[Image 1] Peripheral nerve junction

These nerves are part of the peripheral nervous system but originate from spinal nerve roots that exit the spinal cord through intervertebral foramina [Image 1]. Through the brachial plexus, these nerves combine and branch out to innervate different parts of the upper limb.

Thus, while these nerves are peripheral nerves, their roots originate from the cervical segments of the spinal cord, making them spinal nerves at the level of the spinal cord.

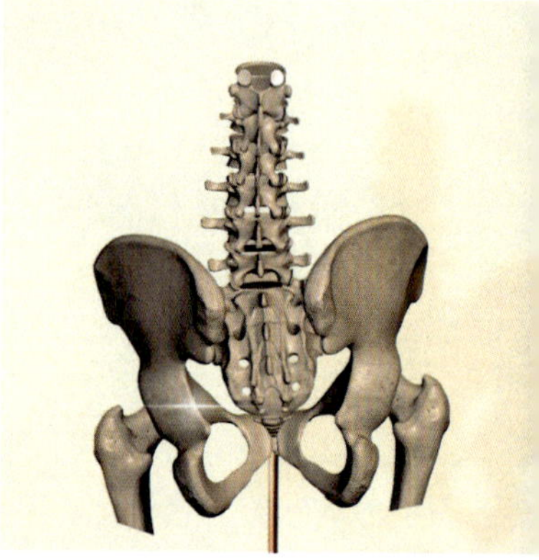

[Image 2] Lumbar scoliosis

Lumbar Scoliosis

Lumbar scoliosis is a condition characterized by an abnormal lateral curvature of the lower back [Image 2]. This condition can cause various symptoms and complications depending on the severity of the curvature and its impact on surrounding structures.

After years of experience in adjusting the atlas vertebra, it has been found that lumbar scoliosis often has its roots in the improper positioning of the atlas vertebra. The atlas, the first cervical vertebra, plays a crucial role in maintaining the balance of the head and the correct alignment of the spine. When the atlas is subluxated, meaning it is tilted to the right or left (lateroflexion), it causes a series of problems that can lead to scoliosis of the entire spine, including the lumbar region.

The atlas vertebra supports the head, which on average weighs between 5.5 and 6 kilograms. When the atlas is subluxated (lateroflexed), the weight of the head is not evenly distributed. The improper position of the head creates additional pressure on one side of the atlas, leading to uneven load distribution. This load is then transferred in a domino effect to all other vertebrae in the spine.

As a result, the spinal column attempts to compensate for this imbalance. The vertebrae shift from their natural positions, leading to the curvature of the spine known as scoliosis [Image 1]. This curvature can affect all parts of the spine, including the lumbar region, which often suffers due to the additional load and improper positioning.

Diagnosis and Treatment Process

When a patient presents with symptoms of lumbar scoliosis, a detailed examination often reveals that the problem originates from the atlas. Diagnosis is made using various methods, including physical examination, X-rays, and other diagnostic tools [Image 2].

After identifying the subluxation of the atlas, the treatment focuses on returning the atlas to its correct anatomical position. This procedure requires precision and expertise to ensure that the atlas assumes its natural position without additional stress on the surrounding structures in just one initial treatment.

After a successful atlas adjustment, patients often notice improvements not only in symptoms related to lumbar scolio-

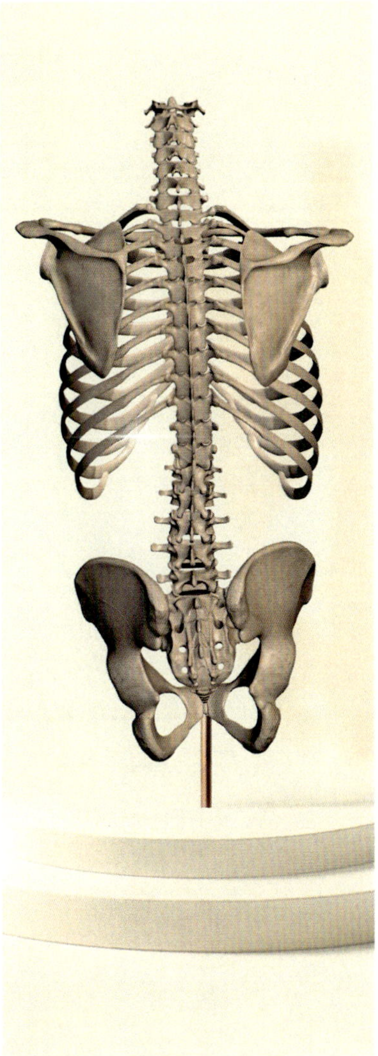

[Image 1] Spinal curvature

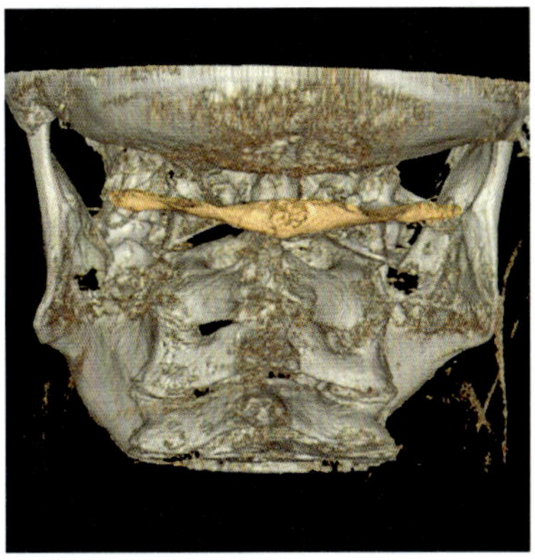

[Image 2] 3D scanner diagnosis

sis but also in overall body posture and balance immediately after treatment. By restoring the atlas to its correct position, the spine has the opportunity to return to its natural shape, with existing lumbar disc herniations retracting. This reduces or completely eliminates spinal curvature, alleviates pain immediately, and improves the patient's quality of life, keeping them away from surgical procedures for disc herniation that disappear with the adjustment of the atlas vertebra [Image 2].

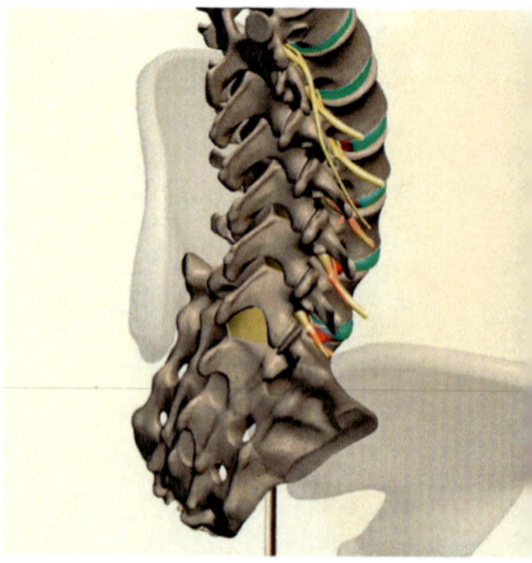

[Image 1] Scoliosis disc herniation

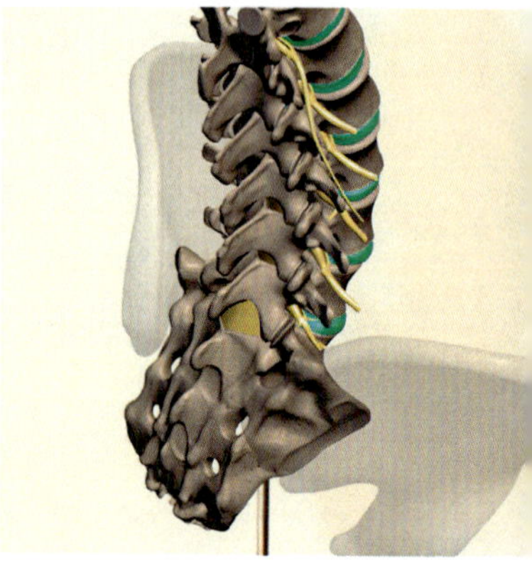

[Image 2] After atlas adjustment

Complications of Lumbar Scoliosis

If untreated, lumbar scoliosis can lead to serious complications that significantly impact the quality of life. Key complications include [Image 1]:

Chronic Pain: Lumbar scoliosis often leads to persistent lower back pain. This pain arises from muscle tension trying to compensate for the spine's abnormal curvature and nerve root compression. Chronic pain can be constant and intense, limiting daily activities and reducing the quality of life.

Spinal Instability: As scoliosis worsens, the spine becomes increasingly unstable. This instability can increase the risk of falls and injuries as the body's balance is compromised. Reduced spinal stability makes it difficult to maintain proper body alignment, increasing the risk of further complications and injuries.

Progressive Deformity: Without adequate treatment, the spinal curvature can progressively worsen. This progressive deformity leads to more pronounced physical deformities, affecting the body's appearance and function. Progressive scoliosis can cause severe breathing problems and internal organ issues due to chest deformation.

Nerve Damage: Constant nerve root compression can result in permanent nerve damage. Nerve compression can cause chronic pain, numbness, or weakness in the lower extremities. For example, compression of the L5 nerve root can cause weakness in foot dorsiflexion (foot drop) and pain in the top of the foot, while compression of the S1 nerve root can cause weakness in standing on the toes (plantar flexion) and pain in the outer foot and little toe.

Impact of Sedentary Occupations

A sedentary lifestyle, typical of many modern occupations, can have serious consequences for spinal health and the muscular system. Prolonged sitting leads to the shortening of femoral muscles (thigh muscles) and gluteal muscles (buttock muscles), which can accelerate the development of lumbar scoliosis and cause lower back pain.

Prolonged sitting, especially in sedentary jobs, can lead to shortening of the quadriceps (front thigh muscles) and gluteal muscles [Image 1]. This shortening significantly affects the health of the lumbar spine and can accelerate the development of scoliosis and cause lower back pain.

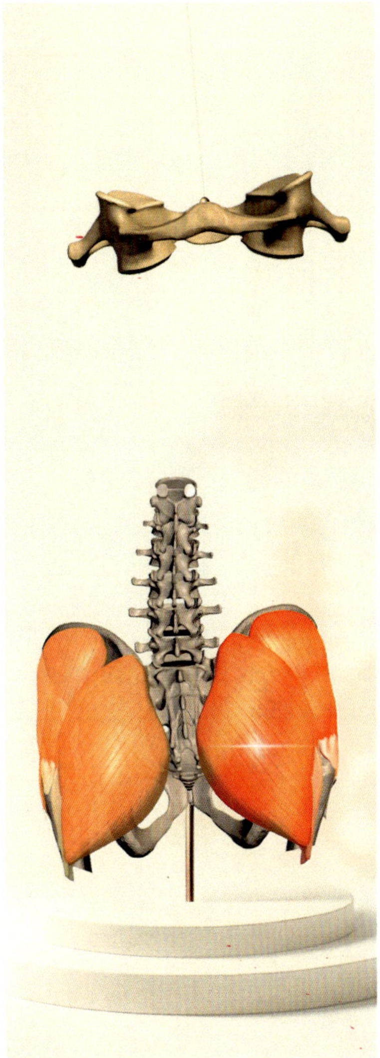

[Image 1] Gluteal inflammation

When a person sits for long periods, the quadriceps and gluteal muscles become shortened and stiff. This shortening places additional pressure on the lumbar spine for several reasons:

Muscle Imbalance: Shortened femoral and gluteal muscles create an imbalance in the muscle system supporting the spine. This imbalance can lead to improper positioning of the pelvis and lower spine, contributing to spinal curvature or scoliosis. When the front thigh and buttock muscles are not balanced, the spine experiences asymmetrical loading, leading to pain and additional complications.

Postural Changes: Prolonged sitting with shortened muscles can cause the pelvis to tilt forward (anterior tilt) [Image 1]. This increases the lordosis (curvature) of the lumbar spine, further stressing the lower back. Increased lordosis places pressure on intervertebral discs and joints, leading to pain and degenerative changes.

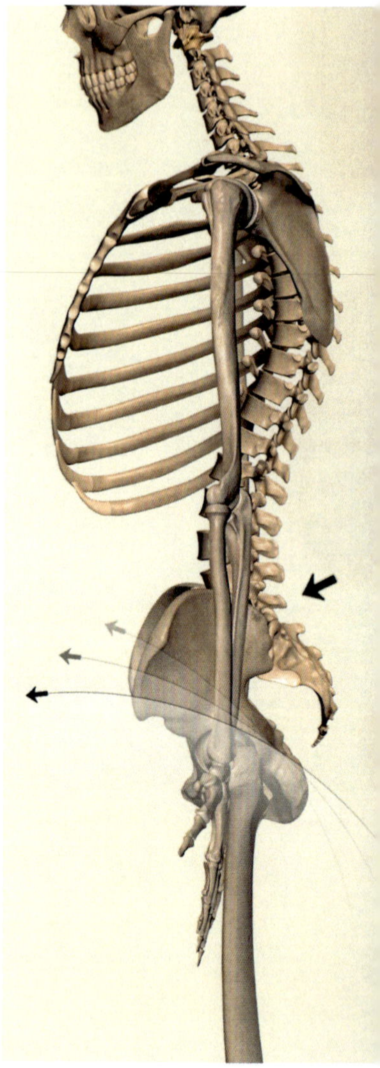
[Image 1] Anterior pelvic tilt

Weak Gluteal Muscles: Shortened and inactive gluteal muscles lose their strength, reducing support for the lower back and pelvis. Reduced support contributes to the development of scoliosis and lower back pain. When the gluteal muscles are not strong enough to support the pelvis and spine, the lumbar region experiences additional strain, leading to pain and increased risk of injury.

Lower Back Pain

Lower back pain is a common problem for people with a sedentary lifestyle. Prolonged sitting can lead to the shortening of femoral and gluteal muscles, significantly impacting the health of the lumbar spine. Here are some key factors contributing to this pain:

Tension in Lumbar Muscles: When femoral and gluteal muscles are shortened due to prolonged sitting, the lower back muscles must take on a greater workload to maintain spinal stability. This additional tension can cause pain and stiffness in the lower back. The lumbar muscles work harder to compensate for the lack of flexibility in the front thigh and buttock muscles, leading to chronic pain and fatigue.

Increased Pressure on Discs: Improper positioning of the pelvis and lumbar spine, caused by shortened muscles, can create increased pressure on the intervertebral discs. This increased pressure can lead to degenerative changes, such as disc herniations, often accompanied by intense back pain [Image 1]. Degenerative changes can further reduce spinal functionality and increase the risk of serious injuries.

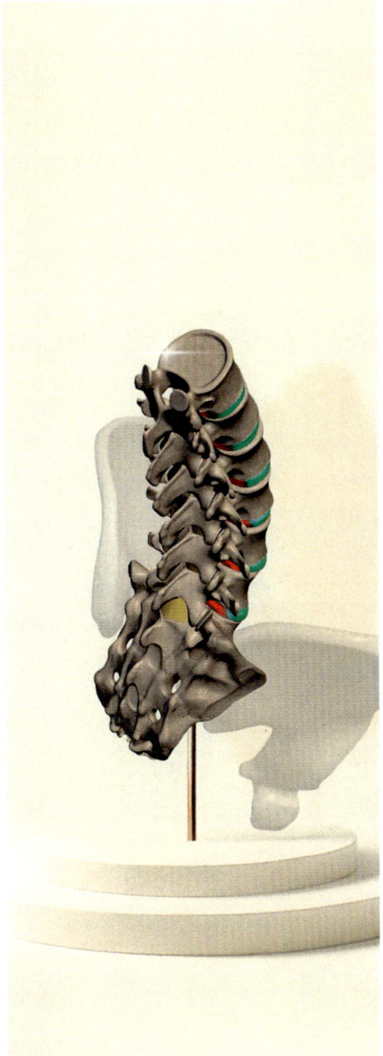

[Image 1] Disc Pressure

Reduced Flexibility: Shortened muscles reduce overall flexibility in the lower body, limiting movements and placing additional strain on the lumbar spine during daily activities. Reduced flexibility means a person cannot properly bend and twist their body, increasing the risk of injuries and additional stress on the lower back.

Prevention of Back Pain

To prevent or alleviate lower back pain caused by a sedentary lifestyle, the following preventive measures are recommended:

Regular Stretching: Stretching exercises for the femoral and gluteal muscles are crucial for maintaining their flexibility. Regular stretching can reduce tension in the lumbar spine and help prevent pain. Flexible muscles allow for better load distribution on the spine, reducing the risk of injuries and degenerative changes.

Strengthening Gluteal Muscles: Strengthening the gluteal muscles is essential for the stability of the pelvis and lower back. Strong gluteal muscles provide support to the spine and help maintain proper body alignment. Regular exercises to strengthen the gluteal muscles can reduce the risk of developing scoliosis and alleviate lower back pain.

Ergonomic Workspace: Proper adjustment of the workspace plays an important role in preventing lower back pain. A chair with lumbar support, a desk at the correct height, and a monitor at eye level can help maintain proper body alignment during work. An ergonomic workspace reduces spinal pressure and helps prevent muscle tension.

Active Breaks: During the workday, it is important to take regular breaks for movement and stretching. Active breaks improve circulation, reduce muscle tension, and help maintain flexibility. Short walks and stretching exercises every hour can significantly reduce the risk of lower back pain and improve overall health.

Common Regions of Lumbar Disc Herniations

Disc herniations are a common problem in the lumbar spine or lower back. Lumbar vertebrae bear most of the body's weight and are subjected to significant pressure, making them prone to degenerative changes and injuries. Disc herniations most commonly occur in the following lumbar regions:

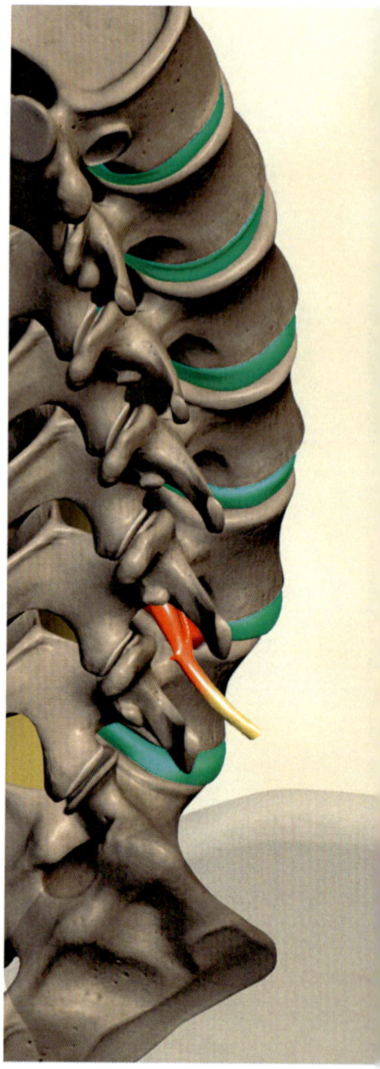

[Image 1] L4 - L5 disc herniation

L4-L5 Region

One of the most common locations for disc herniation in the lumbar spine is between the fourth and fifth lumbar vertebrae (L4-L5) [Image 1]. This region is subjected to significant pressure due to its crucial role in stabilizing and moving the lower back. A disc herniation in this region can cause a variety of symptoms that significantly impact the quality of life.

Lower Back Pain: Lower back pain is a common symptom of disc herniation in the L4-L5 region. This pain is often localized but can radiate to the hips and buttocks, sometimes causing significant discomfort. The intensity of the pain can vary from mild to severe, making daily activities difficult and reducing mobility.

Sciatic Pain: One of the characteristic symptoms of disc herniation in the L4-L5 region is sciatic pain. This pain spreads down the leg along the sciatic nerve, often to the knee or even the foot. Sciatic pain can be intense, often described as a burning or sharp sensation, and is frequently accompanied by tingling or numbness. These symptoms can significantly limit mobility and the ability to perform daily activities.

Weakness and Numbness: Disc herniation in the L4-L5 region can lead to weakness and numbness in the legs and feet. These symptoms occur due to pressure on the nerves that control the muscles of the legs and feet. Weakness can affect the ability to walk or stand, while numbness can reduce the sensation in the legs, increasing the risk of falls and injuries.

L5-S1 Region

Another common location for disc herniation in the lumbar spine is between the fifth lumbar vertebra (L5) and the first sacral vertebra (S1) [Image 1]. This region is crucial for transferring loads between the spine and pelvis, making it highly susceptible to injuries and degenerative changes. A disc herniation in this region can cause a range of symptoms that can significantly impact daily life.

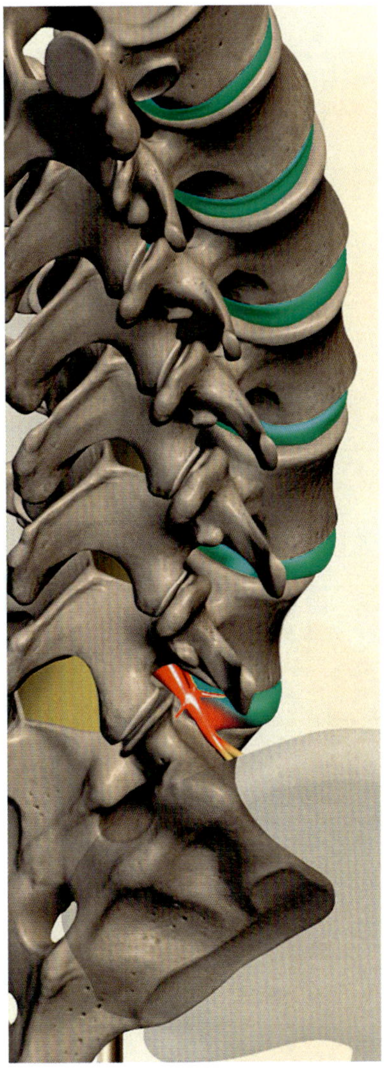

[Image 1] L5 - S1 disc herniation

Intense Lower Back Pain: Intense lower back pain is a common symptom of disc herniation in the L5-S1 region. This pain can radiate to the buttocks and lower leg, often worsening with sitting, bending, or lifting heavy objects. The pain can be constant and exhausting, interfering with daily activities and the quality of life.

Sciatic Pain: Disc herniation in the L5-S1 region often causes sciatic pain, which spreads down the leg, often to the foot and toes. This pain can be sharp, burning, or similar to an electric shock, and can worsen with coughing, sneezing, or prolonged sitting. Sciatic pain can be accompanied by tingling or numbness, further complicating normal movement.

Weakness and Numbness: Compression of nerve roots in the L5-S1 region can cause weakness and numbness in the lower leg and foot [Image 1]. These symptoms can significantly affect walking, especially lifting the front part of the foot (known as foot drop). Weakness can make it difficult to stand on the toes, while numbness can reduce sensation in the foot, increasing the risk of falls and injuries.

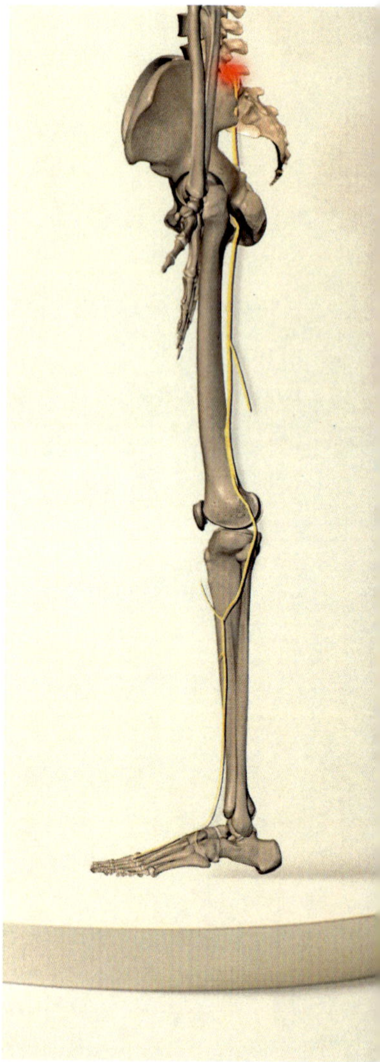

[Image 1] Sciatic nerve

Nerves That Can Be Compressed

L4-L5 Region

The L4-L5 region, located between the fourth and fifth lumbar vertebrae, is one of the most common locations for disc herniation. This region is crucial for stabilizing the lower back and bearing a significant portion of the body's load. A disc herniation in this region can lead to compression of the L5 nerve root, causing a range of symptoms that significantly impact the quality of life.

When a disc herniation occurs between the fourth and fifth lumbar vertebrae, the L5 nerve root can be compressed. Compression of this nerve root can cause the following symptoms:

Lower Back Pain: One of the first symptoms of L5 nerve root compression is lower back pain. This pain is often intense and can be constantly present, making daily activities difficult and reducing the quality of life.

Pain Radiating Down the Leg: The pain can radiate along the side of the leg, often to the top of the foot. This pain is known as radiculopathy or sciatic pain and can be very intense, similar to an electric shock. The pain increases with walking, sitting, or bending.

Weakness in Foot Dorsiflexion: Compression of the L5 nerve root can cause weakness in the muscles responsible for lifting the front part of the foot, known as dorsiflexion. This can make walking difficult, as the foot may "drop" during stepping (foot drop) [Image 1]. This symptom can significantly limit mobility and increase the risk of falls.

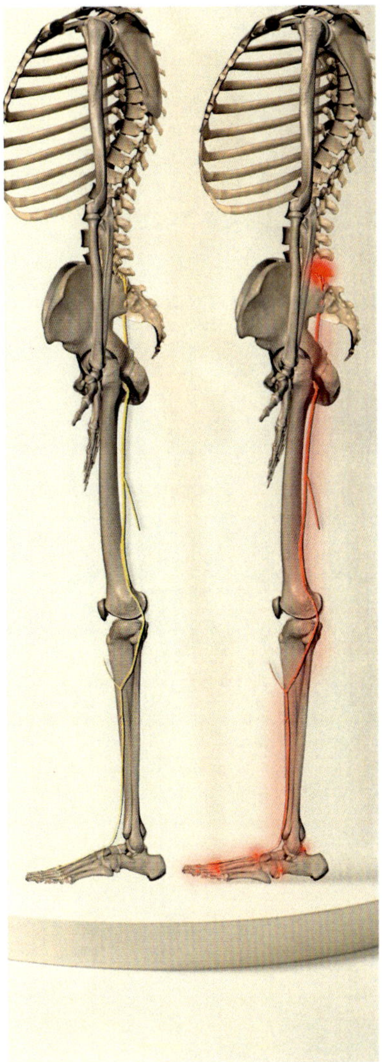

[Image 1] Foot drop

Numbness or Tingling: Numbness or tingling in the top of the foot and big toe are common symptoms of L5 nerve root compression. These symptoms can reduce the sensation in the foot, making walking difficult and increasing the risk of injuries.

L5-S1 Region

The L5-S1 region, between the fifth lumbar vertebra (L5) and the first sacral vertebra (S1), is one of the most common locations for disc herniation. This region is crucial for transferring loads between the spine and pelvis. A disc herniation in this region can cause compression of the S1 nerve root, leading to various symptoms that can significantly impact daily life.

When a disc herniation occurs between the fifth lumbar and first sacral vertebrae, the S1 nerve root can be compressed. Compression of this nerve root can cause the following symptoms:

Lower Back Pain: One of the primary symptoms of S1 nerve root compression is lower back pain. This pain is often intense and can radiate to the buttocks and lower leg, making daily activities difficult.

Pain Radiating Down the Back of the Leg: The pain can radiate down the back of the leg, often to the heel and outer side of the foot. This pain, known as sciatic pain, can be very intense and similar to burning or an electric shock. These symptoms often worsen with sitting, walking, or bending.

Weakness in Plantar Flexion: Compression of the S1 nerve root can cause weakness in the muscles responsible for plantar flexion. This weakness can make it difficult to stand on the toes, which is essential for walking and many other activities. Patients may have difficulty lifting their body on the toes of one or both feet, reducing stability and increasing the risk of falls.

Numbness or Tingling: Numbness or tingling in the lower leg and little toe are common symptoms of S1 nerve root compression. These symptoms can reduce sensation in the lower leg and foot, increasing the risk of falls and injuries.

Other Nerves That Can Be Compressed

In some cases, a disc herniation can also affect the L4 nerve root, especially if the herniation is located between the third and fourth lumbar vertebrae (L3-L4). Compression of the L4 nerve root can cause a range of symptoms that significantly impact daily life and mobility.

Compression of the L4 nerve root often causes pain in the lower back and hip. This pain can be constant and exhausting, interfering with daily activities and reducing the quality of life. The pain can radiate to the front of the thigh and knee. This type of pain is known as radiculopathy and can be very intense, making walking and standing difficult. The pain often increases with bending, lifting heavy objects, or prolonged sitting.

Compression of the L4 nerve root can cause weakness in the quadriceps, the muscles at the front of the thigh [Image 1]. This weakness can make it difficult to straighten the knee and walk, significantly reducing mobility and balance.

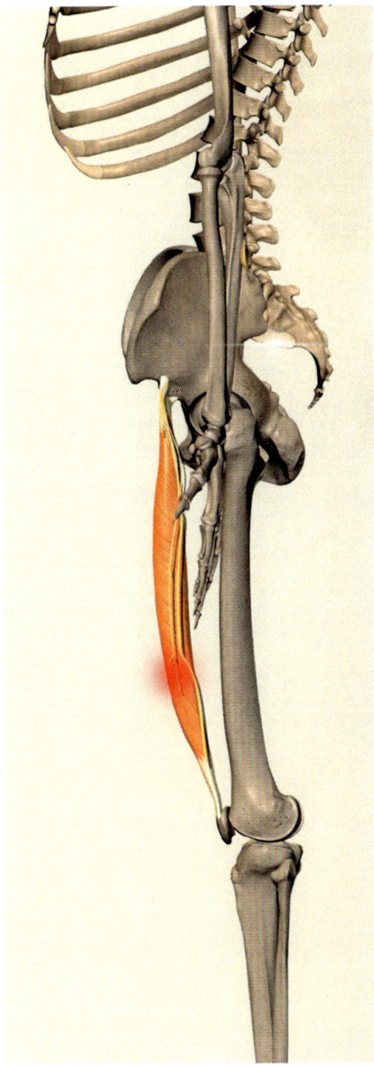
[Image 1] Quadriceps muscle pain

Numbness or tingling in the front of the thigh and knee are common symptoms of L4 nerve root compression. These symptoms can reduce sensation in the front of the leg, increasing the risk of falls and injuries. Tingling and numbness can be constant or occasional but always interfere with normal functioning.

Nerves

Disc herniations in the lumbar spine can cause compression of certain nerve roots, leading to various neurological symptoms. These nerve roots form peripheral nerves with specific functions that affect motor and sensory activity in the lower extremities. One of the most important nerve roots that can be affected is the L4 nerve root.

Femoral Nerve

The femoral nerve is one of the largest and most important peripheral nerves in the human body [Image 1]. It plays a crucial role in the motor and sensory functions of the front of the thigh and the inner side of the lower leg. When the L4 nerve root is compressed, the femoral nerve is often affected, causing symptoms that significantly impact daily life.

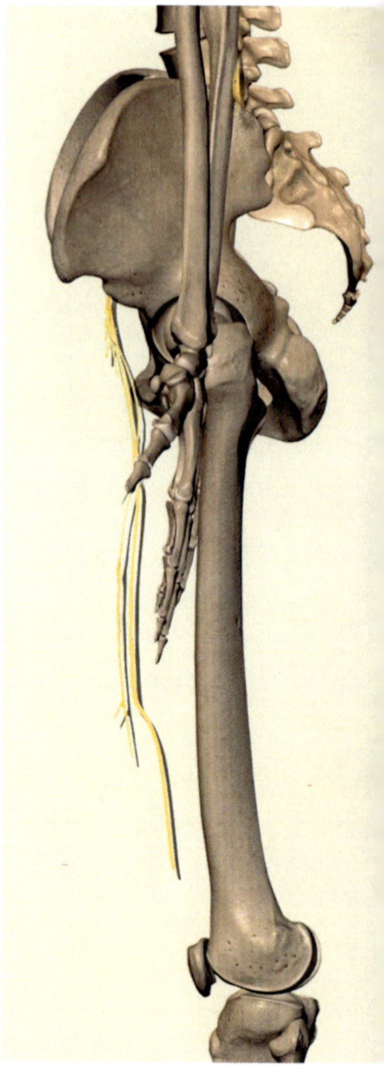
[Image 1] Femoral nerve

The femoral nerve innervates the quadriceps, a group of muscles located at the front of the thigh. The quadriceps consist of four main muscles: rectus femoris, vastus lateralis, vastus medialis, and vastus intermedius. These muscles are responsible for knee extension, which is essential for walking, running, standing, and many other daily activities. When the femoral nerve is compressed, weakness in the quadriceps can occur, making it difficult to straighten the knee and move normally.

In addition to motor functions, the femoral nerve provides sensory innervation to the front of the thigh and the inner side of the lower leg. This nerve enables the sensation of touch, pain, and temperature in these parts of the leg. When the femoral nerve is compressed, pain, numbness, or tingling can occur in the front of the thigh and the inner side of the lower leg, significantly reducing sensation and mobility.

Peroneal (Fibular) Nerve

The peroneal (fibular) nerve, also known as the common peroneal nerve, plays a crucial role in the motor and sensory functions of the lower leg. This nerve is essential for foot and toe movements and for sensation in the top of the foot and the big toe. When the L5 nerve root is compressed, the peroneal nerve can be directly affected, causing a range of symptoms that impact daily life.

The peroneal nerve innervates muscles responsible for dorsiflexion of the foot, lifting the front of the foot. These muscles include the tibialis anterior, extensor hallucis longus, and extensor digitorum longus. Dorsiflexion is essential for normal walking, as it allows lifting of the toes and front part of the foot, preventing them from dragging on the ground [Image 1]. In addition to dorsiflexion, the peroneal nerve is responsible for toe extension, allowing them to straighten.

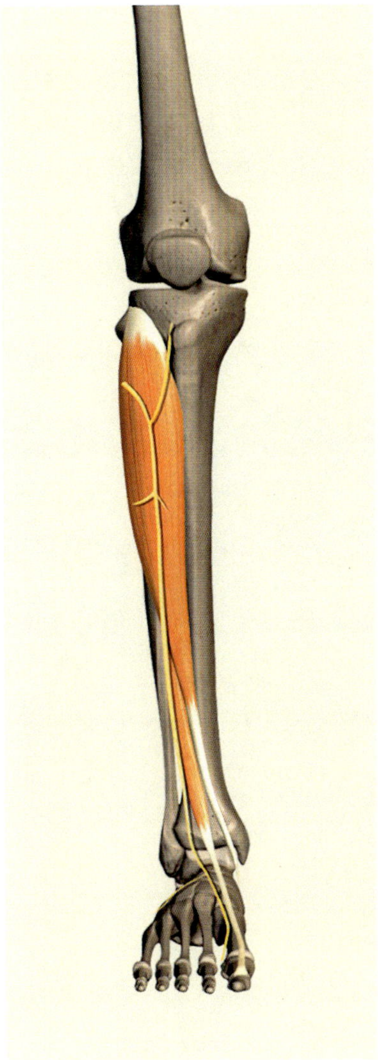

[Image 1] Fibular nerve function

The peroneal nerve provides sensory innervation to the top of the foot and the big toe. This nerve enables the sensation of touch, pain, and temperature in these parts of the foot, which is crucial for maintaining balance and preventing injuries.

Tibial Nerve

The tibial nerve is one of the main nerves in the lower leg, playing a crucial role in the motor and sensory functions of the foot and lower leg. When the S1 nerve root is compressed, the tibial nerve can be affected, causing a range of symptoms that significantly impact daily activities and mobility.

The tibial nerve innervates muscles responsible for plantar flexion, meaning bending the foot downward. These muscles include the gastrocnemius, soleus, tibialis posterior, flexor digitorum longus, and flexor hallucis longus. Plantar flexion is essential for activities such as walking, running, and standing on the toes. These muscles allow for the bending of the foot and toes, providing the stability and strength needed for movement.

In addition to motor functions, the tibial nerve provides sensory innervation to the outer side of the foot and the little toe. This nerve enables the sensation of touch, pain, and temperature in these parts of the foot, which is important for maintaining balance and protecting against injuries.

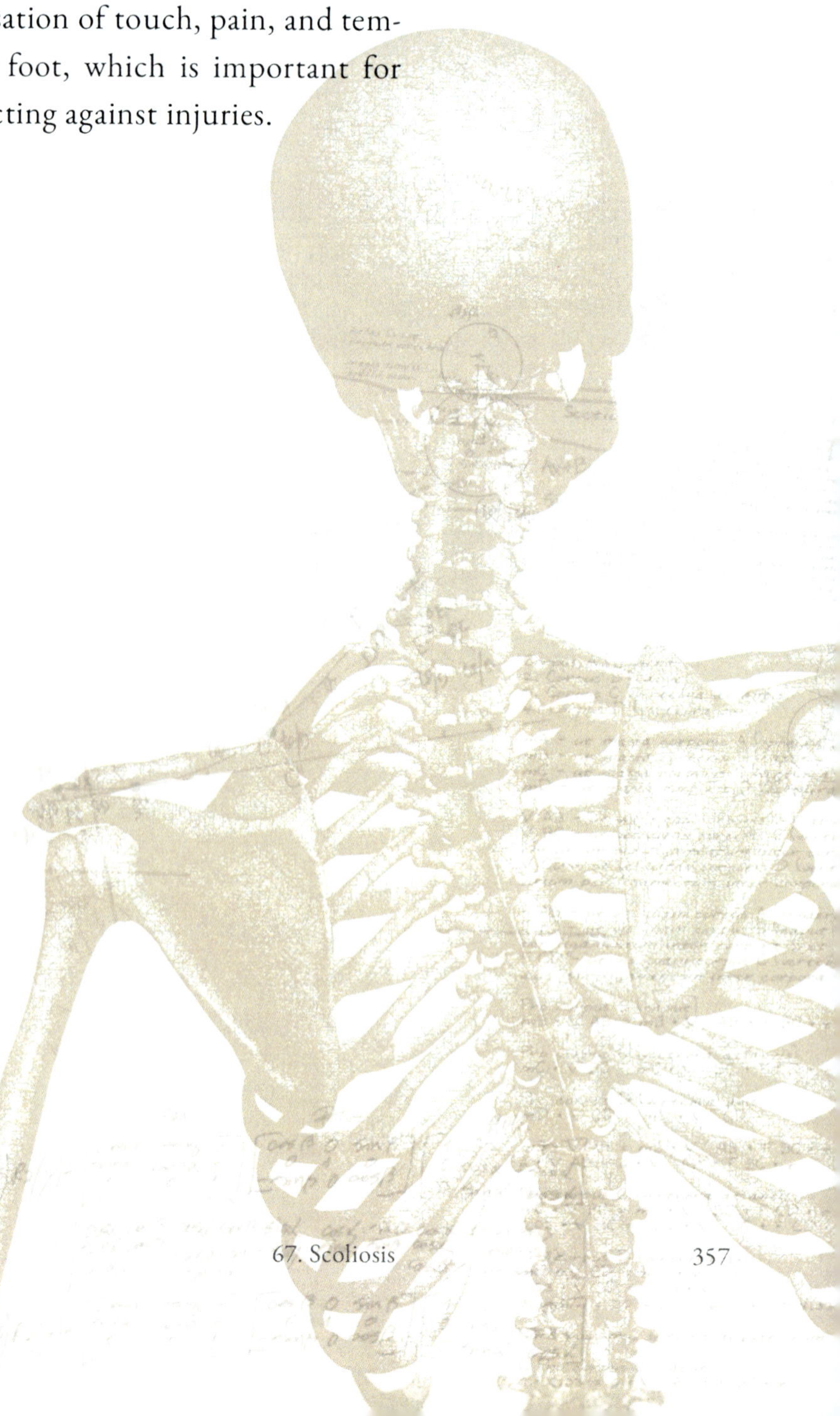

Kyphosis

Kyphosis, particularly in the thoracic region, is a spinal disorder characterized by excessive forward bending of the head, leading to a hunched posture [Image 1]. A forward tilt of the atlas vertebra in relation to the axis can be a significant contributing factor to the development of this condition. When the atlas is abnormally tilted forward, it disrupts the natural alignment of the cervical spine. This misalignment forces the head to shift forward, a condition often referred to as "forward head posture."

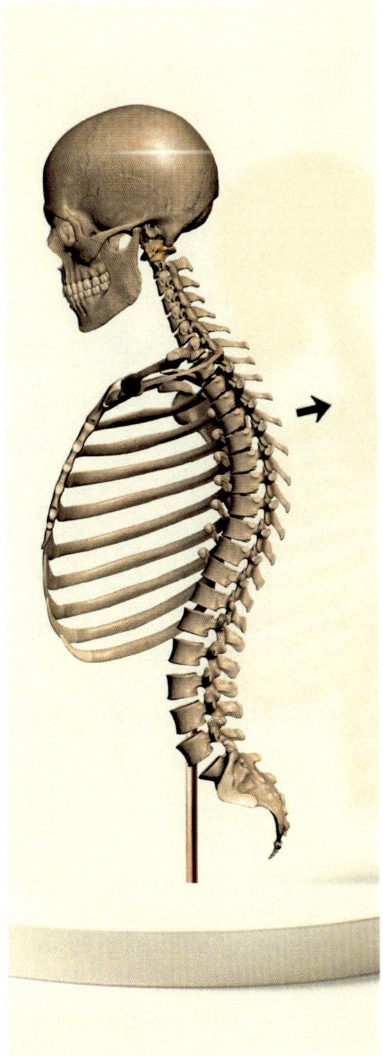

[Image 1] Thoracic kyphosis

As the head moves forward, it changes the center of gravity, placing increased weight and strain on the vertebrae of the neck and upper back [Image 2]. The human head can weigh between 10 to 12 pounds, and as it extends forward, the muscles of the neck and upper back must work harder to support this weight. This situation can lead to mechanical overload, where constant strain to sustain the head in this unnatural position causes muscles to become overstretched and fatigued.

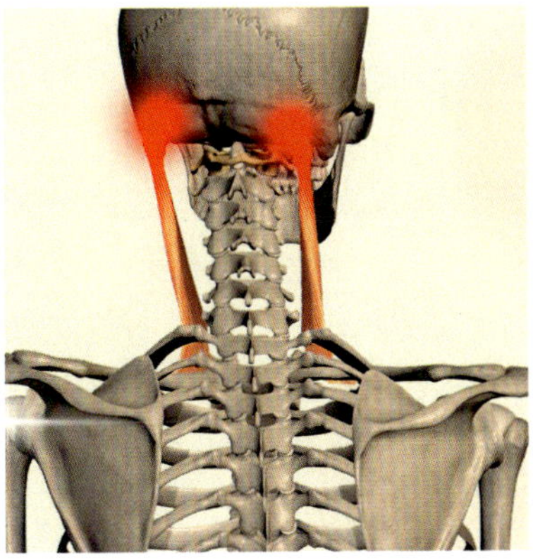

[Image 2] Mechanical muscle overload

This forward position of the head and resultant curve of the spine significantly increase the pressure on the intervertebral discs and can lead to their premature degeneration. Over time, this can cause the vertebrae to compress and become more kyphotic. Additionally, the forward curvature can pinch or compress the nerves emerging from the spinal cord, which can lead to pain and neurological issues such as numbness or tingling in the arms.

The continuous forward tension and pressure not only affect the bones and nerves but also lead to chronic changes in the muscles and ligaments. The muscles in the front of the neck may become shortened, while those in the back are elongated and weakened. This imbalance contributes further to the kyphotic posture. Similarly, in the thoracic region, the constant forward curvature can lead to a stiffening of the spine, making the kyphosis more pronounced and rigid.

Individuals with kyphosis due to forward tilt of the atlas may experience a range of symptoms, including chronic neck and back pain, reduced mobility in the spine, headaches due to nerve compression, and even difficulties with breathing if the thoracic spine is severely affected. The visual appearance of a hunched back and the obvious forward tilt of the head can also affect posture and lead to further musculoskeletal issues.

The improper position of the atlas can significantly impact breathing, especially when thoracic kyphosis is present. Rotation or tilting of the atlas disrupts postural balance, reducing chest mobility and preventing the diaphragm from functioning properly. This leads to shallow breathing and decreased lung capacity, resulting in a lack of oxygen in the body (cellular respiration in the mitochondria – glucose breakdown into ATP molecules) and chronic fatigue. Additionally, tension in the chest and neck muscles further exacerbates discomfort and reduces mobility.

Forward tilting of the atlas can also affect the blood supply to the head and neck, compressing the blood vessels that deliver oxygen to the brain. This may lead to headaches, dizziness, and reduced concentration. Impaired circulation negatively affects tissues and the nervous system, potentially causing muscle weakness and balance issues.

Kyphosis in the thoracic spine is always accompanied by a straightening of the cervical lordosis and an increase in lumbar hyperlordosis. This combination of deformities further complicates spinal curvature issues, creating an imbalance that affects overall postural stability.

Lordosis and Hyperlordosis

Lordosis refers to an increased inward curvature of the lumbar spine, often resulting in a pronounced arching of the lower back. While this condition typically affects the lumbar segment, misalignments in higher parts of the spine, such as the atlas vertebra, can indirectly contribute to or exacerbate the condition of lordosis. When the atlas is displaced from its optimal position, it can trigger a chain reaction throughout the spine, including the cervical, thoracic, and lumbar segments. Improper alignment of the atlas can disrupt spinal balance and load distribution, potentially causing or worsening hyperlordosis [Image 1].

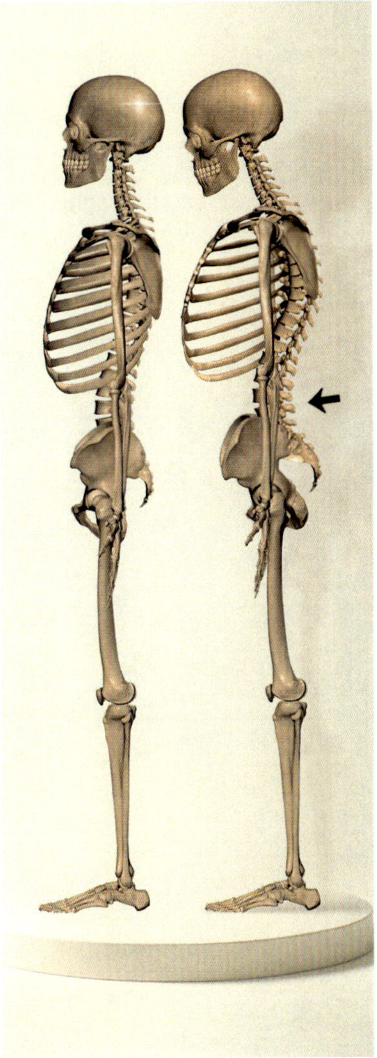

[Image 1] Lordosis and Hyperlordosis

When the atlas is misaligned, particularly if it tilts backward, it can cause a compensatory increase in the curvature of the lumbar spine to maintain head balance and body alignment. This change can further strain the lumbar vertebrae, exacerbating or even inducing lordosis. Additionally, a displaced atlas can affect muscle tone and tension along the spinal column, leading to imbalances that support the development of lordosis.

Symptoms of lordosis associated with a misaligned atlas may include lower back pain, reduced flexibility, and general discomfort during prolonged sitting or standing.

In cases of lordosis and hyperlordosis, the lumbar spine is subjected to additional strain, which can lead to muscle overloading and nerve compression, particularly if lumbar disc herniation is present. The muscles that may be under stress include the erector spinae (responsible for straightening the spine), quadratus lumborum (which helps stabilize the spine and bend the trunk), and the iliopsoas (which attaches to the lumbar vertebrae and assists in hip flexion). These muscles play a crucial role in maintaining posture and movement of the lumbar region, but in hyperlordosis, due to the exaggerated curvature, they often become overworked and painful.

In addition to muscle strain, the nerves that emerge from the lumbar spine can be compressed, especially if disc herniation is present. The most commonly affected nerves are:

The sciatic nerve, which originates from the L4, L5, S1, S2, and S3 nerve roots. Compression of this nerve can cause pain radiating down the leg, known as sciatica.

The femoral nerve, which arises from L2, L3, and L4. Compression of this nerve can lead to pain in the front of the thigh and problems with hip flexion and knee extension.

The obturator nerve, also originating from L2, L3, and L4, may be affected by disc herniation, causing pain and weakness in the inner thigh.

The conclusion is that the root cause of the problem, often found in a misaligned atlas vertebra, must be addressed in order to achieve lasting correction of lordosis and hyperlordosis in the lumbar spine. Only by returning the atlas to its correct anatomical position can the natural balance of the spinal column be restored, reducing excessive pressure on the lumbar vertebrae and allowing the spine to gradually return to its natural alignment. When the atlas is properly realigned, the strain on muscles and pressure on nerves along the spine are relieved, leading to reduced pain, improved flexibility, and long-term stabilization of the lumbar region. This holistic approach, which focuses on the underlying cause rather than just the symptoms, is the key to achieving a permanent solution for lordosis and hyperlordosis.

Torticollis

Torticollis, also known as wry neck, is a condition characterized by prolonged or persistent contraction of the neck muscles, causing the head to remain in a twisted or tilted position [Image 1]. The atlas, which allows a wide range of motion, including tilting and rotating the head, plays a critical role in neck mobility. However, when it undergoes abnormal rotation, it can lead to mechanical disruption of the balance of neck muscles and uneven pressure on nerve structures.

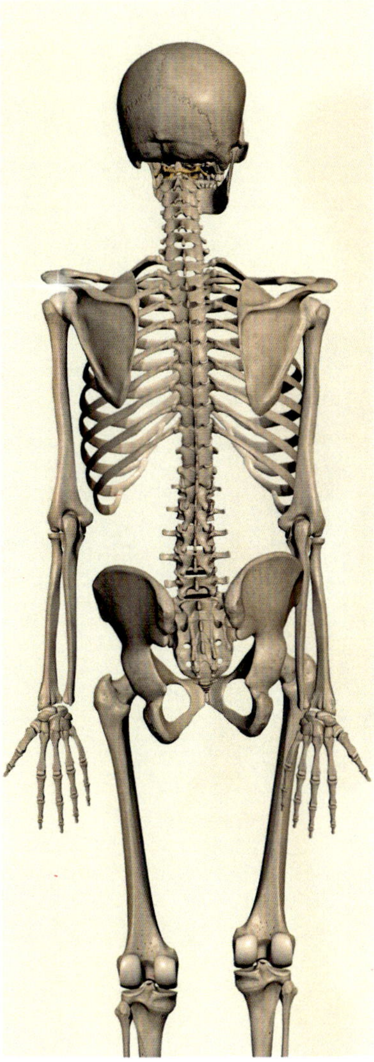

[Image 1] Torticollis

When the atlas is rotated, the muscles on one side of the neck may become overstrained or overstretched, while the muscles on the opposite side are too relaxed or shortened. This imbalance can lead to the head involuntarily tilting or twisting to one side.

A rotated atlas can also exert pressure on or irritate the nerve roots that emerge from the cervical spine. This irritation can cause pain, which further contributes to reflexive muscle spasms to minimize pain, creating a vicious cycle that maintains the abnormal head position.

Additionally, the atlas vertebra is crucial for proprioceptive signals that help the brain understand the position of the head in space. The rotation of the atlas can lead to incorrect information being sent to the brain, causing it to react by attempting to correct the perceived but inaccurate head position. This complex interaction not only disrupts normal neck function but can also have broader implications for overall posture and spinal health.

The paravertebral muscles on both sides of the spine are most affected, as they ensure its stability and mobility. Multifidus muscles, responsible for fine movement control, can also endure extra stress and develop microtraumas.

Disk herniation

Subluxation of the atlas, which refers to the partial displacement of the first cervical vertebra from its normal position, can significantly affect the biomechanics of the entire spine. Although it is not often directly associated with disk herniation, disorders in the position of the atlas can indirectly affect the health and function of the disks, particularly those in the cervical and lower back regions.

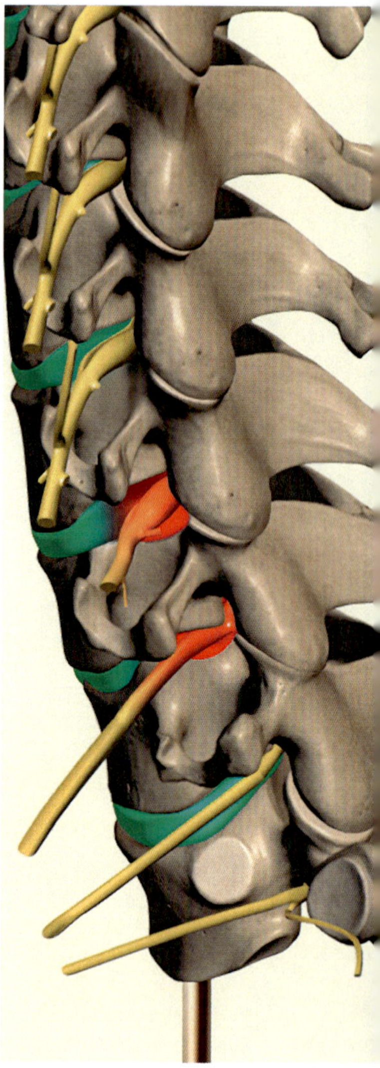

[Image 1] Cervical disc herniation

The atlas is crucial for the proper alignment of the head and neck. When the atlas is subluxated, it can lead to disturbances in the natural posture and alignment of the spinal column. This imbalance can place excessive stress on specific parts of the spine, particularly the cervical and lumbar disks, which are especially vulnerable due to their roles in movement and shock absorption.

When the atlas is subluxated, the load on the disks increases as they must compensate for the altered mechanics of movement and position. This can accelerate disk wear, increasing the risk of disk degeneration and eventually leading to disk herniation.

Improper alignment of the atlas can affect how the weight of the head and upper body presses on the lower segments of the spine. This increases the pressure on the lumbar disks, which can cause or exacerbate a disk herniation.

Disk herniations most commonly occur in the lower back (lumbar spine) and the neck (cervical spine) [Image 1]. These areas are under the greatest pressure due to the biomechanical functions of the body, such as movement, lifting loads, and maintaining balance.

The lumbar area carries the majority of the body's weight

and is subject to significant pressure during daily activities such as walking, sitting, running, and lifting loads. Herniations in this part of the spine are the most common and usually cause pain in the lower back, which can spread to the legs.

Cervical disk herniations in the neck region result from neck strain, which is associated with atlas subluxation. Symptoms may include neck pain, headaches, as well as pain radiating to the arms and fingers.

and is subject to significant pressure during daily activities such as walking, sitting, running, and lifting loads. Herniations in this part of the spine are the most common and usually cause pain in the lower back, which can spread to the legs.

Cervical disk herniations in the neck region result from neck strain, which is associated with atlas subluxation. Symptoms may include neck pain, headaches, as well as pain radiating to the arms and fingers.

Timely diagnosis of atlas displacement is crucial, as atlas misalignment is often the root cause of various issues. Early detection of the displacement can significantly shorten the period of acute and chronic inflammation. When atlas displacement is diagnosed promptly, treatment can begin before the condition worsens, preventing long-term disc degeneration and associated complications. Timely diagnosis allows for quicker intervention, addressing not only the symptoms but also the underlying cause of discomfort. This approach leads to faster recovery, reduces the need for prolonged treatments, and helps restore overall health and well-being more efficiently.

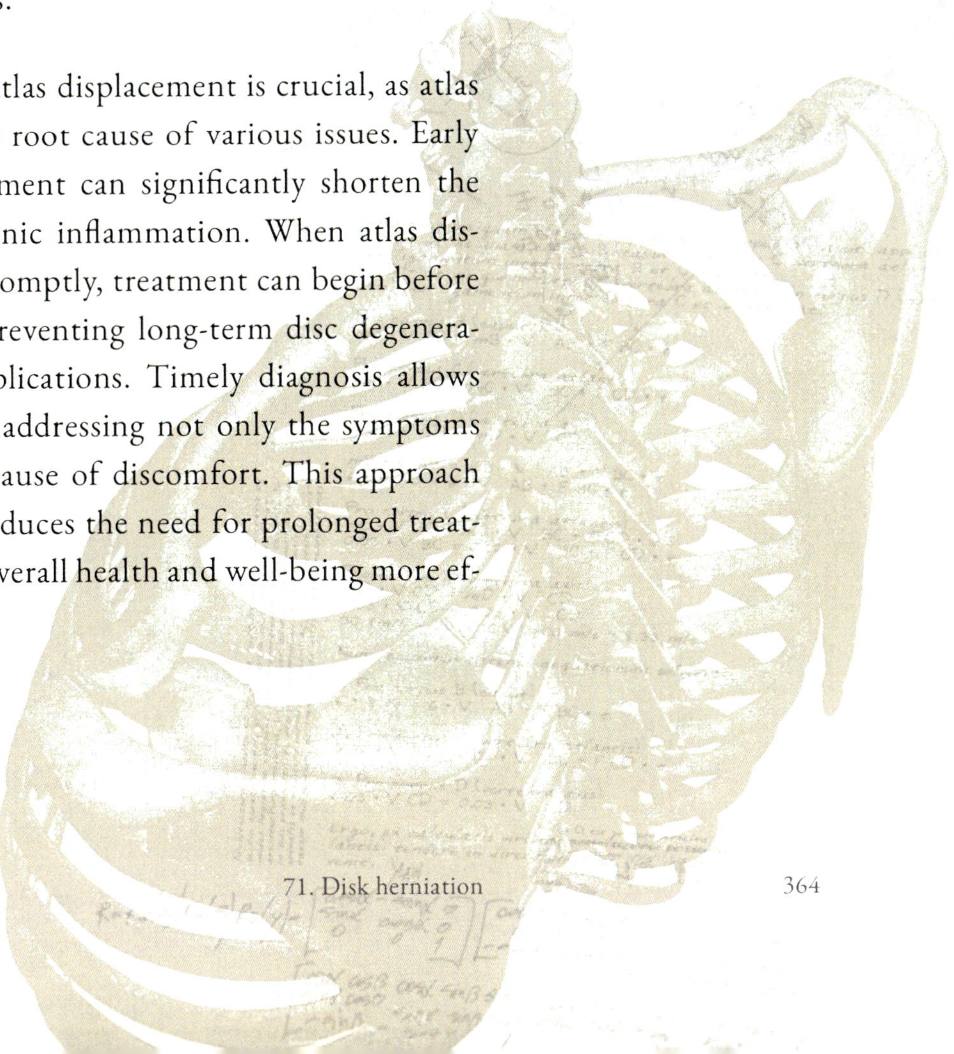

Atlas Subluxation and Digestive Health

Irritable Bowel Syndrome (IBS) is a functional gastrointestinal disorder characterized by chronic symptoms such as abdominal pain, bloating, and changes in bowel habits without visible abnormalities in the intestinal tract. IBS is one of the most common disorders affecting the digestive system. Although it can be very uncomfortable, it does not lead to more serious diseases like cancer or inflammatory bowel diseases.

The most common symptoms occur in the lower abdomen and can be relieved after bowel movements. Symptoms include diarrhea, constipation, or a combination of both, often with variable stool form and consistency. These symptoms can be particularly pronounced and cause significant discomfort. Patients may experience an urgency to use the toilet or feel that the bowels are not completely emptied.

The vagus nerve is crucial for regulating many functions of the digestive tract, including peristalsis (intestinal movements), secretion of digestive juices, and management of inflammatory processes within the intestines. If the vagus nerve is damaged or compressed, which can be caused by the subluxation of the atlas vertebra, it can significantly impact the functions of the digestive system and manifest symptoms similar to IBS.

The vagus nerve plays a key role in controlling the rhythmic contractions of the intestinal walls, which help move food through the digestive tract. If the vagal nerve is compromised due to atlas subluxation, intestinal motility can become irregular, resulting in symptoms such as constipation and diarrhea, commonly seen in IBS.

Moreover, the vagus nerve has a role in modulating inflammatory processes in the body, including the intestines.

Dysfunction of this nerve can lead to exacerbation of inflammatory conditions in the intestines, which can worsen IBS symptoms or even trigger their onset.

The vagus nerve, one of the most important nerves in the human body, is essential for the proper functioning of many organs, including those in the gastrointestinal tract. As part of the parasympathetic nervous system, it plays a significant role in regulating digestion, including the release of bile and the activity of digestive enzymes. When the vagus nerve is compromised, whether due to mechanical pressure or damage, it can affect many bodily functions.

This nerve stimulates the stomach muscles to churn and push food through the digestive tract. It also signals the stomach to secrete acid and enzymes crucial for food digestion. Regarding bile, the vagus nerve encourages the gallbladder to contract, releasing bile into the duodenum to aid in the breakdown of fats.

The atlas vertebra, located very close to the base of the skull, is an area through which the vagus nerve passes. Subluxation of the atlas can lead to mechanical pressure on the vagus nerve, disrupting its normal function. This pressure can cause a reduced ability of the gallbladder to properly contract and release bile, leading to digestive problems with fats. Additionally, it can disrupt the normal secretion of stomach acid and enzymes, resulting in poorer digestion and nutrient absorption.

Symptoms associated with such a disorder may include bloating, abdominal pain, changes in stool consistency and frequency, and a general feeling of discomfort in the abdomen.

Breathing Disorders

Subluxation of the atlas, or the partial displacement of the first cervical vertebra from its normal position, can have a broad range of effects on various bodily functions, including breathing. The medulla oblongata, a part of the brain located in the brainstem, houses vital centers for the regulation of breathing. Therefore, any anomalies in the position of the atlas can directly impact the function of this respiratory center, potentially causing breathing disorders.

The atlas vertebra not only supports the head but also plays a crucial role in maintaining the structural integrity of the neck and protecting neural pathways that pass from the brain to the rest of the body. When the atlas is subluxated, it can cause compression or irritation of neural pathways, including those leading to the medulla oblongata.

The medulla oblongata contains the respiratory center that automatically regulates the rhythm and depth of breathing. Disorders in this region can lead to various symptoms, such as apnea, which is a temporary cessation of breathing during sleep; hyperventilation, which involves excessively rapid or deep breathing; and dyspnea, which is difficulty breathing or shortness of breath.

Patients with breathing disorders caused by atlas subluxation may experience symptoms including irregular breathing rhythms, labored breathing, shallow breathing, a sensation of tightness in the chest, and frequent pauses in breathing during sleep. Diagnostic procedures may include radiographic imaging or 3D scanning of the cervical spine to determine if there is a subluxation of the atlas, along with detailed respiratory tests such as spirometry or sleep studies to assess respiratory function.

Tension Headaches

Tension headache syndrome, the most common type of headache, is characterized by mild to moderate pain typically described as a pressing or tightening sensation, often likened to wearing a tight band around the head. These headaches can last from 30 minutes to several days, and the frequency and intensity may vary from person to person.

The main symptoms include a constant, pressing pain that is not pulsating. The pain usually affects both sides of the head and can extend to the neck or even the shoulders. The pain may be accompanied by sensitivity of the scalp, neck, and shoulders to touch, and a general feeling of fatigue or irritability may accompany the headache.

An improper position of the atlas can cause biomechanical imbalance which increases tension in the neck and scalp muscles. This tension can lead to constant pressure on the occipital nerves, located at the back of the head. The occipital nerves pass near the atlas, and any pressure or irritation of these nerves can cause pain that spreads from the neck, over the back of the head, to the eyes. The pain is usually dull and pressing, which is characteristic of tension headaches.

Headaches caused by the compression of the occipital nerves and subluxation of the atlas typically cover the area that includes the back of the head, often radiating upwards to the top of the head or towards the eyes. In some cases, the pain may also affect the temporal region (temples).

Tension headaches can diminish concentration and cause persistent mental fatigue, which negatively impacts daily activities and overall quality of life. If left untreated, chronic neck and scalp tension may worsen, leading to migraines or other more severe headaches.

Final Thoughts

Complex combined subluxation of the atlas encompasses a series of conditions that involve the abnormal positioning of the first cervical vertebra. This condition has significant consequences on neurological functions, the structural integrity of the spinal column, and the overall health of the patient. The presence of multiple types of subluxations—including inclinational, anterolisthesis, posterior, lateral, and rotational-highlights the complexity of these disorders and the need for detailed diagnostics and targeted therapeutic approaches.

Each of these subluxations requires careful consideration and a specialized treatment approach that includes methods for adjusting the atlas vertebra to return it to its correct anatomical position and reduce or completely eliminate symptoms. It is crucial to emphasize the need for an individualized therapeutic plan that takes into account the specific subluxations and associated symptoms of the patient.

In conclusion, the complex combined subluxation of the atlas presents challenges for both diagnosis and treatment. Understanding the different forms of subluxations and their impact on functionality and health is key to effectively managing this condition and improving the quality of life of patients.

A precise diagnosis is important, but it doesn't address the root cause of the problem. Until the cause is addressed-specifically the correction of the atlas vertebra, whose misalignment triggers these subluxations—the cycle remains incomplete, leaving us trapped in a labyrinth of symptoms caused by atlas displacement. Without correcting the atlas, we are merely treating the symptoms rather than resolving the underlying issue, which leads to further biomechanical disturbances in the spine and continued health problems.

Complex Combined Atlas Subluxation

Complex Combined Atlas Subluxation results from early trauma that disrupts body statics over time, tilting the head forward, rotating the shoulders and pelvis, and altering spinal curves. In its chronic phase, it causes symptoms like dizziness, headaches, arrhythmias, muscle pain, and digestive issues.

Atlas is displaced and tilted forward, rotated backward on the right side, and lowered on the right side.

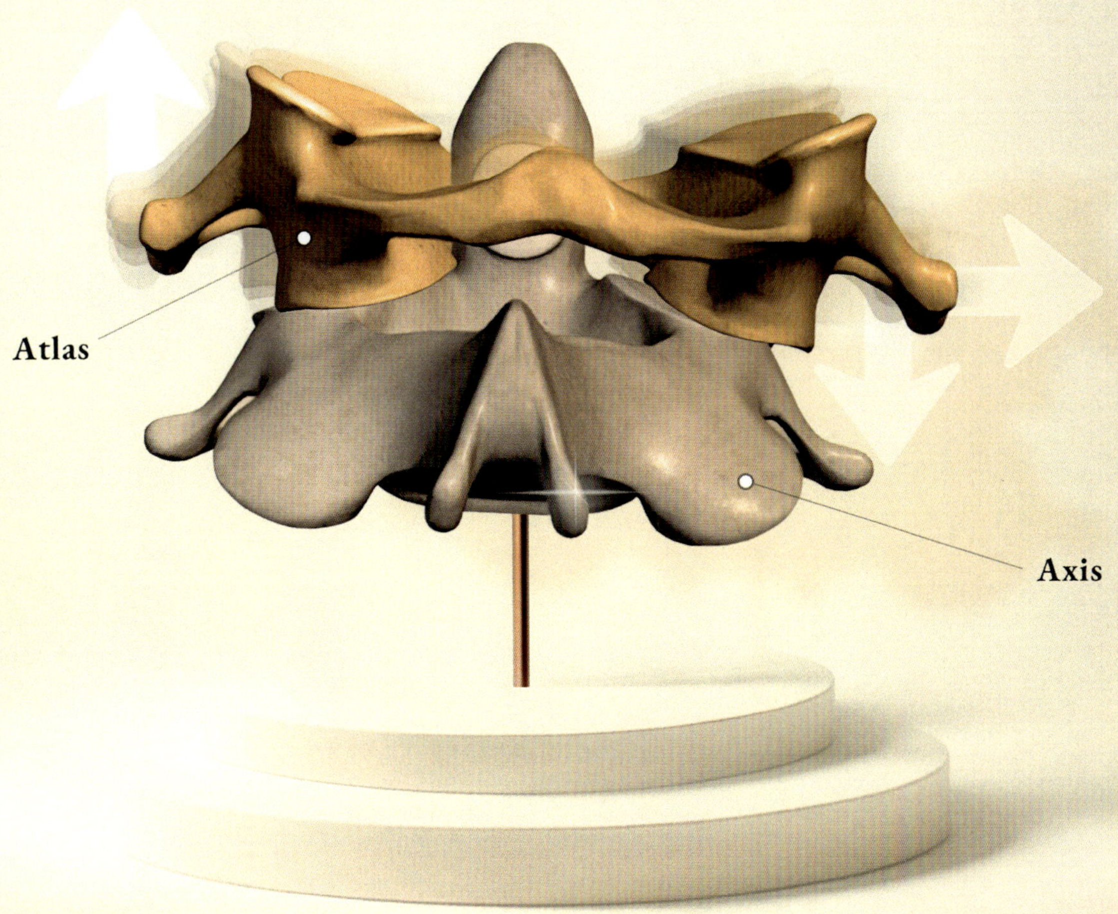

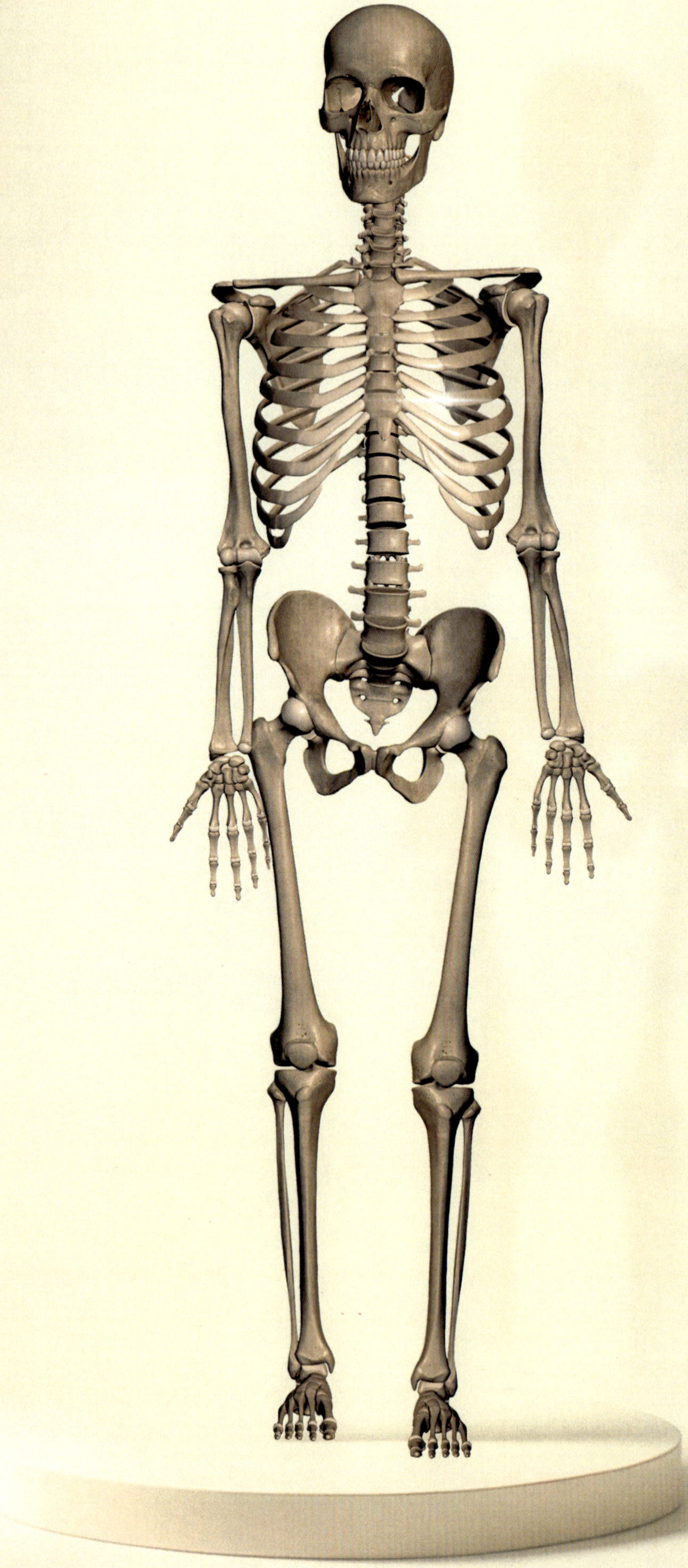

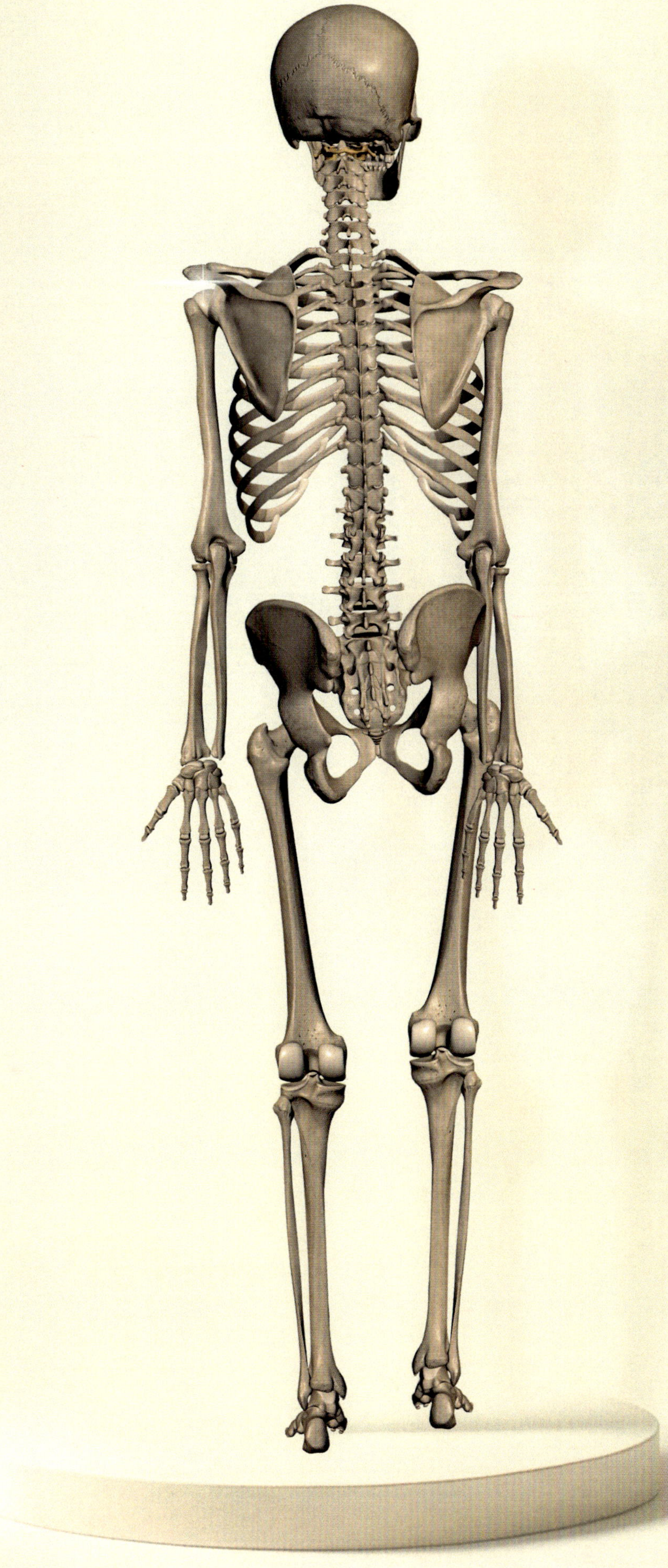

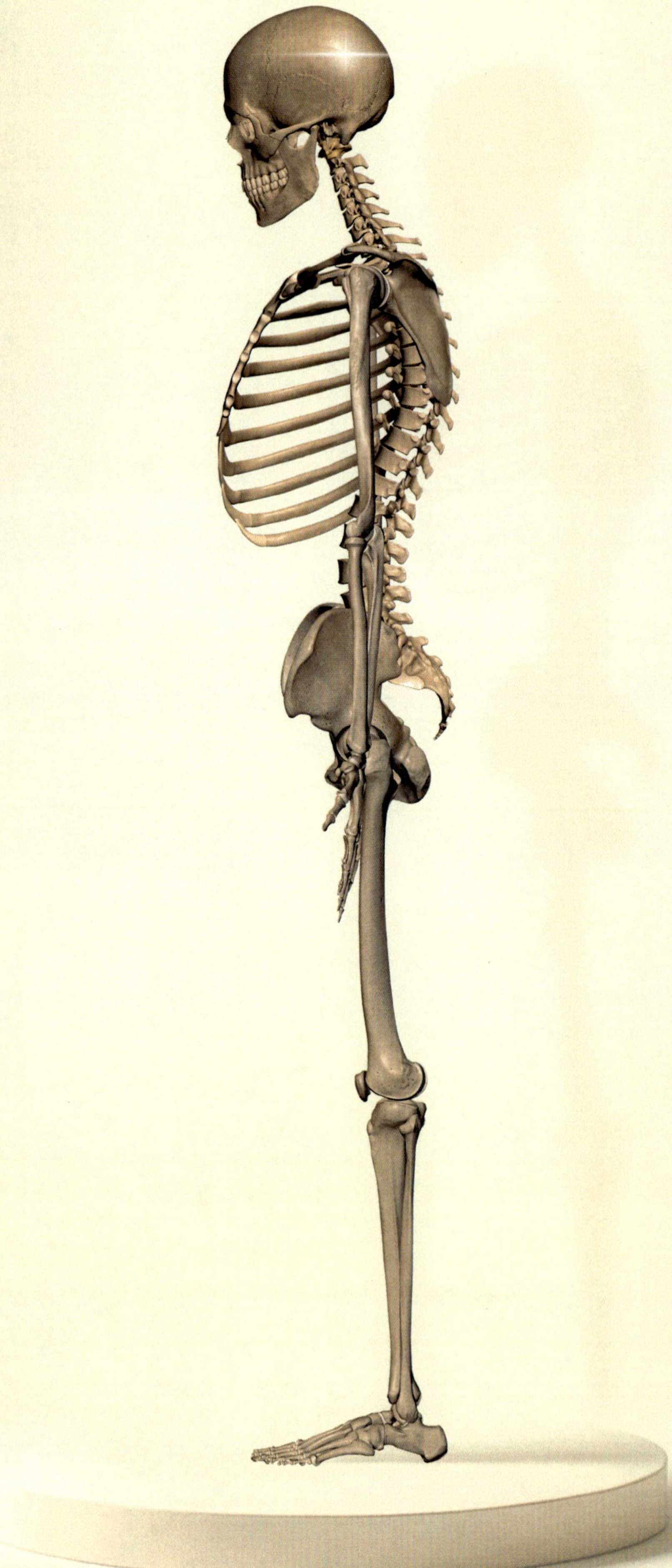

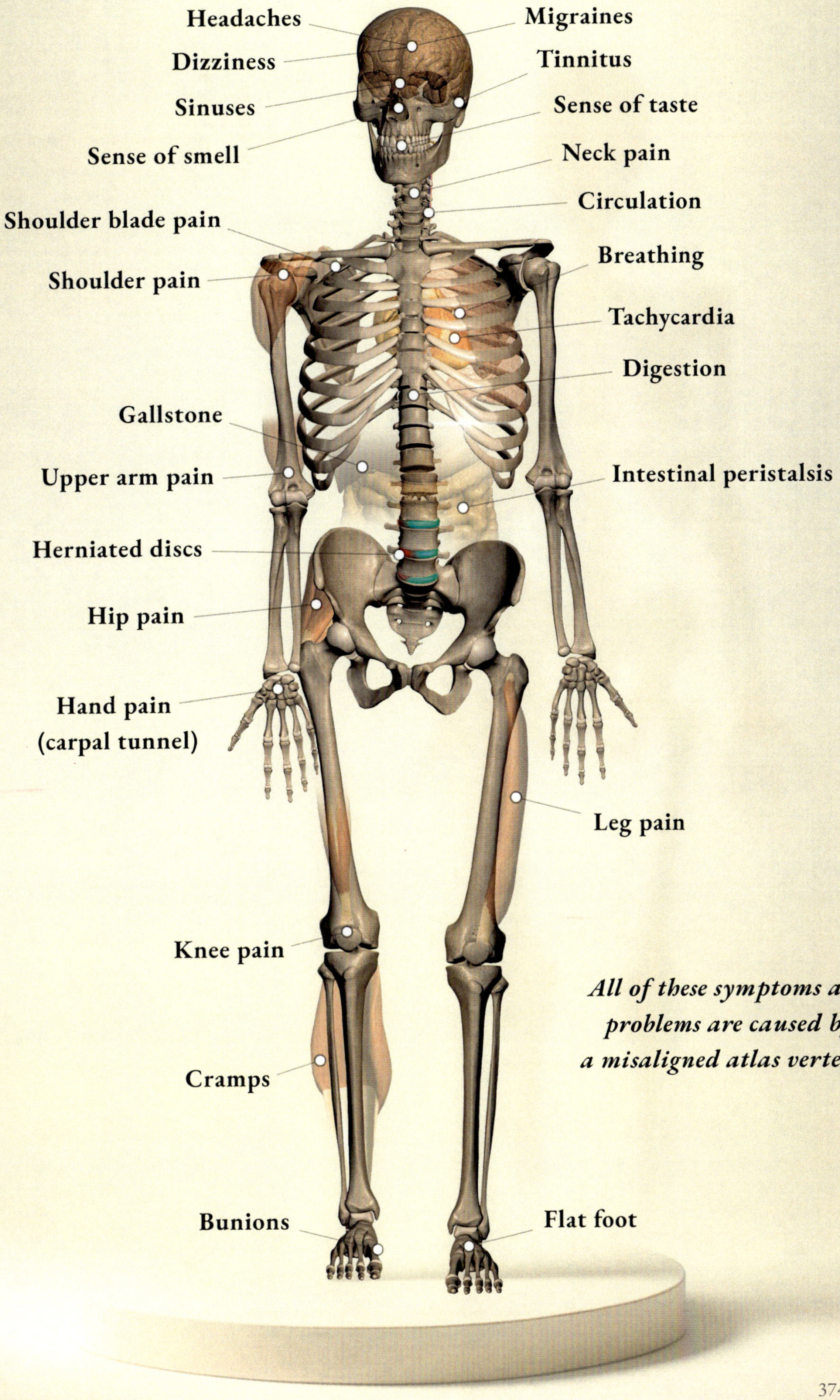

All of these symptoms and problems are caused by a misaligned atlas vertebra.

Chapter 9

Atlas adjustment method "Harmonious Balance"

Harmonious Balance Method

The atlas adjustment technique known as "Harmonic Balance" represents a sophisticated approach in medical practice aimed at restoring the optimal position of the first cervical vertebra. The significance of this technique lies in its holistic approach, which not only deals with the adjustment of the atlas itself but also encompasses the overall condition of the patient, from initial diagnosis to post-treatment education and prevention. This introductory text provides insight into the various aspects of the "Harmonic Balance" process to illustrate its comprehensive impact on patient health.

1. Patient Diagnosis Analysis

The process begins with a detailed collection of anamnestic data, which includes discussions with the patient about their current symptoms, medical history, and previous treatments. This step is crucial for understanding the underlying causes of issues and tailoring the treatment to the specific needs of the patient.

2. Patient Examination

Following the initial diagnosis, a thorough examination ensues, assessing the mobility of the neck, postural deviations, and asymmetries in structure. This phase is necessary to identify specific areas that require intervention and to ensure that the adjustment technique will be customized to the individual characteristics of the patient.

3. Preparation for Treatment

Creating a calm and supportive environment is essential for the success of the treatment. Preparation includes placing the patient in a comfortable position and applying relaxation techniques to reduce anxiety and optimize the body's response to treatment.

4. Atlas Adjustment Massage Technique

"Harmonic Balance" utilizes specially designed massage techniques and adjusted pressures for atlas adjustment. These techniques are carefully developed to ensure maximum treatment efficacy with minimal stress for the patient, while also promoting long-term stability and alignment of the atlas.

5. Results and Follow-up Procedures

After the treatment, it is important to assess its effectiveness through monitoring the symptoms and functionality of the patient. This step may involve additional sessions or adjustments to the therapeutic plan, depending on the individual response of the patient to the treatment.

6. Patient Education

The last, but no less important segment is educating patients on ways to maintain the health of the neck and spine, as well as techniques for preventing future injuries. This includes advice on proper posture, ergonomics, and exercises that patients can perform independently.

Overall, "Harmonic Balance" is not just an adjustment technique; it is a comprehensive treatment process that promotes the general well-being and health of patients. Through a combination of precise diagnostics, carefully executed treatment, and continuous education, this atlas adjustment method has proven to be key in providing long-term solutions for neck and spine issues. This method not only helps alleviate current symptoms but also proactively acts to prevent future health problems related to the spinal column and neurological functions.

Maintenance of Results and Post-Treatment Support

A crucial aspect of the "Harmonic Balance" is the maintenance of achieved results through continuous monitoring and post-treatment support. This includes regular follow-up examinations, where atlasologists can monitor the stability of the atlas and the overall condition of the spine. These checks help in the early identification and intervention in case of any deviations or the recurrence of symptoms, ensuring that patients maintain optimal health and functionality.

Integration with Other Therapeutic Modalities

"Harmonic Balance" is often used in conjunction with other therapeutic modalities to achieve the maximum therapeutic effect. This may include physiotherapy, relaxation massages, or relaxation techniques such as hydrotherapy and music therapy, which further support patient recovery and well-being. By integrating different approaches, patients receive a holistic treatment that addresses not only the physical but also the mental aspects of their health.

Importance of Education and Self-Help

In addition to professional treatment, a significant emphasis in "Harmonic Balance" is placed on educating patients about self-help methods they can practice at home. This includes stretching exercises, self-massage, and ergonomic practices that patients can use to maintain the health of their neck and spine. By providing these tools, patients become active participants in their treatment and recovery process, contributing to the long-term preservation of their health.

Conclusion

The atlas adjustment technique "Harmonic Balance" represents a revolutionary approach in the treatment and prevention of spinal column diseases and related neurological functions. With its comprehensive approach that integrates precise diagnostics, specialized treatment, and continuous education and support, "Harmonic Balance" offers patients not only relief from current problems but also strategies for a healthier and more active life.

Patient Diagnosis Analysis

In the context of the "Harmonic Balance" atlas adjustment technique, patient diagnosis analysis is foundational for successful treatment. This process is multilayered and requires detailed understanding to achieve the best possible outcomes for each individual patient. The diagnosis analysis encompasses several key steps focused on a deep understanding of the patient's health status and history, enabling precise targeting of therapeutic interventions.

The first step in diagnosis analysis is the comprehensive collection of anamnestic data. Conversations with the patient about current symptoms, the duration, and intensity of pain or discomfort can reveal how symptoms impact the patient's daily activities and overall quality of life.

A detailed interview with the patient is a fundamental step in the diagnostic process, especially in approaches like "Harmonic Balance," which focuses on holistic treatment and rehabilitation. This phase allows physicians to gain deeper insights into the patient's health condition, which is crucial for creating an effective and personalized treatment plan.

Discussing current symptoms, the duration, and intensity of pain or discomfort is more than just collecting medical data; it is a process that helps understand how a disease or disorder manifests in the patient's life. This information is vital for comprehending the severity of the condition and its impact on daily activities and the quality of life of the patient.

In addition to discussing symptoms with the patient, it is essential to conduct a thorough physical examination to assess the condition of the spine, muscles, and nervous system. If needed, the patient may be referred for 3D scanning, offering a detailed view of atlas position and potential subluxations.

Detailed Interview Aspects

1. Collecting Information on Symptoms:

The physician starts with detailed questions about the type of symptoms, including pain, fatigue, limited movement, or any other sensations that the patient may experience. It is crucial to identify when the symptoms began, their frequency, duration, and any triggers that may worsen or alleviate them.

2. Assessing Intensity and Frequency:

The intensity of pain is often assessed using pain rating scales, such as the Numeric Rating Scale (NRS) or the Visual Analogue Scale (VAS). These scales allow for the quantification of pain, which can help in monitoring changes over time.

3. Impact on Daily Activities:

Understanding how symptoms affect the patient's ability to perform daily activities such as work, hobbies, and family interactions is key to the overall assessment. This includes the impact on employment, social activities, the ability to care for oneself, and the overall emotional and psychological status.

4. Emotional and Psychological Aspects:

Pain and discomfort can significantly affect a patient's emotional state. Stress, anxiety, or depression can both be a cause and a consequence of chronic pain. These aspects must be part of the conversation to ensure a holistic approach to treatment.

These steps are essential for giving the physician a full understanding of the patient's health. Detailed symptom assessment is key for accurate diagnosis and creating a personalized treatment plan.

Integrating Treatment Plans

The information gathered during a detailed interview enables the medical team to develop a personalized treatment plan that addresses not only physical symptoms but also supports the emotional and psychological well-being of the patient. For example, patients experiencing high levels of stress might benefit from the inclusion of relaxation techniques or counseling as part of their treatment.

A detailed interview is indispensable in the diagnostic and treatment process. Through this approach, physicians can not only identify and treat current symptoms but also develop strategies to manage or eliminate the long-term causes of pain and discomfort. This thorough understanding of a patient's condition forms the basis for effective treatment and lasting improvement in the patient's quality of life.

With the help of a detailed interview, the medical team can identify not only current symptoms but also potential risks that could lead to future health problems. This enables the development of a proactive approach that focuses not just on treatment but also on prevention. For instance, patients at risk of degenerative changes in the spine might receive recommendations for specific exercises, lifestyle changes, or ergonomic adjustments at work, which can slow down or even halt the progression of the condition.

A detailed understanding of each patient's individual characteristics allows physicians to tailor therapeutic interventions to be as effective as possible. For example, some patients may respond better to gentler adjustment techniques or specific types of massage, while others may require more intensive therapies. The information gathered can also help determine the frequency and duration of treatments that will best suit the needs and capabilities of the patient.

As therapy progresses, information obtained during initial interviews can assist in the ongoing monitoring of treatment effectiveness. This includes regular reassessment of symptoms and adjustment of the therapeutic plan in response to changes in the patient's condition. Such a tailored approach not only increases the chances of a successful outcome but also enhances patient engagement and satisfaction, which are crucial for the success of long-term treatment.

A detailed interview is not just a tool for gathering information; it is the foundation for building trust between the patient and the medical team, a key component of any successful therapeutic relationship. Investing time in understanding the patient as a whole person, with all their medical, emotional, and social aspects, lays the groundwork for a holistic approach to treatment that can significantly improve outcomes and help patients lead healthier and more fulfilling lives.

A multidisciplinary approach to patient care is ideal for comprehensive and effective therapy, especially for complex conditions that involve both physical and psychological aspects of patient recovery. Specialists such as physiatrists, orthopedic surgeons, neurologists, therapists, and psychologists collaborate to provide optimal care, each contributing their specific expertise.

Physiatrists focus on motor function recovery, orthopedic surgeons monitor improvements in musculoskeletal issues, neurologists assess neurological functions, while therapists work on muscle strengthening and posture improvement. Psychologists provide support in emotional recovery. Together, they ensure a well-rounded approach that addresses both the physical and mental aspects of healing, creating a tailored treatment plan for each patient.

Medical History Review

Reviewing a patient's medical history is also a crucial component of the diagnostic and treatment planning process in medical practice. This step allows physicians to gain detailed insights into the health challenges a patient has faced previously, which is essential for creating an effective and safe treatment plan.

The medical history review includes a comprehensive collection of data about all previous health problems, interventions, surgeries, as well as medications and therapies used. This review also involves analyzing family medical history, which can indicate genetic predispositions affecting the risk of developing certain diseases. This information helps in identifying potential health risks that may not be immediately apparent, allowing for a more targeted and personalized approach to treatment.

By understanding a patient's past medical events and family health patterns, physicians can anticipate possible complications or interactions and tailor their therapeutic strategies accordingly. This can significantly improve the outcome of treatments by preventing adverse effects and ensuring that the interventions are both safe and specifically suited to the patient's unique health profile.

Developing personal methods for analyzing medical history is essential, as diagnoses can sometimes be inaccurate. Relying on one's own knowledge, experience, and observations of the patient's current condition allows for decisions that align with specific circumstances. This approach avoids blindly following authoritative opinions, which may be incorrect, and ensures a more accurate and effective treatment strategy. By applying critical thinking and adapting to each case, physicians provide care that better meets the patient's needs.

Medical History Components

1. Previous Medical Issues:

Doctors review all past diagnoses and health issues the patient has encountered. This includes chronic diseases such as diabetes, hypertension, heart diseases, as well as any acute or episodic health issues like infections or injuries. A thorough understanding of these conditions helps in crafting a comprehensive treatment plan that takes into account the long-term health trends and needs of the patient.

2. Surgical Procedures:

It is crucial to gather information about all past surgical interventions, including the dates of the surgeries, the types of procedures performed, and their outcomes. Understanding a patient's surgical history helps physicians anticipate potential complications or limitations in treatment, ensuring that any new interventions are safe and appropriately tailored to the patient's specific medical background.

3. Previous Treatments:

Details of previous medical treatments, including medications, physical therapy, alternative therapies, and any other relevant medical interventions, are vital for understanding how the patient has responded to different therapeutic approaches in the past. This knowledge can guide future treatment options and help avoid repeating ineffective or harmful strategies.

4. Family Medical History:

Reviewing the health problems of close relatives can reveal patterns or risks for hereditary diseases, such as cardiovascular diseases, certain types of cancer, or genetic disorders.

These insights are crucial for risk assessment and planning preventive measures. They enable the medical team to advise the patient on lifestyle adjustments, screening tests, and other proactive strategies tailored to their specific genetic risks.

Overall, a comprehensive medical history review is not just about gathering data; it's about building a deep and nuanced understanding of a patient's health journey. This holistic approach ensures that treatment decisions are informed, precise, and aligned with the patient's unique health context and life circumstances.

Previous medical issues and surgical procedures can provide important insights into the condition of the spine, particularly regarding the position of the atlas vertebra. Many health problems are often a consequence of a misaligned atlas, which causes the spinal column to twist and leads to symptoms or illness as a result. For example, if a patient has had gallbladder issues, a hernia operation, and pain in the lumbar region, we can immediately conclude that the atlas is shifted to the right and tilted on the right side. These symptoms clearly indicate the presence of scoliosis and a problem with the body's static posture, especially on the right side.

Additionally, if the patient's right shoulder is rotated forward and they experience chest pain along with tingling or weakness in the left arm, it can be predicted that the atlas is rotated, with its right side shifted backward. This detailed analysis allows for a more accurate diagnosis and treatment adjustments, directly improving the patient's health and well-being. Such observations come from years of experience and knowledge gained through practice, and they can greatly aid not only in diagnosis and treatment but also in predicting future health improvements for the patient.

Collecting Medical History

The process of collecting medical history begins with a conversation between the doctor and the patient. The doctor asks detailed questions to clarify every aspect of the patient's health history. The questions are usually structured to cover all important aspects of health, from general questions about well-being and functionality to specific inquiries about symptoms and treatments.

Understanding the medical history is essential for developing a personalized treatment approach that considers all potential variables that could affect the patient's health. A well-documented medical history also facilitates communication between various healthcare professionals involved in the patient's care, ensuring that all relevant medical data can be easily transferred and used for optimal management of the patient's health condition.

A thorough knowledge of a patient's medical history allows doctors to tailor therapeutic approaches to the specific needs and conditions of the patient. For example, a patient with a history of allergic reactions to certain medications will have a customized treatment regimen that avoids those medications and minimizes the risk of allergic complications.

The review of medical history also plays a key role in prevention. Understanding genetic predispositions and past health challenges can help doctors take steps to detect and treat diseases early before they become more serious problems. For instance, if a patient has a family history of heart disease, the doctor might recommend regular cardiovascular screenings and interventions aimed at reducing risk.

The review of medical history provides an opportunity to educate patients about their health conditions and potential risks. Doctors can use this chance to inform patients about the importance of adhering to therapeutic plans, healthy lifestyle habits, and preventive measures that can reduce the risk of future health issues.

The review of medical history is not just a procedural step; it is the foundation for building a comprehensive and effective treatment plan that is tailored to the unique needs of each patient. It ensures that all aspects of a patient's health are considered with care and expertise, which is crucial for achieving optimal treatment outcomes and improving the overall quality of life of patients. Through thorough analysis and careful monitoring, the medical team can effectively manage even the most complex health challenges, affirming the value of a comprehensive approach in contemporary medical practice.

Collecting medical history involves several key aspects for a comprehensive understanding of the patient's health. Social history, including habits, diet, and stress levels, helps in more precise treatment planning. Mental health, such as anxiety and depression, impacts physical health and adherence to therapy. Information about supplements and alternative treatments is crucial to avoid potential drug interactions. Regular updating of medical history allows for better monitoring of the patient's condition, while social support enhances the success of treatment. These factors enable personalized and effective care, improving treatment outcomes.

Additionally, a thorough medical history helps identify early signs of potential health risks, allowing for timely interventions. Proper documentation also ensures smooth communication between healthcare providers, ensuring continuity of care across various treatments.

Reviewing Past Treatments

Analyzing the treatments a patient has undergone plays a crucial role in medical practice, especially in the context of managing chronic conditions or long-term therapies. This process not only provides insights into a patient's treatment history but also allows doctors to develop a personalized and often more effective treatment plan based on past experiences.

Reviewing previous treatments enables doctors to identify which therapies had a positive effect and which did not yield the expected results. This step is particularly important because each patient responds differently to treatment; what works for one patient may be ineffective or even harmful for another.

Steps in Analyzing Previous Treatments

1. Data Collection:

The physician begins by thoroughly questioning the patient about all previous therapies, including medications, surgical interventions, physiotherapies, alternative treatments, and any other forms of treatment the patient has utilized.

2. Evaluating Reactions and Outcomes:

For each therapy, the effects – both positive and negative – are considered. This includes improvements in symptoms, adverse effects, and the patient's satisfaction with the treatment.

3. Identifying Patterns:

By analyzing the effectiveness of past treatments, physicians can identify patterns that may indicate how the patient's body reacts to certain types of treatments. For example, if a patient consistently responds well to a particular medication or therapeutic method, similar approaches might be preferred in future treatments.

4. Considering Patient Preferences:

It is also important to consider the patient's personal preferences and experiences. Patients who have had negative experiences with certain therapies may be more cautious or even refuse similar approaches in the future, which can affect their compliance with the treatment plan.

Implications for Future Treatments

The analysis of previous treatments not only informs the effectiveness of various therapeutic approaches but also enables physicians to tailor treatments in a way that minimizes risks and maximizes the chances for success. For instance, if a patient has a history of negative reactions to certain medications, those drugs can be excluded from future treatment regimes.

The process of reviewing past treatments is essential for achieving optimal outcomes in a patient's care. This approach not only helps in creating a more personalized treatment plan but also increases patient safety and satisfaction, thereby improving the overall treatment experience. Through careful evaluation and adjustment, doctors can more effectively manage a patient's health conditions, prevent potential complications, and ensure that therapeutic strategies are as successful as possible.

Furthermore, integrating a patient's feedback about previous therapies enhances the quality of medical practice.

Actively involving the patient in the decision-making process about their treatment increases their trust and satisfaction, which further motivates patients to adhere to recommended treatments and participate in their own healing process.

The analysis of previous treatments also serves as a platform for educating patients about the various therapeutic options available and possible outcomes. This education helps patients understand how certain treatments work, their benefits and risks, and how they can proactively manage their health.

By reviewing and considering past treatments, physicians can also anticipate a patient's future health needs. Based on previous responses to treatments, it is possible to develop long-term strategies aimed at minimizing recurrences, managing chronic conditions, and maintaining optimal health status.

Ultimately, the process of analyzing previous treatments is an indispensable element in providing high-quality healthcare. It not only informs the current approach to treatment but also provides a foundation for continual improvement and adaptation of medical practices. With proper application and understanding, this process can significantly enhance treatment outcomes and contribute to the overall improvement of patients' quality of life, ensuring they receive support that is tailored not just to their medical, but also to their emotional and social needs.

Patient Examination

A thorough examination of the patient's neck, spine, and surrounding tissues is a crucial component in assessing and managing musculoskeletal conditions. This detailed evaluation allows healthcare professionals to assess mobility, identify postural deviations, detect the presence of asymmetry, and other anatomical abnormalities that are relevant for planning therapeutic interventions.

Steps in the Patient Examination Process:

1. Visual Examination:

The examination begins with visual inspections of the neck and spine as the patient assumes various positions (standing, sitting, and lying down). The clinician looks for any visible signs of asymmetry, abnormal curvatures (such as scoliosis or kyphosis), or other irregularities that may indicate underlying issues.

2. Palpation:

Palpation involves using the hands to feel the spinal structures, muscles, and surrounding tissues. This technique helps identify areas of tenderness, swelling, muscle spasm, or other tactile indicators of pathology. Palpation is crucial for precisely locating specific areas that may contribute to the patient's discomfort or functional limitations.

3. Range of Motion Assessment:

The patient's range of motion in the neck and back is tested through various movements. This assessment helps evaluate the spine's flexibility and potential movement restrictions. Standard movements include flexion, extension, rotation, and lateral bending of both the cervical and lumbar regions. Any deviation from the normal range of motion can indicate stiffness, injury, or other musculoskeletal problems.

4. Posture Assessment:

Evaluating the patient's posture provides insights into spinal alignment and potential stresses on the musculoskeletal system. Poor posture can lead to or exacerbate conditions such as neck and back pain. The alignment of key anatomical landmarks is examined to determine if there are postural imbalances that require intervention.

5. Neurological Examination:

A neurological exam may be conducted to check nerve function and reflex integrity, especially if there is suspicion of nerve compression or damage. This part of the examination includes testing reflexes, muscle strength, and sensory perception, which can help identify neurological deficits associated with spinal abnormalities.

6. Special Tests:

Depending on the initial findings, specific orthopedic or neurological tests may be performed to further assess the integrity of particular structures. These tests aid in diagnosing conditions such as disc herniation, nerve compression, or ligament injuries. Examples include the straight leg raise test for lumbar disc herniation or Spurling's test for cervical radiculopathy.

A detailed examination of a patient's neck, spine, and surrounding tissues is fundamental for establishing an accurate diagnosis and formulating a comprehensive treatment plan. It enables healthcare professionals to integrate clinical findings with the symptoms reported by the patient and their medical history, leading to a holistic approach to patient care. This process not only aids in diagnosing the underlying causes of pain and dysfunction but also guides therapeutic interventions that will be most effective for the individual patient.

A thorough examination is essential for identifying specific issues that may require urgent medical intervention, such as severe neurological compromises or structural abnormalities. It also helps prevent future complications by recognizing early signs of potential problems and allows doctors to suggest lifestyle modifications or therapeutic exercises that can improve functional status and reduce pain.

Through this comprehensive examination, doctors can establish a foundation for the long-term monitoring of the patient, which is crucial for managing chronic conditions. This includes regularly re-evaluating the patient's condition to monitor the effectiveness of treatments and timely adjusting therapeutic strategies in response to changes in the patient's health status.

Ultimately, a detailed patient examination is not just a diagnostic tool; it is essential for building trust between the patient and the healthcare team, a key component of any successful therapeutic relationship. Investing time and expertise in thoroughly understanding every aspect of a patient's physical condition lays the groundwork for a holistic approach to treatment that can significantly improve treatment outcomes and contribute to the overall improvement of patients' quality of life.

Palpation of the Atlas Vertebra: The Most Effective Method

Palpation of the atlas vertebra is a key element in precisely determining its position within the cervical segment of the spine. This method allows physicians to manually feel and assess the position of the first cervical vertebra, particularly in relation to significant landmarks such as the lower jawbone and the mastoid bone of the skull.

The atlas vertebra, or C1, plays a fundamental role in supporting the head and enabling its movement. Its unique anatomy and position at the top of the spinal column require precise assessment methods to ensure proper alignment and function. Through palpation, physicians can directly feel the lateral masses of the atlas and their relationship with surrounding structures, including the articular processes of the second cervical vertebra (axis) and bones of the head.

Focus on the Lower Jawbone and Mastoid Bone of the Skull

The lower jawbone, known as the mandible, serves as a key reference point due to its proximity to the atlas and its mobility, which can affect cervical biomechanics. By palpating between the atlas and the lower jawbone, physicians can assess whether there is any subluxation or abnormal pressure that could impact optimal mobility and function.

On the other hand, the mastoid bone of the skull, located just behind the ear, provides another critical landmark. Palpating this area can reveal deviations in the position of the atlas, especially when considering rotation or lateral deviation. This information is vital for diagnosing and correcting torsional abnormalities that can lead to headaches, dizziness, and other neurological symptoms.

The Importance of Precise Palpation

Precise palpation is not only important for diagnosing existing conditions but also for planning effective therapeutic interventions. Understanding the exact position of the atlas allows physicians to tailor adjustment techniques, which can significantly improve treatment outcomes and accelerate patient recovery. Additionally, accurate assessment of the atlas position through palpation can help prevent future complications associated with improper alignment of the cervical spine.

Ultimately, palpation of the atlas vertebra, focused on its relationship with the lower jawbone and the mastoid bone of the skull, not only provides a thorough insight into the current status of the patient's cervical anatomy but also sets the foundation for a comprehensive approach in diagnosing and treating disorders related to the cervical spine.

If palpation of the atlas vertebra reveals specific irregularities in its position or the position of other structures in the cervical region, accompanied by unusually rare symptoms, further diagnostics using 3D scanning is recommended. This type of diagnostic testing provides a detailed and in-depth visual representation of the atlas and surrounding structures, offering key information that is not available through palpation alone.

The Importance of 3D Scanning in the Diagnosis of the Atlas Vertebra

1. Precision in Visualization:

3D scanning provides high-quality, detailed images that allow for the precise depiction of anatomical details in the cervical region. This technology can identify subtle anomalies and irregularities that may not be detectable with standard radiographic methods.

2. Detailed View of Structural Features:

3D scanning enables a detailed view of the atlas's position relative to other cervical vertebrae, as well as insights into the condition of intervertebral discs, ligaments, and nerve structures. This is particularly important for diagnosing the causes of unusual symptoms such as chronic headaches, dizziness, or neurological deficits.

3. Detection of Complex Disorders:

A 3D scanner can detect complex disorders such as fine rotational shifts, anterolisthesis (forward movement of a vertebra), or retrolisthesis (backward movement), conditions that can have significant implications for patient functionality and treatment options.

4. Therapy Planning and Monitoring Results:

The precise information obtained from scanning is invaluable for planning therapeutic procedures. Additionally, 3D images allow for effective monitoring of changes over time, which is crucial for assessing the effectiveness of the chosen therapy.

The precise information obtained from scanning can be invaluable for planning therapeutic procedures. Additionally, 3D images enable the effective monitoring of changes over time, which is crucial for assessing the efficacy of the chosen therapy.

The use of 3D scanning in diagnostics represents an important step in the treatment process when palpation reveals abnormalities that require a deeper understanding and more precise analysis. This technology not only improves the accuracy of the diagnostic process but also allows for the customization of treatments that specifically target the unique needs and conditions of the patient, thereby increasing the chances of a successful treatment outcome.

Treatment Preparation

Preparation for Treatment

Preparation for treatment is a crucial step in the healing process that directly affects the success of therapeutic interventions. This segment of treatment requires carefully creating a comfortable and relaxed environment, which can significantly reduce patient anxiety and increase their receptiveness to the upcoming atlas vertebra adjustment therapy. Detailed preparation involves several important aspects:

1. Communication:

Adequate and open communication between the healthcare provider and the patient is fundamental for establishing trust. The doctor should clearly explain all the steps that will be taken during the treatment, as well as the expected outcomes and possible sensations the patient may experience. It is also essential to address any questions the patient may have and address any concerns regarding the atlas vertebra adjustment treatment.

2. Comfortable Positioning of the Patient:

Proper positioning of the patient is vital for the success of the therapy. The patient should be placed in a way that they feel completely comfortable and secure. This may include adjusting treatment tables, pillows, or supports to suit the patient's individual needs, reducing physical stress and allowing easier access to the treated areas.

3. Application of Relaxation Techniques:

Relaxation techniques, such as deep breathing or listening to soothing music, can be beneficial in reducing anxiety and stress in the patient before and during the treatment.

These techniques help reduce muscle tension and promote an overall state of calm, which can enhance the effectiveness of the therapeutic intervention for atlas vertebra adjustment.

4. Creating a Pleasant Atmosphere:

The ambiance in the treatment room should be pleasant and calming. This can include controlling the temperature, lighting, and noise levels, as well as using aromatic oils or diffusers to further contribute to a relaxing experience. A pleasant environment can help the patient relax and mentally prepare for the treatment.

5. Patient Education:

Informing the patient about steps they can take before coming to the treatment, such as wearing comfortable clothing or avoiding heavy meals, can further contribute to the therapy's success. Additionally, educating the patient on what to expect after the treatment can help minimize any reactions.

Preparation for treatment is, therefore, a multifaceted process that requires careful implementation to maximize therapeutic effects and ensure the patient has the most positive experience during the entire healing process.

The First Touch

Preparation for treatment involving atlas vertebra adjustment begins with creating a favorable atmosphere for the patient, where particular emphasis is placed on the first touch between the healthcare provider and the patient. The first touch is crucial as it sets the tone for the entire treatment experience and can significantly influence the patient's perception of the therapy. Since the treatment is performed while the patient is seated, with the atlasologist approaching from behind, it is important that each contact is made with great care and empathy.

Gentle and Friendly First Touch

The first touch should be gentle and friendly. The atlasologist should lightly place their hands on the patient's shoulders, conveying a sense of security and support. This approach not only helps reduce patient anxiety but also encourages relaxation of the neck and shoulder muscles, which is crucial for the treatment's effectiveness. A gentle pressure on the shoulders can also serve as an introduction to further therapeutic processes, preparing the patient for deeper and more specific technical interventions that will follow.

The Importance of Continuous Gentleness in Touch

All touches during the treatment, whether it involves further palpation or specific atlas vertebra adjustment techniques, should be performed with care. When manipulating the cervical region, where the atlas is located, the atlasologist should use stable yet extremely gentle movements to maintain the patient's comfort. Gentleness in touch not only reduces any discomfort but also strengthens the trust between the patient and the therapist.

Patient Comfort and Safety

During the treatment, it is particularly important to ensure that the patient feels comfortable and safe at all times. This includes properly supporting the patient's head and neck, using pillows or rolls for additional support, and carefully handling all movements performed during the treatment. Maintaining constant verbal contact during the treatment can also help the patient feel informed and involved in the process, contributing to a general sense of security and satisfaction.

Preparation for treatment and the first touch are essential for the therapy's success. Through a gentle and friendly approach, the atlasologist can establish trust and create a positive experience for the patient, thus not only improving the chances of treatment success but also increasing the likelihood of the patient's satisfaction and willingness to cooperate throughout the entire healing process.

Prior to the Atlas Vertebra Adjustment Treatment

Thorough preparation and detailed patient education are crucial for achieving optimal results and ensuring the patient's comfort and trust in the process. Effective communication between the patient and the atlasologist involves explaining every aspect of the treatment, including the steps it will encompass and the expected results. Here is how this process might look:

Introductory Explanation After Palpation

The atlas vertebra adjustment treatment begins with an introductory explanation following careful palpation. The atlasologist uses this moment to inform the patient about the current position of the atlas, its function, and the importance of correcting its position for overall health and well-being. In this conversation, the doctor highlights how the continued improper position of the atlas can negatively affect neurological functions and the musculoskeletal system.

The patient is thoroughly informed about what to expect after each step of the treatment, including pain reduction or increased mobility. The atlasologist also mentions potential improvements in posture, reduction of headaches, or dizziness if present, which may occur and resolve during the treatment. The possibility of adjusting the treatment based on the patient's response is emphasized, ensuring maximum comfort and therapy efficiency.

An important aspect of the treatment is educating the patient on how they can contribute to the success of the atlas vertebra adjustment process. The atlasologist guides the patient on ways to independently support the therapy and proper posture during the treatment, contributing to a more comfortable and effective execution of the treatment.

Transparent communication and thorough explanation of all aspects of the treatment are key to building trust and ensuring the therapy's success. It is important for the patient to feel like an active participant in their healing. By providing detailed information and empowering the patient, the atlasologist lays the foundation for long-term improvement in the patient's quality of life and health.

Mechanical Vibrations

Mechanical Vibrations in Ligament Therapy

Mechanical vibrations represent an innovative approach in physical therapy and rehabilitation, offering numerous benefits for the health and functionality of ligaments. This method relies on the use of specialized devices that emit vibrations of a specific frequency, intensity, and duration to directly affect tissues. When applied to ligaments, vibrations not only improve blood and lymph circulation in the treated area but also stimulate metabolic processes within the cells themselves.

The effect of vibrations on the ligaments is multifaceted. First, they help increase local circulation, leading to better tissue nourishment and more efficient removal of metabolic waste. This is particularly useful in accelerating the recovery process after ligament injuries. Additionally, mechanical vibrations can help increase ligament elasticity, reducing the risk of future injuries by enhancing the tissue's ability to withstand mechanical stress.

Furthermore, regular application of vibration therapy can reduce pain and stiffness, allowing patients to more easily perform daily activities and participate in rehabilitation exercises. Vibrations work by activating sensory receptors in the skin, which can help block the transmission of pain signals to the brain, known as the gate control theory of pain.

Due to these advantages, mechanical vibrations have become a valued tool in modern rehabilitation, providing a non-invasive, effective, and pleasant way to enhance the health and functionality of ligaments. All these benefits make vibration therapy an essential part of comprehensive therapeutic programs aimed at maintaining and improving musculoskeletal health.

Principles of Mechanical Vibrations Affecting Ligament Relaxation

Mechanical vibrations affect ligament relaxation through several physical laws and principles, the most important of which are:

1. Law of Frequency and Resonance: Every object, including tissues in the human body, has its natural resonance frequency. When the vibration applied to the ligament matches its natural frequency, resonance occurs. Resonance can increase the amplitude of oscillations within the tissue, contributing to greater relaxation and relief of tension within the ligaments.

2. Biomechanical Principles: Vibrations affect the mechanical properties of tissues, such as elasticity and viscosity. Through cyclic stretching and relaxation, vibrations can help reduce mechanical stress, increase circulation, and improve lymphatic drainage in the treated area.

3. Thermal Effects: Mechanical vibrations can generate mild heat due to internal friction between tissue molecules. This heat can enhance elasticity and relaxation of the ligaments, facilitating manual treatments and reducing the risk of injury.

4. Effects on Microcirculation: Vibrations can stimulate microcirculation within tissues, increasing the flow of blood and the availability of oxygen and nutrients. This can help speed up the recovery process and reduce inflammation.

5. Gate Control Theory of Pain: This theory suggests that vibrations can stimulate sensory nerves that transmit signals faster than nerves that carry pain, effectively "closing the gate" for pain signals traveling to the brain. This can reduce the perception of pain in patients.

Application of Mechanical Vibrations in Atlas Vertebra Adjustment

The method "Harmonic Balance" utilizes mechanical vibrations to achieve optimal relaxation and correct positioning of the atlas vertebra, thus improving the overall health and functionality of the entire body.

Principles of the "Harmonic Balance" Method

The "Harmonic Balance" method employs specially designed devices that produce mechanical vibrations at targeted frequencies optimal for stimulating the ligaments of the atlas. The vibrations work by relaxing and elongating the ligaments, reducing their rigidity, and allowing the atlas to move back to its natural position. This process not only restores structural balance to the cervical spine but also enhances neurological function, as proper alignment of the atlas can significantly affect cerebral circulation and neural pathways.

Safety and Efficacy

Unlike traditional adjustment methods that may use forceful and often painful manipulations, "Harmonic Balance" offers a non-invasive, gentle, and pleasant alternative. The vibrations are gentle enough to avoid causing additional discomfort, making the method suitable even for patients who are sensitive to pain or have a fear of manual manipulation.

Long-Term Benefits

Continuous use of this method can help maintain the correct position of the atlas and prevent future issues related to its position. Regular treatments can lead to gradual improvements in posture, reduction of symptoms associated with subluxation, and overall enhancement in quality of life.

Patient Education and Trust

An important aspect of the "Harmonic Balance" method is educating patients about the importance of maintaining cervical spine health and the potential consequences of neglecting symptoms. Transparent communication and detailed explanations about the treatment process help build trust and patient engagement, which is crucial for therapy success.

Advantages Over Traditional Methods

Mechanical vibrations offer several advantages over traditional ligament treatment methods, such as strikes, sudden pressure changes, or ligament stretching through bone manipulation. These advantages make mechanical vibrations particularly attractive in the context of rehabilitation and ligament health maintenance.

1. Non-Invasiveness and Safety:

Mechanical vibrations are extremely non-invasive compared to methods involving bone manipulation or direct pressure on ligaments. This approach minimizes the risk of injury and complications that can arise from more aggressive treatments.

2. Increased Circulation Without Additional Stress:

Vibrations stimulate blood and lymph fluid circulation in the treated area, which is crucial for tissue nourishment and recovery. Unlike sudden pressure changes or strikes, which can cause microtraumas or further tissue damage, vibrations achieve this in a gentle and controlled manner.

3. Promotion of Tissue Flexibility and Strength:

While aggressive methods like stretching or manipulation can sometimes overstrain ligaments, leading to potential tears or other damage, mechanical vibrations can help increase tissue elasticity without the risk of overextension or damage.

4. Pain Reduction and Recovery Acceleration:

Mechanical vibrations can effectively reduce pain through the gate control theory of pain, suggesting that vibrations can block pain signals traveling to the brain. This method not only alleviates pain but also allows patients to progress more quickly in their rehabilitation programs.

5. Improvement of Proprioception:

Proprioception, or the sense of body position in space, can be improved through the use of mechanical vibrations. This is particularly useful after ligament injuries, where re-establishing neuromuscular coordination is often necessary.

6. Increase in Range of Motion:

Unlike methods that force movement through direct manipulation, vibrations can help naturally increase the range of motion through stimulation and relaxation of tissues, avoiding the risk of injury due to excessive pressure or sudden movements.

Conclusion

The "Harmonic Balance" atlas adjustment method represents a significant advancement in spinal treatment, especially those related to the atlas. This technique not only offers a gentle and effective solution for correcting atlas positioning but also provides patients with an opportunity to experience comprehensive improvement in both physical and mental health. Through this method, patients receive not only treatment but also the tools for long-term maintenance of health and well-being, proving that "Harmonic Balance" is more than just therapy – it is a pathway to a better, healthier life.

By integrating mechanical vibrations, therapists can offer treatment that is not only effective but also safe, comfortable, and less stressful for patients, making it an ideal choice for long-term ligament health management.

Specialized Training Importance

The technique of adjusting the atlas vertebra is a sophisticated and precise medical procedure that requires specialized training and a deep understanding of anatomy, biomechanics, and pathophysiology, particularly the anatomy of the cervical region. This process cannot be effectively or safely performed without detailed professional knowledge, which is acquired through rigorous education and practice.

The encyclopedia on atlas vertebra adjustment before you is based on a rich decade of experience and encompasses thousands of cases of adjusted atlas vertebrae. The information contained in this work provides not only an insight into the various techniques and approaches used in practice but also a deeper understanding of the impact that proper atlas adjustment has on the overall health of patients.

The importance of training and expertise in this field cannot be overstated. Each adjustment procedure requires precision and care, as improper execution can lead to serious complications. Through the analysis of thousands of cases, practitioners gain the necessary knowledge and skills that allow for effective and safe treatment, as well as the adaptation of treatment methods to the individual needs of each patient.

This encyclopedia is an essential resource for all healthcare professionals who are involved or wish to be involved in atlas vertebra adjustment techniques, providing them with access to valuable information that can enhance their practice and improve treatment outcomes for patients worldwide. Through this work, professionals gain insights into best practices and methods that are confirmed by years of experience and expert knowledge.

Although atlas vertebra adjustment may appear simple to an observer, merely watching how the method is performed in no way qualifies an individual to attempt this technique independently.

Any attempt to adjust the atlas vertebra without appropriate medical training can result in serious, permanent injuries. Adjusting the atlas without adequate knowledge and experience can cause complications such as nerve damage, vascular issues, or even permanent spinal cord damage. Therefore, it is imperative that these types of treatments are left exclusively to trained healthcare professionals who have undergone rigorous training and certification programs.

In addition to medical training, practitioners who adjust the atlas must have a comprehensive understanding of the various techniques and methods used in this procedure, as well as the ability to tailor the treatment to the specific needs of each patient. Education in this field also includes learning about potential risks and how to minimize them, as well as understanding ethical standards that ensure patients receive the highest level of healthcare.

Thus, it is important for individuals considering atlas vertebra adjustment to seek services exclusively from licensed professionals who have acquired their knowledge and skills through accredited training programs and who regularly participate in professional development to stay up-to-date with the latest scientific advancements and practices in their field.

Chapter 10

" Holistic Path to Health "

Recapitulation of Key Concepts

In the book "The Renaissance of Healing Art," the emphasis is on the importance of the atlas vertebra in maintaining overall health. Understanding its anatomy and function is crucial because the unique structure of the atlas allows for mobility and stability, supporting the head and enabling various movements. This integrity is vital for the proper functioning of the nervous, circulatory, and lymphatic systems.

Central to the book is the "Harmonic Balance" method, a comprehensive approach to correcting atlas imbalances. This method integrates detailed diagnostic steps, patient examination, and preparation for treatment, aiming to restore internal balance and promote healing. The impact of proper atlas alignment goes beyond physical health, influencing aesthetics and an individual's self-confidence by enhancing overall well-being and beauty.

The "Harmonic Balance" method uses mechanical vibrations that act on the ligaments of the atlas, allowing them to relax and properly position the atlas. Through this technique, balance in the cervical spine is achieved, improving not only physical health but also the neurological function of the body.

The book introduces advanced diagnostic techniques such as 3D scanning and observation of body statics. These methods allow for precise identification of atlas subluxations and help tailor treatments to individual needs. Understanding these innovative approaches can empower readers to seek comprehensive diagnostic options that go beyond superficial symptom relief.

Encouragement to Take Action

"The Renaissance of Healing Art" is not just a guide but an invitation to embark on a journey toward inner harmony and vitality. The author encourages readers to embrace the challenge of exploring a new dimension of health and healing. By taking action, whether through seeking treatment, adopting preventive measures, or pursuing education, readers can unlock the power within themselves to transform their health and well-being.

The author's personal journey highlights the transformative potential of holistic healing. By sharing experiences and knowledge, the book aims to inspire readers to explore new approaches to health. The belief in the body's ability to heal itself when given proper support and care is central to this message. Harmony between the body, mind, and spirit is essential for maintaining health and well-being, and readers are encouraged to consider these interconnected aspects in their health practices.

A holistic perspective is not merely an aesthetic ideal but a practical approach to achieving optimal health. The historical context enriches this perspective, tracing the evolution of healing practices from ancient civilizations to modern integrative medicine. The author's personal journey underscores the importance of holistic methods, particularly in adjusting the atlas, which transcends conventional symptom-focused treatments.

We invite you to embark on this journey, exploring methods and techniques to achieve lasting health and inner peace. Through proactive action and continuous learning, you can achieve true transformation and improvement in your life. Start your journey toward holistic health and discover the potential within you.

Gratitude and Invitation

As we conclude this journey through "The Renaissance of Healing Art," I want to express my deep gratitude to all the readers who have joined me on this path. Your dedication to exploring and applying holistic approaches to health is crucial for achieving optimal well-being and inner harmony.

First and foremost, thank you for the time and attention you have dedicated to reading this book. Your openness to learning about the "Harmonic Balance" method and holistic health approaches demonstrates your commitment to better health and quality of life. I believe that through this journey, you have gained new insights and knowledge that will help you enhance your health and well-being.

This is just the beginning of your path to holistic health. This book is designed to provide you with tools and knowledge that you can apply in your daily life, but true transformation comes through continuous learning and application. I encourage you to continue exploring and learning about various holistic health approaches.

Explore other holistic methods and therapies that can contribute to your health. Learn about the importance of proper posture, ergonomics, and exercises that support neck and spine health. Join communities that share your passion for holistic health. Sharing experiences and knowledge with others can be extremely beneficial and inspiring. There is always something new to learn. Keep up with the latest research and innovations in the field of holistic health. Regularly attend seminars, workshops, and lectures to continue expanding your knowledge.

I believe that it is important not only to treat symptoms but also to explore the deeper causes of health problems.

This book aims to inspire you to take an active role in your health journey. By applying holistic principles and methods such as "Harmonic Balance," you can achieve a deeper understanding of your body, mind, and spirit, and thereby achieve lasting changes in your health and well-being.

As our understanding of health and healing evolves, new opportunities for exploring and applying holistic approaches emerge. The "Harmonic Balance" method is just one of many ways you can achieve balance and harmony in your life. I hope this book will serve as a guide and inspiration on that journey.

Thank you once again for your trust and dedication. Continue to explore, learn, and apply the knowledge you have gained, and may your journey toward health and harmony be filled with joy and success.

With gratitude and best wishes for your future exploration and health,

Doctor Oljaca

Epilogue

As we reach the end of this journey through the world of medical science and holistic health, it's important to reflect on the core principles that have guided us from the start. The goal of this book was not merely to provide information or impart knowledge but to inspire a transformation in how we perceive and care for our health.

Throughout the topics covered, we have emphasized the importance of maintaining a peaceful life, the correct positioning of the atlas vertebra, and a healthy spine. These elements are the pillars of our well-being. A calm and balanced life allows us to reduce stress, which is often the root of many health issues. The proper alignment of the atlas vertebra not only enhances the overall function of the body but also prevents numerous ailments that may arise from misalignment in this crucial part of the spine. A healthy spine is the foundation of our body, the bearer of vitality and energy, enabling us to walk through life firmly and steadily.

Health is not just the absence of disease; it is a complex balance between body, mind, and spirit. Recognizing this holistic approach, we become more aware of the importance of the daily decisions we make—from our diet and physical activity to the emotional and mental states we cultivate. Caring for the spine and atlas vertebra is not just about physical health, but about the overall energy and vitality that allows us to achieve a long and fruitful life.

Through this text, I hope to have illuminated the paths that lead to a better understanding of your body and the processes within it. I encourage you to continue exploring, to not be afraid of asking questions, and to always seek the most holistic solutions for your health needs. Your health is in your hands, and only you can make the decisions that will improve the quality of your life. Let this book inspire you to take the first step towards that goal and always strive to fulfill the potential within you.

Thank you for the precious time you've dedicated to reading this book. For those who wish to become direct participants in improving the health of many patients, I invite you to join the Doctor Oljaca Academy and become a specialist in atlas vertebra realignment. See you at the Academy!

Thank you for placing your trust in me by reading this book. I hope its messages will serve as a guide in the future, helping you find balance, peace, and health in your everyday life.

Acknowledgments

1 Corinthians 15:3-4

For I delivered unto you first of all that which I also received, how that Christ died for our sins according to the scriptures;

And that he was buried, and that he rose again the third day according to the scriptures.

Ephesians 2:8-9

For by grace are ye saved through faith; and that not of yourselves: it is the gift of God:

Not of works, lest any man should boast.

Romans 5:1

Therefore being justified by faith, we have peace with God through our Lord Jesus Christ.

Titus 3:5

Not by works of righteousness which we have done, but according to his mercy he saved us, by the washing of regeneration, and renewing of the Holy Ghost.

Author Biography

Dr. Oljaca is a dedicated practitioner of natural medicine who has devoted a significant portion of his time to researching the technique of atlas vertebra realignment. After two years of intensive research, he developed a unique method for adjusting the atlas vertebra, which has brought relief to thousands of satisfied patients. With over a decade of experience, he has transformed countless patients' pain into smiles. This book, which also serves as a textbook, is the culmination of his knowledge and experience, generously shared with his readers and future students of the Doctor Oljaca Academy.

Doctor Oljaca Academy

Doctor Oljaca Academy was established with the goal of providing thorough education and specialized training in the field of atlas vertebra realignment, one of the key techniques in natural medicine. The Academy was created in response to the growing need for experts who can offer patients effective and safe solutions to various health issues caused by atlas vertebra misalignment.

The training program at the Academy is carefully designed to give students a deep understanding of anatomy, biomechanics, and the specific techniques necessary for successfully realigning the atlas vertebra. Through a combination of theoretical lectures, practical workshops, and supervised clinical practice, students acquire the essential knowledge and skills to become top specialists in this field.

Our mission is to contribute to improving the health and quality of life of patients worldwide through the education and training of new generations of specialists. Participants in our Academy not only gain technical knowledge but are also equipped to provide a holistic approach to treatment, considering the overall health of the patient. Doctor Oljaca Academy is where theory and practice come together to achieve the highest standards in patient care.

All information about this academy can be found on our official website ***doctoroljaca.com***, or you can contact us directly via the contact form for additional details.